Health Observation of School Children

Health Observation of School Children

A GUIDE FOR HELPING TEACHERS AND OTHERS
TO OBSERVE AND UNDERSTAND THE SCHOOL CHILD
IN HEALTH AND ILLNESS

GEORGE M. WHEATLEY, M.D., M.P.H.
Third Vice-president, Health and Welfare,
Metropolitan Life Insurance Company

GRACE T. HALLOCK
Coauthor of Health for Better Living Series,
Understanding Health, Health Heroes Series,
and other health books

Illustrations by BARBARA PFEIFFER

Second Edition

THE BLAKISTON DIVISION
McGraw-Hill Book Company, Inc.
New York   Toronto   London   *1956*

Preface

Success in teaching depends largely upon the ability of the teacher to help her children to realize their individual potentialities for healthy physical, mental, emotional, and social growth. An invaluable, indeed a practically indispensable, aid in this important part of the work of teaching is an understanding both of what it means to be healthy and of the significance of deviations from good health. In the light of this understanding, the teacher forms her concept of each child as a whole and exercises her happy privilege of providing educational experiences geared to his individual needs and capabilities.

In the preface to the first edition of this book, published in 1951, emphasis was given to the importance of the strategic position occupied by the teacher in the health observation of school children. At that time, school and health authorities had long recognized that teachers through their day-by-day association with their children could be of the greatest possible help in identifying children in need of the professional services of specialists on the school-health-service staff.

Experience had shown, however, that the usefulness of the teacher in her role of health observer was necessarily limited both by the amount of briefing she had received during her student days on what to look for and by her interest in applying her knowledge and skills for the benefit of her children in actual classroom situations. Several excellent starts had been made in giving teachers the background information which would help them to understand the health problems of individual children. Among these pioneer enterprises had been the preparation by the Metropolitan Life Insurance Company of a filmstrip and booklet on teacher observation. The enthusiasm with which these materials were received by the schools, together with impressions gained through conversation and correspondence that a more comprehensive approach would be welcomed, led to the writing of this book.

Since its publication it has found its way into a growing number of schools and colleges whose programs are devoted wholly or in part to the education of future teachers. Furthermore, teachers in service are gradually discovering the usefulness of the book, not only as a guide in observing significant deviations from the usual appearance or behavior of individual children but also in finding answers to many of the questions

which arise in their efforts to make health as a way of life seem meaning-
ful and worth working for to children and their parents. There is evidence, too, that nurses serving the schools are using the book as a source
of suggestions for ways of interpreting to teachers and parents medical
information about the health status and needs of individual children.

The book was originally designed to give knowledge that would be
helpful to teachers and others who are concerned with the health observation and guidance of school children. But their own health is rightly
of no less concern to teachers than is that of their students. And experience has shown that they can use much of the knowledge in the book to
gain an understanding of their own health and its ups and downs.

In the second edition there has been no change in the lines of approach. In general these lines have two major objectives. The first is furnishing teachers with knowledge which will help them to understand
what they see in observing children. It is necessary to get a picture of
health before it is possible to gain skill in recognizing deviations from it.
In this book, therefore, teachers are given information about ways in
which healthy children grow and develop, how the healthy body maintains the conditions necessary for ordinary effective living and prepares
itself to meet emergencies, and how the healthy mind works in making
the adjustments required to deal successfully and happily with the vicissitudes of everyday life.

Although most student teachers are given courses in physiology and
psychology, the knowledge gained is seldom related as directly or as
closely as we have tried to relate it to the health observation of school
children. Moreover, there is not much material available to help teachers
and other lay observers understand the physiological basis of the signs
and symptoms that they are asked to look for and report. It is not necessary to know what peculiar combination of conditions sets in action the
forces within the body which produce signs and symptoms in order to
understand how those forces work. A motorist may not know what caused
the leak in a tire, but he knows that the tire is flat because a collapsible
rubber tube deflates when the air has escaped. Exactly what atmospheric
conditions resulted in a rainbow or a sunset at a particular hour and.
place the casual observer does not know, but that ignorance does not
keep him from understanding the mechanics of rainbow and sunset
formation. Just so, the teacher may not know what combination of causative factors has produced particular signs and symptoms in a particular
child, but she can understand the action of the forces within the body
which produce such signs and symptoms.

In this book many different signs and symptoms are explained with
reference to the parts of the body with which they are associated—

bleeding gums, boils, a cough, a running ear, for example. But even to understand the mechanics of such localized evidences of trouble, it is necessary to have some knowledge of the systems of the body—how they work together for the good of the whole and how they cooperate in measures of defense against actual or impending evil. In gaining this understanding the teacher will acquire a scientific background for her observations of the child.

The second major emphasis is on the various disorders and physical defects that are most prevalent among school children. Practically all educational and health authorities agree that teachers should be familiar with the signs and symptoms at onset and the methods of control of the common communicable diseases of childhood. There are many other conditions, such as defects of vision and hearing, malnutrition, accidental injuries, tooth defects, emotional disturbances, digestive troubles—to name a few of the chapters in the forever-to-be-continued story of the ailments and mishaps of the young—with which everyone who is with children for any length of time will have to deal.

The descriptions of such ailments and mishaps are in no case intended to furnish the teacher with grounds for diagnosis. The information given is only that which any intelligent layman who has a responsibility for children would wish to have. Parents also will find this information helpful in spotting early changes from the usual appearance and behavior of their children.

The teacher's responsibility as a lay observer ends with the reporting of her observations to the proper person in the school-health-service setup. There is no end, however, to her responsibility as a teacher for each child's welfare. Her knowledge of the health status of each child is bound to contribute to her success in teaching as measured by her ability to help him realize his potentialities for good health in the broadest sense of this term.

It often happens that the task of convincing parents of the need for taking the action recommended by the physician falls on the teacher or nurse or on both working together. Knowing something about a disease or defect, if medical diagnosis indicates that a child has it, will be helpful in interpreting the physician's findings and recommendations to the parents and sometimes to the child himself. The teacher who has this knowledge will be able to cooperate intelligently with the physician and the parents in any follow-up procedures required. And she will realize the importance of making sure that the child does what he should do— wear his glasses or his hearing aid, for example—while he is under her supervision.

To increase the usefulness of the book in institutions which have teacher-education programs, tests designed to help the students make sure that important information is remembered and understood are included at the end of each chapter. The popularity that quizzes of various kinds enjoy justifies the assumption that the readers will get pleasure from testing themselves. Also included are suggestions for activities that may be carried out by student teachers in their laboratory or practice schools or by teachers in service in their own classrooms.

Selected references for further reading on the various subjects covered are given at the end of each chapter. For the second edition these references have been thoroughly revised so as to include helpful new books and pamphlets published within the last few years. A list of organizations mentioned in the text may be found at the end of the book together with their current addresses.

For the sake of clarity, we have used the device of referring to the teacher as "she" and to the child as "he," except when a girl is specifically indicated.

The format and arrangement of chapters in the second edition of this book remain the same as in the first edition. Several changes and additions have been made, however, to keep pace with progress in medical science and public health and with changes in the statistical picture as it helps to clarify the most important health problems in the school ages. All statistical charts and tables giving mortality or morbidity figures have been revised according to the latest information available.

Increased emphasis has been given to the accident situation in childhood and youth and to the need for intensifying safety education in the schools. The discussions of infectious disease reflect the most recent scientific knowledge regarding the nature and methods of control of those diseases still matters of concern to teachers, nurses, and parents. A brief description of infectious mononucleosis has been added, as this disease seems to be on the increase among young people.

The immunization timetable has been set up according to the latest recommendations of the American Academy of Pediatrics and the American Public Health Association, and all other tabulated information on communicable diseases and orthopedic impairments has been revised to bring it up to date. The text on poliomyelitis has been entirely rewritten in order to supply teachers and nurses with the latest news in the field of polio research and with an evaluation of the results that may be expected from the development of the Salk vaccine for the prevention of paralytic polio.

The section on dental caries has been emended to call attention to the favorable reports from dental and public health authorities on the effectiveness of the fluoridation of communal water supplies in reducing the occurrence of this very common childhood disease.

Growing interest in the medical and surgical uses of blood and its products made it seem desirable to add a new section on blood grouping with special reference to the Rh factor.

We have enjoyed picking up and amplifying from many helpful, but scattered and not readily available, sources the why, the what, and the how of observing school children in health and illness. We hope that this book will continue to serve a useful purpose in helping teachers to co-operate effectively with parents, physicians, nurses, and all others who are concerned with the health of the school child.

GEORGE M. WHEATLEY
GRACE T. HALLOCK

Acknowledgments

It is a pleasure to acknowledge our indebtedness to colleagues and friends who reviewed portions of the text in manuscript and gave us information and advice of inestimable value. If we have failed to interpret and use their criticisms and suggestions aright, the fault is wholly ours.

We wish especially to thank Mrs. Donald B. Armstrong, psychotherapist, New York; Miss June Bricker, Director, Home Economics Bureau, and Miss Marjorie L. Craig, Director, School Health Bureau, Metropolitan Life Insurance Company; Dr. Franklin Foote, Executive Director, National Society for the Prevention of Blindness; Dr. J. T. Geiger, Assistant Medical Director, Metropolitan Life Insurance Company; Miss Sally Lucas Jean, former Consultant in Health Education, National Foundation for Infantile Paralysis; Dr. Milton Levine, Assistant Professor of Pediatrics, New York Hospital-Cornell Medical Center; Dr. Ely Perlman, Adjunct Physician in Allergy and Research Assistant, Department of Bacteriology, Mount Sinai Hospital, New York; Miss Nina Ridenour, Director, Division of Education, National Committee for Mental Hygiene; Dr. Norman C. Wetzel, pediatrician, Cleveland Heights, Ohio; and Miss Pauline Brooks Williamson, Secretary, American Association for Gifted Children.

For valuable assistance in revising the charts, tables, and references for the second edition, our thanks go to the following friends in the Metropolitan Life Insurance Company: Mr. Herbert Marks, Manager, Medical Statistics, Statistical Bureau; Miss Eugenie Glatzl, Library; Mrs. Emily Hammond, School Health Bureau; and Mrs. Sophia C. Dertz, Health and Welfare Editorial Bureau.

We wish also to acknowledge the courtesy of those who furnished many of the illustrations that appear in the text. Our thanks go especially to the Metropolitan Life Insurance Company for permission to use the colored photographs (Plates 1–16) from "What Teachers See," and numerous statistical charts and tables throughout the book; to the National Foundation for Infantile Paralysis for permission to reproduce the diagram and posters in the section on poliomyelitis; to Dr. Howard V. Meredith, Professor, School of Health and Physical Education, University of Oregon; Dr. Harold C. Stuart, Head of the Department of

Maternal and Child Health, School of Public Health, Harvard University; Dr. Norman C. Wetzel; and the American Medical Association for permission to reproduce the charts and tables credited to them in the section on measuring physical growth and development; to the National Society for the Prevention of Blindness for permission to reproduce the Snellen test charts in the section on vision testing; and to Dr. Charles H. Best, Banting and Best Department of Medical Research, University of Toronto, for permission to adapt the diagram of the cochlear canal in the section on the structure of the ear from the diagram in Best and Taylor's "The Human Body and Its Functions."

We wish also to thank Dr. Morton A. Seidenfeld, Director of the Division of Psychological Services and Public Education, National Foundation for Infantile Paralysis, for reviewing the text on poliomyelitis prepared for the second edition.

In the sixth century a "false judgment" given against Columba, an Irish saint, by Diarmuid, King of Ireland, in a dispute over a book is said to have been the cause of a famous battle. St. Columba borrowed a book from a gentleman named Finnian and copied the gospel out of it without Finnian's knowledge. Whereupon "Finnian said that it was to himself belonged the son-book which was written from his book, and they both selected Diarmuid as judge between them. This is the decision that Diarmuid made: that to every book belongs its son-book, as to every cow belongs her calf." [1]

This book, too, is a son-book, for many books and pamphlets, far too numerous to name, have gone into the making of it. But looking around among those with which we have lived for many months before they are finally dispersed, we should be ungrateful indeed not to mention specifically Best and Taylor's "The Physiological Basis of Medical Practice"; Cannon's "The Wisdom of the Body"; Thorner's "Psychiatry in General Practice"; Zinsser's "Textbook of Bacteriology" (revised by Smith, Martin *et al.*); Kahn's "Man in Structure and Function"; The American Public Health Association's "Control of Communicable Diseases in Man"; O'Hara's "Air-borne Infection"; and Davison's "The Compleat Pediatrician."

[1] Quoted in Henry Osborn Taylor's "The Mediaeval Mind," p. 136, Macmillan, New York, 1914.

Introduction

The movement to enlist teachers as observers of the health of school children gained momentum when the bacteriological discoveries of the last quarter of the nineteenth century furnished educational and public health officials with reason for hoping that something might conceivably be done about controlling the spread of infection in the schools. Systems of medical inspection were set up in the schools of several large cities, and part of the responsibility for reporting evidence of infection fell upon the teachers.

In New York City, in 1897, for example, the Department of Health assigned medical inspectors to call at three or four different schools every day, to *ask the teachers* whether any of their children seemed ill, and to inspect those whom the teachers reported for signs of communicable disease. As it worked out, many inspectors did not go to the schools at all but questioned the teachers over the telephone. When an obviously infected child was found, the only measure taken was to exclude him from school. Infectious eye and skin diseases were found in so many thousands of children that the schools in many sections of the city became practically deserted. Lillian Wald's suggestion in 1902 that public health nurses working with the school medical inspectors might help to clear up some of these conditions led eventually to the establishment of the public health nurse as an invaluable member of the school-health-service team.

As the thicket composed of cases of gross physical neglect was cleared away, many other menaces to the health of school children began to stand out more clearly. These were, for the most part, medical problems—for example, focal infections, defects of the eyes and teeth, and malnutrition—which called for more refined techniques than simple observation. School health services, in most places where they were set up, were considered to be the sole responsibility of physicians, nurses, and dentists, and great reliance was placed upon the periodic school medical examination as a means of finding children in need of professional attention.

However, the results of concentrating on the purely medical aspects of the school health service were disappointing. Generally speaking for the country as a whole, in most schools routine health examinations became little more than cursory and superficial inspections of the students to meet the demands of legislation or to assure the public of the school's interest in the health of the children. Certainly there was little educational value either for the students or their parents in such hurried inspections. Moreover, it sometimes happened that children in serious need of attention were not discovered, and the records of a substantial proportion of children known to have severe uncorrected defects were lost somewhere in the shuffle of inefficient filing systems.

The importance of putting the teacher back into the observation post from which she had been withdrawn in the advancing front of the routine medical examination was first publicly recognized in 1924 by Dr. James Frederick Rogers, then Consultant in Hygiene of the United States Office of Education. In his pamphlet "What Every Teacher Should Know about the Physical Condition of Her Pupils," [1] Dr. Rogers paid tribute to the "unique, first-line position" of the teacher in the health observation of school children and pointed her out as "the 'keystone' of the health examination service." The practical information given in this historic pamphlet for use as a guide in the continual health appraisal of children by their teachers has since been amplified and presented in many different forms in other publications.

In the early thirties, an increasing number of educational and health authorities felt that something was wrong somewhere along the straight pathway which ideally should have led from the detection of remediable defects in school children to their correction. This uncomfortable feeling was crystallized in the report of a study [2] made in 1932–1933 in the New York City schools. The situation pictured in this report was recognized as reasonably representative of the situation in the country as a whole—at least in the large urban centers. The recommendations made in this and earlier studies were given successful field testing in the Astoria Health District demonstration study [3] sponsored by the Department of Health and the Board of Education of New York City.

In the four-year Astoria study, interest was focused on the role of the teacher in the school-health-service program. New York City teachers were already expected to observe children for departures from good health and to refer those in obvious need of attention to the nurse or

[1] Pamphlet No. 68 (Revised 1945), Federal Security Agency, United States Office of Education.

[2] "Physical Defects—the Pathway to Correction," American Child Health Association, New York, 1934. (A study of physical defects among school children in New York City, conducted by the research division of the American Child Health Association in cooperation with the Department of Health and the Department of Education, supervised by a special advisory committee, and financed by the Metropolitan Life Insurance Company.)

[3] Nyswander, Dorothy B., "Solving School Health Problems," Commonwealth Fund, New York, 1942.

the physician serving the school. Building on this foundation, methods were worked out for making the teachers' continuing observations a vital part of the school program for maintaining and improving the children's health. As a result, the health observation of school children became teacher-centered rather than physician-centered or nurse-centered. Instead of the routine periodic medical examination of all children, the "Astoria plan" of school medical service calls for the examination of each child when he enters school, either by the school physician or his family physician, and thereafter only when the observations of teacher or nurse, or both, indicate that he is in need of further medical attention. It was found during the study that examinations by physicians of children referred by teachers as needing medical attention showed that eight out of ten such children actually had health problems. This was a striking demonstration of the efficiency of alert, informed teachers in recognizing "something wrong" when they see it.

The Astoria plan is now used in the New York City elementary schools and has influenced school health programs in many parts of the United States and Canada. The fundamental role of the teacher in the school health program is currently emphasized on the value-defining, policy-making level by national organizations interested in school health.[4] Furthermore, it would be difficult now to find a manual on school health services or school health examinations issued by state health or educational authorities, or both, which does not emphasize the value of the teacher's observations in detecting signs and symptoms that indicate the need for medical, dental, or other specialized care.

Recognition of the strategic position of the teacher as an observer who may be depended upon to find children with health problems led the Advisory Educational Group of the Metropolitan Life Insurance Company to recommend the production of a sound filmstrip in color which would help teachers to visualize both the evidence of good health in their children and also some of the signs that should be looked on with suspicion as indicating departures from good health. This filmstrip, entitled "Teacher Observations of School Children," was prepared in 1945 under the general direction of one of the authors of this book (Dr. Wheatley) with the guidance of a subcommittee of the Advisory Educational Group consisting of Dr. C. E. Turner, Professor Emeritus of Public Health, Massachusetts Institute of Technology; Miss Julia Wade Abbot, former Director of Early Childhood Education in the Philadelphia public schools; and Dr. Charl O. Williams, Director of Field Service

---

[4] See "Suggested School Health Policies," a report of the National Committee on School Health Policies, formed in 1945 by the National Conference for Cooperation in Health Education.

of the National Education Association. The color photographs were taken by the late Dr. Lewis Henry Koplik in the children's clinic of the New York Hospital—Cornell Medical Center, and at the Hunter College Elementary School in New York City. Later these photographs with further explanatory text were reproduced in the Metropolitan booklet "What Teachers See." As indicated in the Preface, the encouraging reception given to the filmstrip and booklet led the authors of this book to believe that teachers would welcome an opportunity to broaden their understanding of children's health needs as they go forward to write new chapters in the history of the health observation of school children.

Contents

Preface   v

Acknowledgments   xi

Introduction   xiii

Chapter 1. SEEING THE CHILD AS A WHOLE   1
              The Art of Observing Children   1
              The Chief Health Problems of Childhood   13
              The Child as a Whole   20

Chapter 2. THE GROWING CHILD   31
              Physical Growth and Development   31
              Measuring Physical Growth and Development   42
              Mental Growth and Its Measurement   64
              Emotional and Social Development   71

Chapter 3. THOUGHTS AND FEELINGS,
              ACTIONS AND REACTIONS   86
              Ins and Outs of the Nervous System   86
              Observations Related to Endocrine Activity   92
              Defense Reactions of Physical Origin   99
              Psychogenic Reactions   114
              Organic Disorders of the Nervous System   121
              Mental Illness of Psychogenic Origin   136
              Identifying Children with Emotional
                and Social Problems   141

Chapter 4. WHAT TO KNOW ABOUT THE HEART,
              BLOOD, AND LYMPH   154
              Circulation Survey   154
              Signs and Symptoms of Circulatory Disorders   159
              Rheumatic Fever   161
              Blood and Its Composition   164
              Blood Disorders   170

Tissue Fluid   173
What to Do in Case of Circulatory Emergencies   178
Diseases Spread by Blood-sucking Insects   183

Chapter 5. ON THE AIR ROUTE   192
The Respiratory Passages   192
Respiratory Infections in General   197
Respiratory Infections in Particular   201
Respiratory Allergies   218
The School and Respiratory-disease Control   220
What to Do in Respiratory Emergency   224
Speech Difficulties   228

Chapter 6. ALONG THE ALIMENTARY ROUTE   249
Preparation of Food for the Body's Use   249
Signs and Symptoms of Gastrointestinal Disorders   257
Gastrointestinal Infections   264
Observations about the Mouth   274
Observations about the Teeth   278
How the Body Uses Food Materials   288
Meeting the Food Needs of School-age Children   295
The Kidneys and Their Work   302

Chapter 7. THE BODY'S ENVELOPE   312
Topography and Functions of the Skin, Hair,
    and Nails   312
Observing Cutaneous Deviations from Normal   319
Observing Deviations from Normal Mirrored
    by the Skin   326
Skin Infections   329
Skin Infestations   340
Skin Injuries   343

Chapter 8. STOP! LOOK AND LISTEN   349
What "Meets the Eye" in Observing Eyes   349
Seeing Right and Seeing Wrong   356
Vision Testing   367
Observations about the Ears   374
Hearing Right and Hearing Wrong   378
Hearing Testing   384

Chapter 9.   ON GROWING STRAIGHT   393
                Bones and Muscles   393
                Why Muscles Can Work Together in Moving
                    and Balancing the Body   406
                Posture and Its Appraisal   410
                Crippling Defects in School Children   419
                Common Bone, Joint, and Muscle Injuries   424
                Observing Children for Orthopedic Defects   430

Addresses of Organizations   437

Visual Aids   439

Index   455

Chapter 1   SEEING THE CHILD AS A WHOLE

The Art of Observing Children
The Chief Health Problems of Childhood
The Child as a Whole

THE ART OF OBSERVING CHILDREN

In general, observation means the act of noticing or paying attention to things perceived through the senses. We observe the shape and colors of a tree (things seen), the rustle of leaves (things heard), the odor of a rose (things smelled), the savor of salt (things tasted), the texture of cloth (things felt). Everything we know about the outside world and the people in it, all the experiences that teach us and guide us, come to us through observation.

Practically all of us observe the appearance and behavior of others and form opinions based on our observations. "He looks tired," "She looks happy," "He acts scared," "She's too fat," "He's too thin"—these are only a few of the things we think or say which show that we are constantly appraising someone's state of health or state of mind.

But what are such observations worth? Do they serve any useful purpose? That depends upon what makes an observation worth while. Is it vague or specific? Is its significance understood and appreciated? Is it an idle observation or one that can be put to work for the benefit of the person observed?

A woman sitting opposite a child on a bus might think to herself, "That child looks pale and thin." But this observation has no value in getting something done for the child, because the child means nothing to the observer.

A visitor in the home of identical twins might say to their mother, "My, those children look so much alike that I don't see how even you can tell them apart." And the mother might find it difficult to explain why it is that she can easily tell Johnny from Jimmy. "If they were your children," she might say, "you would notice many ways in which they are different." In effect she would be saying that her powers of observation have been sharpened by her love and interest. It is interest in a particular child, then, that largely determines whether the things we

1

notice about that child are specific enough to convey a real meaning for us. But even interest is helpless if the knowledge and understanding necessary for intelligent observation are lacking.

Standards of Comparison

A little girl on first hearing the story of the creation exclaimed, "My, Adam must have been happy that first morning when he saw the sun come up." She had grasped the idea that Adam, observing the first sunset, had no way of knowing there would be a sunrise. And we cannot appreciate the significance of what we observe in children without something to go on—some standard of comparison based on knowledge and experience. Of course, we have a general idea of the look of health—rosy cheeks, bright eyes, glossy hair, firm flesh, rounded contours, sturdy legs, good posture. We speak of "radiant health," or of a person being "aglow with health," and think we know what we mean when we say it. But if we come right down to cases, how can we be fairly sure that the plump rosy-cheeked child is healthy and the thin pale child undernourished? What do we have to go on? Suppose we look at Tommy Brown through the eyes of his mother, his teacher, and his doctor.

The Mother's Yardstick. To his mother, Tommy is unique. She does not compare him objectively with other children, because to her there is no comparison. However, she has learned how Tommy looks and behaves when he is healthy and happy, or, as she might say, when he is "like himself," and that knowledge furnishes her with a yardstick for checking up on what she observes. Either Tommy is *like himself*—as he is when she knows that he is well and happy—or *unlike himself*—as he is when he is ailing and fretful.

The Teacher's Yardstick. Tommy's teacher, like his mother, has an opportunity to become familiar with his appearance and behavior from day to day. Through constant association the child makes a distinct impression on her. She forms an opinion of his learning ability, his attitude toward his work and his playmates, his behavior in the classroom and on the playground. She is in a position to note changes for the worse in her picture of the child at his best. But she also has a more objective yardstick than that of his parents. Tommy shares her interest and attention with 30 children or more. She is sensitive not only to changes that make Tommy look or act unlike himself, but also to individual differences that may or may not throw him too far out of line with what she has learned through training and experience to expect of children of approximately his age in the way of behavior and learning ability.

The Physician's Yardstick. The physician's interest in a child who is brought to his attention for a routine medical examination or because of a particular illness or physical defect is based largely on his obligation to deliver the professional verdict and recommendations for which he is consulted. Is Tommy physically sound and well nourished? Or is there something wrong? And, if so, what? In making his examination the physician constantly compares his findings with what he knows to be normal for healthy children of approximately that age. There are, for example, normal chest sounds, normal body temperature, normal vision, and so on. And there are typical sets of signs and symptoms to guide him in making a diagnosis if he finds any marked departures from normal.

Of the value of the physician's observations there can be no doubt. Just as an astronomer with a telescope can make many more observations about the heavens and learn far more about a particular star than the casual stargazer can, so the physician with his trained eyes and ears and finger tips and precision instruments and tests can make many more observations about the body and learn far more about the physical condition of a particular child than a layman can. And not only that—what he observes means far more to him than it would to the untrained observer. Anyone can listen to heart sounds through a stethoscope, but only a physician can *interpret* the meaning of those sounds. Anyone can observe visible signs of trouble in the body, but only a physician can identify a particular disease or defect and tell it apart from any number of others that may resemble it.

The Value of Teacher-Parent Observations

In the last analysis, the only way in which we can be sure of getting the correct answer to our question, "Is this child healthy?" or, if he seems ill, "What is the matter with him?" is to ask the doctor.

What then are the observations of parents and teachers worth? Are they to be considered unemployable or may they be put to work?

Getting Medical Attention for Children Who Need It. First of all, how is a child to get to the doctor when he needs medical attention? Under ordinary circumstances the family physician depends almost entirely on parental observation as a means of reaching his child patients when they need him. For that reason alone, parents should know what to watch for in the way of specific signs and symptoms as a means of sharpening the natural keenness of observation occasioned by their love and interest. And when the child goes to school, still another "seeing eye" is focused on him.

The chief value of the teacher's observations, as far as getting a child to the doctor for needed medical attention is concerned, lies in the fact that they are likely to be more objective than those of the parents. A mother may actually be too close to a child to notice a slowly developing defect. Progressive loss of hearing is commonly referred to as a "thief in the night," creeping up on one unawares. The same may be said of the insidious development of nearsightedness or of malnutrition or of certain diseases, such as rheumatic fever, tuberculosis, and diabetes. Also, children like everyone else have little personality quirks, and these are often so familiar to parents that they may quite effectively disguise a developing defect. "But he has always been like that—he never pays attention," a mother might say in reply to the suggestion that lack of attentiveness may indicate loss of hearing. Even obvious signs of trouble, such as decayed teeth (especially "baby teeth"), poor posture, chronic "sniffles," excessive overweight, and behavior difficulties of various kinds, may be disregarded at home either because "familiarity breeds contempt" or because such conditions do not seem to have any appreciable direct effect on the child's general health.

At school, on the other hand, an objective measure of accomplishment is set up in the welter of emotions that surrounds practically all children. A teacher is bound to be puzzled if a particular child does not seem to be making the progress he himself has led her to expect of him, or if he seems to be out of his class as compared with others in his group. And she has the welfare of the whole class to think of as well as the welfare of each child in it. Is the behavior of one or two children upsetting the morale of the group? Is Tommy's running nose or the sore at the corner of Jane's mouth "something catching"?

In a school with a well-organized health service, the teacher has an opportunity to discuss all such problems with the school nurse or school physician. In schools without such facilities, she may carry her concern directly to the parents. In either case she is able to perform a real and lasting service for a child by calling attention to departures from good health which might otherwise have been neglected.

Helping the Doctor to Understand the Child. The second important contribution of the observations of parents and teachers to a child's welfare is the light they throw on the doctor's search for the best way to help the child.

The human body has often been compared to a machine, which can be checked by a doctor as a piece of machinery can be checked by a skilled mechanic to make sure that there is "no sand in the gearbox," no loose or missing or damaged parts. But the comparison breaks down when we think of the body as made of living stuff subject to the innumerable delicate adjustments occasioned by the interplay of body, mind, and spirit. This interplay is what makes us individuals—each one of us a person unlike all other persons—whose health status cannot be determined simply by objective measurements like urinalyses and blood tests and measurements of heart capacity and reactions to the knee-jerk test, and so on.

The difference between the human body in general and the human body in particular is what makes the difference between the study of medicine as a science and the practice of medicine as an art. And that is why unlikeness to self—to the way in which a person usually looks and acts—is an important finding from a medical practitioner's point of view. No patient likes to be treated as if he had been newly created in the waiting room to satisfy a doctor's curiosity. And no physician can do his best for a patient who is a closed book in everything that cannot be determined by rule of thumb. But the modern physician often does not have the opportunities open to the old-time family doctor to know his patients inside out. He has to depend more than his predecessors did on secondhand observation to get the information that will enable him to do his best for us and our children; he has to ask questions, and we have to know the answers!

Any mother who has been present at a medical examination of her child knows the sort of questions the doctor asks: "When did you begin to notice that she was losing weight?" "How is his appetite?" "Has his face always twitched like that?" "Is he naturally pale?" "Does his head ache in the morning or at night?" "How long has he been troubled with constipation?" And so on. The doctor is trying to get a picture of the child as he usually looks and behaves so that he can appraise the importance of what he observes. And for that he must depend upon those who are constantly with the child.

The teacher can perform for the school nurse and school physician the same services that the mother performs for the family physician, not only in selecting children who need medical check-ups, but also in giving information that she is in a good strategic position to obtain. Also she may be of great service in getting needed information to the family physician by sharing her observations with the parents. Upon the information given by those who know the child well, coupled with what he finds out for himself, the doctor bases his diagnosis and decides on the treatment. And just as the mother at home cooperates best with the doctor when she knows what he hopes to accomplish, so the teacher is best able to give the child the supervision and guidance he needs in school when she has learned from doctor and nurse what the child's health problems are and how they can be solved.

Learning to Be a Good Observer

In order to decide whether a child who is not obviously ill needs medical attention, training in observation is necessary. This means cultivation of the knack of observing what a person not medically trained can observe.

Practicing Observation. An easy first step in acquiring this knack is to look for just one thing in the children encountered during a day. For example, if you look only for freckles, you will be surprised to find how quickly you become aware of freckles and the pattern of their distribution on the face. You may watch for the color of eyes until you find yourself automatically noticing eye color in children. Other easy exercises in observation, which may be compared to the simple finger exercises one learns when playing the piano, include noting the number of children in a class who wear glasses or the number who write left-handed.

The next step is comparable to playing one's first "piece" on a musical instrument. It consists of the unobtrusive observation of individual children for five minutes or so, with the object of describing afterward from memory each child's face and body build and gait. This method has proved useful in the formal training of teachers in the art of observation. Opportunities are made for a group of teachers and a school physician to watch children for a certain length of time. Then each teacher writes down her impressions of each child. Later in a group conference the physician reviews the teachers' descriptions and points out any significant observations which have been missed.

The final and most important step is practice in observation for the specific purpose of detecting departures from good health. Since this implies familiarity with normal appearance and behavior, it is necessary to define what is meant by "normal."

What Is "Normal"? In a great many different situations, our conception of normality is based upon what is conspicuously familiar. It is a conspicuously familiar fact, for example, that the mean body temperature of the great majority of healthy persons is 98.6°F. (see Defense Reactions of Physical Origin, in Chap. 3). So the "normal" mark is set at 98.6° on our clinical Fahrenheit thermometers.

In a large group of persons of a certain age, the height of the majority will be within a few inches above or below the mean, or average, height of the group. The ordinary range in height at various ages is so familiar that we can tell at a glance whether a person is unusually tall or unusually short. The same is true of weight and body shape. Going on what may be called our feeling for normality, we can readily tell whether a person is unusually thin or unusually fat, unusually well shaped or unusually misshapen. Our conception of what is right and proper in the way of behavior is also based upon our experience with the sort of behavior that is conspicuously familiar at various ages. It is all right—"normal"—for a child to be childish, for example, but not for an adult.

Day-by-day Observation of Particular Children. In observing a child, we use both our familiarity with normality and its standard variations, won by lifelong experience in observing the people around us, and our familiarity with that particular child's *usual* appearance and behavior.

The teacher in her day-by-day association with her children learns how each one looks and behaves when he is well. It may take some time to gain this knowledge, but once acquired it makes a great difference in the ease with which significant changes in appearance and behavior are recognized. To illustrate what is meant by the sort of knowledge that underlies the common expression, "He is not the same child," observe the pictures of Jane in Plates 1 and 2.

In Plate 1 you see Jane as her teacher sees her when she is healthy and happy. Her face glows with life. The color of her skin and lips is good. She looks rested but alert, ready to join eagerly in the day's activities.

By treasuring her impressions of Jane as a picture of health, the teacher has a basis for comparison in her careful and unobtrusive observation of Jane's appearance and behavior from day to day. She knows that as clouds change the look of a sunny landscape, so illness changes the look of a healthy child.

In Plate 2 you see the changes from her usual appearance which her teacher noticed when Jane returned to school after an illness. Her face now looks drawn and tired. Her pink cheeks have become sallow and her clear eyes dull with circles beneath. Her usually glossy hair now lacks luster, and her happy rested expression has been lost. Just by looking at her and observing her behavior, her teacher can tell that she is not yet ready to take full active part in the school program.

Time and Place of Observation

The system of daily health inspection in operation in most schools at the present time is an outgrowth of—we might almost call it a hangover from—the methods adopted in the latter part of the nineteenth century to deal with the appalling prevalence of communicable disease among school children, especially in the larger cities. The control of communicable diseases was then such an imperative problem that practically everything else was ignored. When trachoma, diphtheria, and a host of other dangerous infections were rampant, no one had time to look for or to bother with deviations from good health that were not catching or seriously crippling. It is as if a gardener should come upon a garden choked with weeds, which had to be cleared away before any attention could be paid to less obvious, but no less important, menaces to the health of the flowers.

Those days fortunately are far behind us, thanks to the extraordinarily rapid progress in preventive medicine and to the work of all those who have made it possible for children to benefit by immunization procedures and other measures for controlling the spread of communicable disease. As a result, there is time today to practice a more refined technique—to explore possibilities that would not occur to teachers confronted with cases of gross medical neglect. Tony, who is not making good progress in school, may have no obvious physical condition like trachoma or scabies to explain his backwardness. Yet his teacher, in her concern for Tony's well-being, is on the alert for signs that may indicate that something connected with his health is causing the pendulum of his learning ability to describe a smaller arc than the one that sets the tempo in the group.

Formal Inspection. Although the state of emergency that occasioned the deputizing of teachers as inspectors of school children for signs of communicable disease no longer exists, except possibly in epidemics, the habit of devoting a period at the beginning of each day for the formal inspection of the children by the teacher still persists in many school systems. The inspection is made in a good light and usually while the pupils are seated. Points of observation include the skin of the forearms, hands, face, and neck (for cleanliness, signs of skin infection, rash, signs of scratch marks, etc.); hair and fingernails (for "nits," neatness, and cleanliness); teeth and gums (for cleanliness, bleeding or inflamed gums); ears (for cleanliness, discharge from ear canal); nose (for nasal discharge); and clothing (for cleanliness and neatness, possession of handkerchief or paper tissues).

A daily formal inspection of this kind has its advantages and also its disadvantages. Among its advantages is the guarantee that the children will be observed attentively for at least five minutes or so at the start of the day, just as a formal period of health instruction is a guarantee that provision for guiding children in the ways of health will be included in the curriculum. Probably its chief disadvantage is the chance that it may be embarrassing to individual children. Another is the psychological effect on both teacher and children. Upon its completion it is apt to be dismissed from the mind as something over and done with for the day. The child has "passed" so to speak; the teacher has done her duty—so on to the reading, and writing, and arithmetic.

Informal Inspection. In informal morning inspections, the teacher observes each child as she says "Good morning." She stands with her back to the light and looks at the child unobtrusively, but with a purpose. Just as she notes whether his hair is combed and his face washed, so she makes a quick estimate of his facial expression. Is it happy and smiling? Or is it unusually pale or sad? Does he look tired or rested? Is his nose "running"? Are his eyes clear and bright? or droopy-lidded? or inflamed?

Children who seem to need a closer inspection as evidenced by this quick "once-over" may then be looked at carefully in as good a light as possible. If the teacher notices signs and symptoms which in her opinion require the immediate attention of a doctor or nurse, she will then follow the procedures for referral that are in operation in the school. For example, it may be routine to send the child directly to the nurse or physician serving the school, or to refer him to the principal, who will seek the advice of the physician or nurse, or to send the child home with an explanatory note.

Keeping health inspection informal—not making an issue of it— increases the chances that it will become a continuous process throughout the school day, because there is nothing about it to suggest a dead end—a job done. There are many ready-made opportunities throughout the day to make worth-while observations without involving extra time and effort on the teacher's part. For example, what posture does the child assume as he sits in his seat? Does he slump down or slouch over? How far from his eyes does he hold his book when he reads? Is his position cramped when writing? What does he choose to eat from the menu in the school lunchroom? If he brings his lunch, what are the contents of his lunch box? Does he spend an adequate time in eating? Or does he "swallow his lunch whole" so as to have more time for play? Does he play happily with others? Or is he unduly quarrelsome? Or does he "hang back" from entering group games?

Parental Observation. When the child is in school he is removed for part of his day from the solicitous observations of his parents. However, the times and opportunities for observation open to parents cover many important factors connected with the child's health or health habits. Parents, for example, should "look at" their children carefully, but informally and unobtrusively, while they are eating breakfast. Are their appetites as good as usual? Do they appear rested, alert, ready for the day's activities? Are there any signs of the sniffles which might indicate that they should stay at home? Before they leave for school one question that usually arises is whether they are dressed suitably for weather conditions. After school parents should be on the lookout for signs of unusual fatigue, unhappiness or discouragement, poor appetite at supper, and so on, which might indicate poor adjustment to school or some physical condition that needs medical attention. It is better to learn by indirection how a child feels than by nagging him with direct questions.

The Teacher as a Member of the School-health-service Team

The major aims of a school health service are the health maintenance and the health improvement of school children. Striking a true balance between these two aims depends upon the recognition of two cardinal facts. The first is that no child who has reached the age of reason can be kept healthy and safe solely by what is planned and done for him. His continued well-being depends in large part upon what he himself feels and thinks and does. Upon this fact the teacher bases the health education of her children. She is concerned with the cultivation of correct attitudes toward health and safety and the encouragement of practices that make for health and safety.

The second cardinal fact is that no child can get rid of an already existing physical defect or infection or chronic illness merely by knowing and practicing the rules of healthful living. The child who learns in school that milk is an excellent source of the calcium necessary for building good teeth can drink milk till the cows come home without having a single decayed tooth restored to health. No amount of hand washing and sneezing into a handkerchief are going to cure Johnny's cold. No waiting for the green light will set Mary's broken leg, nor will wearing rubber boots on rainy days repair the damage already done to Frank's heart by rheumatic fever.

Existing departures from good health are hard problems, which health education alone cannot solve. Yet they interfere with the process of education itself. In varying degrees they endanger the child's present—and, possibly, future—well-being. If contagious, they are a menace to the whole group. The need for school health service is based upon the fact that in any school, at any time, there are bound to be children who, for some reason, are not up to par; or who are suffering from a specific disability, such as poor eyesight or loss of hearing; or who appear to be "coming down with something," which may or may not be catching; or who have skinned their knees or cut their fingers or injured some other part of their bodies.

School-health-service activities include complete medical examinations or health appraisals; dental examinations and cleaning of teeth; screening tests for vision and hearing; conscientious follow-up after medical and dental examinations, to assure the correction of any adverse conditions discovered; communicable-disease control; first aid in case of emergencies;

and health counseling and guidance. To provide all the students in a school with everything they need in the way of health care and supervision requires the services of many different professionally trained persons—physicians, public health nurses, dentists, dental hygienists, psychologists, and other specialists. What is provided in actual practice depends upon the resources available in the school and community. The kind and amount of specialized services found in different schools range all the way from complete coverage in a very few large urban school systems to no specialized services in remote, one-room schools.

Responsibility for carrying on the health services in a school varies by states or by different communities within one state. In some places the health department is responsible; in others, the department or board of education; in still others, the health and education departments jointly. Whatever may be the administrative status of the school health service, its operation is closely related to the school program as a whole. The core of our thinking regarding the goals, organization, and functioning of a good school-health-service program is the conviction that health service in a school must be a cooperative undertaking in which members of the teaching staff and members of the health-service staff work together as one team instead of considering themselves as members of two different teams. Also the school team must work with the parents and with organized groups and individuals in the community who are interested in giving school children opportunities to stay healthy or to obtain needed medical, dental, nursing, or other specialized care.

At present, it is agreed that there should be an intimate connection between the work of the teachers in the classroom and the work of the specialists in the school health unit. We have come, full circle, back to the time fifty-odd years ago when the observations of the teachers were a vital link in the system of school medical inspection (see Introduction). The recognition of the strategic position occupied by the teacher in her day-by-day association with her students is making possible the gradual evolution of a more efficient plan for health appraisals than the old one based on the idea that "every child should be given an annual routine health examination." The trend now is to have children examined and given booster immunizations, preferably by the family physician, before they enter school and then to provide three or four additional examinations at important stages in the child's progress through school. For example, these examinations might take place (a) upon entering the intermediate grades (Grade 4); (b) upon entering junior high school (Grade 7); (c) upon entering senior high school (Grade 10); and (d) possibly in the year before graduation from high school. Dental supervision, of course, must be given more frequently.

In between these routine examinations any student whose appearance or behavior suggests to the teacher or nurse, or to both, that medical attention is needed is referred for an immediate interim examination. In many schools the teacher is also responsible for making screening tests of vision, hearing, and speech; for weighing and measuring students; for noting the causes of absences as reported by the parents; and for assisting in the record-keeping and follow-up procedures incident to routine examinations and screening tests. In short, not only is the teacher the key person in the health-education aspects of the school health program as a whole, but also she is often a hard-working member of the school-health-service team.

As a specialist in education, however, the teacher is primarily concerned with ways in which the students' experiences with health-service activities can be used in the classroom to make health education vital and functional. In preparation both for medical examinations and for screening tests of various kinds, there are innumerable opportunities, depending upon the age of the students, for the teacher to correlate previews of the procedures to be followed with the subject matter of history and the biological and physical sciences. After all the returns on examining and testing procedures are in and duly entered on the students' health records, the recommendations of the examiners furnish a rich store of educational leads to the teacher, who, alone or in cooperation with the nurse or health counselor, is responsible for the health guidance of individual students. The small emergencies, like minor injuries, and the big emergencies, like epidemics, which call the forces of the school health service into action are all "good grist at hand" to keep the mill of health education going.

Members of the school-health-service staff are concerned with the health education of individual older students in connection with their health-counseling activities. Also, they have many opportunities to make effective use of health education in their work with all the children and their parents. The health examination of elementary school children furnishes an opportunity of this kind. The parents are notified that their child is to be examined and are invited to attend the examination. Beforehand the nurse confers with the teacher and the mother to secure information that may furnish the physician with valuable leads as he makes his examination. During or after the examination the mother and the teacher have an opportunity to talk over the findings with physician and nurse and to discuss plans for follow-up procedures.

This close working together of all those most intimately concerned with the child's well-being will enable teachers and parents to appreciate the significance of their observations and to gain confidence in their powers of observation. On the other hand it will supply the physician and nurse with clues to guide them in doing their part in safeguarding the health of the child.

The chief concern of the physicians, dentists, nurses, and other professionally trained personnel who are serving the school is rightly the actual carrying on of health-service activities. But they are finding out that they get much better results when they take time to get acquainted with the boys and girls and their parents, to explain what they are doing clearly and simply as they do it, to volunteer praise where it is due, to give reasons for their recommendations to parents, teachers, and others responsible for acting on them, and to develop and maintain effective working relationships with private physicians and other individuals or groups in the community concerned with meeting health and welfare needs.

THE CHIEF HEALTH PROBLEMS OF CHILDHOOD

Child-health problems today are in several respects radically different from those which confronted parents and teachers earlier in the twentieth century. The most important change has been the great reduction in the death rate for school-age boys and girls in the last two decades (Fig. 1).

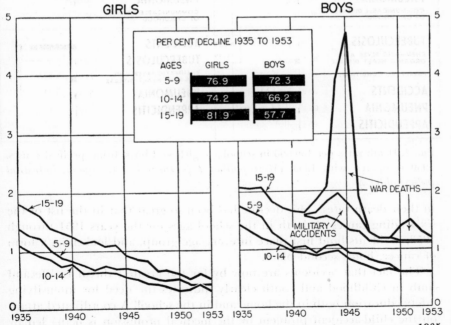

FIG. 1. Death rates per 1,000 in school-age girls and boys, by age groups, 1935 to 1953. (*Metropolitan Life Insurance Company, industrial policyholders.*)

The savings in life represented by this reduction are in large part the
fruits of the amazingly brilliant and productive work done during the
past 50 years in controlling the infectious diseases. Although diseases in
this category are still important causes of death by disease among school-
age children, Figure 2 shows that there has been a very marked decline

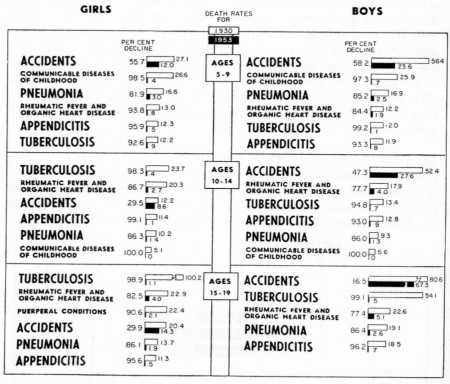

Fig. 2. Death rates per 100,000 in school-age girls and boys, from specified causes,
1930 compared with 1953. (*Metropolitan Life Insurance Company, industrial
policyholders.*)

in their death rates. This decline has been so great that in the list of the
six leading causes of death in the school ages for the years 1951 through
1953, accidents hold first place in every age group, and leukemia, a form
of cancer, holds second place.

The fact that accidents are now by far the greatest threat to life and
limb in childhood and youth clearly indicates the need for intensifying
safety education both in the home and in the school. A coordinated attack
on the child-accident problem by the medical profession is being led by
the recently organized Committee on Child Safety of the American
Academy of Pediatrics.

Success Stories

In the early years of the twentieth century scarcely any child escaped a first infection with tuberculosis, which is recognized by a reaction to the tuberculin test (see Tuberculosis, in Chap. 5). Today fully one-half, and in some places three-fourths, of all our children grow up without acquiring a sensitizing dose of tubercle bacilli. This has been accomplished both by educational programs, which have gained the cooperation of the public in combating tuberculosis, and by organized efforts to find and treat persons with active tuberculosis in time to prevent its spread.

Diphtheria once returned year after year in devastating epidemics, closing schools and inspiring terror in every parent or teacher who heard a child complain of a sore throat. With diphtheria toxoid available for making susceptible children immune from diphtheria, any community, if it wishes, can now ensure the disappearance of this disease. Many large cities where immunization of children has been universally and continuously practiced have proved this point.

Typhoid fever and other milk-borne and water-borne gastrointestinal infections were once high-ranking causes of death in infancy, childhood, and youth. Now they are disappearing, largely as a result of the work of public health sanitarians who have succeeded in safeguarding water and milk supplies over large areas.

Pneumococcal pneumonia, the most dreaded of the acute respiratory infections, is being conquered, both as a result of improved methods of preventing and treating the infections that pave the way for pneumonia and as a result of the means now available—notably chemotherapeutic drugs, such as sulfadiazine, and antibiotics, such as penicillin and aureomycin—for successfully treating pneumonia itself.

These four examples are given merely to illustrate the spectacular change that has taken place in the past twenty-five or thirty years in our thoughts and feelings about children's illnesses. Although there are still several diseases—leukemia, for example—which can make us sick at heart, there is no longer the generally hopeless attitude that prevailed before medical research began to show tangible results. Medical old-timers in their reminiscences have told us of the gloom pervading the medical wards in contrast to the cheerfulness of the surgical wards in the period when medicine was stymied and surgery was forging ahead. Now, the gloom is lifting. There is every reason to believe that the day will come when both medicine and surgery will have the means at hand to deal with most, if not all, of the chief causes of early death.

Tales of Woe

The fact that the death rate is declining among school children does not mean that there has been a comparable reduction in illnesses, physical defects, and accidental injuries. The Paradise of Children would indeed return to earth if there were some way of getting completely rid of colds and sore throats, chickenpox and measles, upset stomachs and broken bones, decayed teeth and impetigo, head lice and poison ivy, and all the other minor and major afflictions of the young. Although many of these afflictions are not ordinarily serious, some of them may interfere with a child's education or lead to worse trouble later on. Others may be blessings in disguise by immunizing children from infections that might have serious consequences later in life.

In efforts to improve physical and mental fitness in the later years of life, physicians are now seeking in the records of the earlier years clues to the infirmities of middle and old age. Who can estimate the effects on body or mind, or both, of the insults and injuries that may have been sustained in bouts with illness, or in unhappy experiences at home or in school, or in substandard nutrition, or in efforts to compensate for some undiscovered physical defect! Children's bodies and minds, by and large, are pretty tough, if the heritage is good, but sometimes unfavorable environmental influences are tougher.

It would be impossible to protect all children from environmental impacts that may or may not leave scars on their developing personalities. What the school can do through health education and health services, in cooperation with home and community agencies, is to reduce the chances of infection, injury, malnourishment, and the development of neurotic trends; recognize and work for the correction of remediable defects and conditions; and help those children who are irretrievably handicapped to make as good an adjustment as possible to life as they must live it.

Leading Causes of Illness and Disability in School Children

Records of absences from school, when carefully kept and analyzed, furnish concrete statistical evidence regarding the causes of illness among school children. Several studies of school absenteeism have been made in recent years. Two of the most recent are (a) a study of school absenteeism made in certain selected classrooms in each of the provinces of Canada during the school year 1946–1947; and (b) a pilot study of school absenteeism carried on in elementary schools in seven California cities from January to June of 1947. Charts summarizing the findings of these two studies regarding causes of absence in terms of per cent of days lost from school in urban areas are reproduced in Figure 3. Other studies indicate that the situation pictured in these charts is reasonably representative of the situation prevailing throughout the country, at least in urban centers.

Respiratory Infections. Respiratory infections are universally recognized as the chief illnesses responsible for school absences. They include the common cold, sore throat, bronchitis, sinus conditions, and pulmonary tuberculosis. Of these, the common cold is by far the worst offender. The picture here has not changed a great deal over the years.

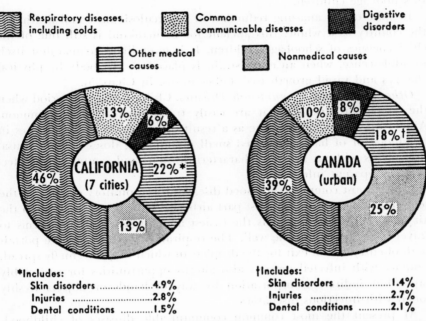

*Includes:
Skin disorders 4.9%
Injuries 2.8%
Dental conditions 1.5%

†Includes:
Skin disorders 1.4%
Injuries 2.7%
Dental conditions 2.1%

Based on studies of school absenteeism in seven California cities (1947) and in Canada (1946-1947).

FIG. 3. Causes of absence in terms of per cent of days lost from school. (*From "Health Bulletin for Teachers," November, 1949, Metropolitan Life Insurance Company.*)

Colds probably cause as many absences today as in the school days of the fathers and grandfathers of the current crop of children. But the bacterial invasions of the lungs which are so often invited by the respiratory virus infections—notably colds and influenza—are not nearly so potentially dangerous to life as they once were. Although pneumonia is still rated among the leading causes of death in the school ages, far fewer children are getting it and dying of it, thanks largely to the use of the sulfonamides and antibiotics in its prevention and treatment.

The sore throats and colds that are caused by certain members of the streptococcal family of bacteria are feared chiefly because they are so often associated with worse trouble. Repeated streptococcal infections of the nose and throat are responsible for lighting up the rheumatic infections that play such havoc with young hearts (see Rheumatic Fever, in Chap. 4). The death toll from acute rheumatic fever and rheumatic heart disease combined is much lower than it was two decades ago. But this combination is still a highly important cause of sickness and death in school-age children.

In spite of the amazing reduction in tuberculosis cases and deaths for the country as a whole, this ancient foe of mankind is still one of the chief enemies of school-age children. It is most likely to manifest itself in adolescence, when an extra strain is placed on the body by physical changes and rapid growth (see Tuberculosis, in Chap. 5).

Other Common Communicable Diseases. Childhood is the period when the contagious diseases that are easily transmitted are most common. Almost all adults are immune as a result of having had such diseases in childhood or of having received small immunizing doses of their causative agents without showing characteristic signs and symptoms of infection (inapparent infection).

All the most common childhood diseases are respiratory diseases in the sense that they are for the most part airborne. Direct passage through the air from person to person is the easiest and quickest way for germs to travel from the sick to the well. The respiratory passages are the portals both of entry and of exit for the droplets in which they are chiefly spread. Contact with infected persons also affords opportunities for reasonably rapid but indirect transportation by way of hands or objects freshly soiled with infectious discharges.

At present the most common communicable diseases of childhood, other than colds, are chickenpox, measles, German measles, whooping cough, and scarlet fever. Mumps is less communicable than measles and chickenpox, and consequently more adults are susceptible to it than to other diseases common in childhood.

Scarlet fever is a streptococcal infection which is feared mostly because of the complications that may follow it, notably acute rheumatic fever (see Chap. 4) and acute glomerular nephritis (see The Kidneys, in Chap. 6). Various substances for giving temporary or long-lasting protection from scarlet fever are available, chiefly for use in epidemics.

More than 95 per cent of the cases of *whooping cough* occur in children less than five years of age. Usually the disease can be prevented by immunization with whooping cough vaccine, beginning at three months of age or earlier.

Measles deaths can now, to a large extent, be avoided through the use of gamma globulin (see Blood and Its Composition, in Chap. 4) to protect babies and young or feeble children temporarily after exposure and to lessen the severity of attacks in older children. It is not considered wise to protect healthy older children completely, because a light attack is a cheap way of gaining immunity from a disease that often has serious consequences in later life.

Teachers may expect that the communicable diseases that are usually much milder in children than in adults—modified measles, German measles, chickenpox, and mumps—will continue to be a leading cause of school absences. Reduction in the sickness rate of these diseases is not a matter of great public health concern and is even considered unwise by some physicians. There is something to be said for the old belief that it is better to let children have ordinarily mild contagious diseases and get them over with rather than to make a great effort to protect them from illnesses that are usually far more serious when contracted later in life. This is particularly true of German measles and mumps. German measles occurring in an expectant mother within the first 3 months of pregnancy may result in serious congenital defects in the child. Mumps occurring after puberty may be complicated by inflammation of the sex glands (see Mumps, in Chap. 6).

Digestive Disorders. Digestive disturbances as a group constitute the third most important cause of illnesses among school children. Stomach-ache, nausea and vomiting, diarrhea, and constipation, to name the most common, are really symptoms that may indicate a temporary gastro-intestinal upset or some more serious condition for which the digestive system may or may not be directly to blame.

Temporary Upsets. Gastrointestinal upsets are very common in child-hood, largely because many children have not learned discretion in eat-ing or drinking or have formed poor eating or bowel habits or have especially sensitive stomachs or bowels. "Green-apple stomach-ache" is symbolic of children's experiments with excessive amounts of indigestible foods. And any adult who has had much to do with children is familiar with the spells of vomiting, or colic, or diarrhea that so often occur after periods of excitement or fatigue or overeating, especially of sweets.

Infections. The principal diseases in the gastrointestinal group for which bacteria or viruses are responsible include bacillary dysentery, infectious hepatitis (acute catarrhal jaundice), and food infections and food poisonings. Appendicitis is not nearly so deadly as it used to be (Fig. 2), but it is still a very common disease among children of school age. Education of the public in "what to do till the doctor comes" when symptoms of appendicitis develop, and the use of sulfonamides and penicillin in combating peritonitis, account largely for the drop in the death rate from this dangerous infection.

Miscellaneous Conditions. A fourth fairly large group of disorders is composed of several different ailments and conditions, each of which is comparatively rare as a cause of absence. The top-ranking disorders in this miscellaneous group, in order of importance, are skin conditions, such as impetigo and ringworm of the scalp; accidental injuries; and dental conditions. A few are serious diseases, such as cancer, meningitis, diabetes, malaria, and undulant fever.

Physical Defects

Death rates shed light on illnesses that terminate fatally in a certain number of cases. Records of absences from school because of illness permit us to sort out and group the illnesses that are most common in the school ages. But such evidence sheds little or no light on the prevalence of defects and disorders which are not a direct threat to life or which do not directly cause loss of time from school.

Both from special studies of physical defects among school children and from our own observation, we know that there are large numbers of children in school today with decayed teeth; defective vision, hearing, and speech; and borderline malnutrition, as well as mild specific nutritional deficiencies. In addition to children with physical disabilities, there are large numbers who show marked deviations from normal behavior which later may lead to serious mental ill health.

We have taken a quick and somewhat casual look at the health problems that are most common in childhood. It is not by any means a complete review of all the ills of the flesh and the spirit to which teachers should be alerted. It is well to remember also that the eyes and the ears of true observers are not blind and deaf to all but the majorities and the averages. It is no comfort to the person with a rare disease or condition to know that it is rare. Knowing from training and experience what can be expected of healthy children in a certain age group in the way of appearance and behavior, the teacher will be guided by what she personally sees and hears, no matter how ordinary or how extraordinary a deviation from the average or normal may be.

THE CHILD AS A WHOLE

At first sight a child is only what he appears to be on the surface. Just as the passengers on a ship, observing an iceberg, see only the unsubmerged tenth, so the teacher meeting a child for the first time observes only the unsubmerged part of his personality—his body build and posture; his facial features and expression; the coloring of his skin, hair, and eyes; his tone of voice and diction. She gets what is called "a first impression," which may be good or bad according to the child's appearance and manner and their impact on her own personality.

First impressions are important if they indicate that a child differs radically from most other children in the group in appearance or behavior (see Identifying Children with Emotional and Social Problems, in Chap. 3). Ordinarily, however, it is as unwise for one human being to trust a first impression of another human being as it would be for a ship's captain to trust the impression that there is no more to an iceberg than what he sees floating on the ocean. Of course, no iceberg can begin to compete with a human being in complexity and uniqueness. To appraise the whole child correctly on better acquaintance—the nine-tenths below the surface as well as the one-tenth above—the teacher must have a working knowledge of human beings in general and what makes them tick, as well as of that particular child.

Individual Uniqueness

By "personality" we mean the person as a whole—body, mind, and spirit working together as a unit. Every child at any one time is the unique product of the personality he inherited from his parents as modified by the dynamic exchanges between himself and his environment.

The Child and Heredity. Every one of the billions of cells in the human body contains in its nucleus 48 chromosomes,[1] which are replicas of the 24 originally passed on by the father and 24 originally passed on by the mother. Chance determined which 24 of each of the parent's 48 chromosomes were transmitted. Furthermore, since both parents inherited their characteristics in the same manner, it is obvious that each child possesses hereditary factors handed down in part from generations of ancestors.

Knowing the laws of inheritance, it is easy to understand why the children in one family may resemble one another closely and the children in another family may differ greatly from one another in hereditary characteristics such as eye color, hair color, skin color, body build, and general level of intelligence. The amazing thing is that no two children (except identical twins) can be exactly the same in their hereditary make-up.

Amram Scheinfeld shows us in his book "You and Heredity" that 16,777,216 different combinations of hereditary factors can theoretically be produced from any one set of 24 chromosomes (the number contributed by each parent to the child). Any child—any human being—is the result of the meeting of a particular sperm with a particular ovum, each

[1] Chromosomes are the minute threadlike structures along which the genes that carry hereditary characteristics are strung like beads.

one of which carried one combination of hereditary factors out of a possible 16,777,216 different combinations. The chance that brought that particular sperm and egg together, Scheinfeld tells us, "could happen only once in some 300,000,000,000,000 times!" [2]

The possibility that one child ever has been or ever will be exactly like another child, so far as the inherited part of his personality is concerned, is practically nonexistent.

The Child and Environment. A child's equipment and potentialities at birth are continually being modified by the forces and things, the people and events, to which he is exposed. Strictly speaking, environment is everything to which a living organism is able to respond. In the case of a human being, it includes all the animate and inanimate sources of stimuli that arouse in him the sensations of seeing (unless he was born blind), hearing (unless he was born deaf), tasting, touching, smelling, pain, heat and cold; the air he breathes, the food he eats, the water he drinks; the customs (things he should do), the taboos (things he should not do), the demands, criticisms, rewards, punishments, promises, and ideals of the people with whom he comes in contact.

If we were not safe in saying that personality is unique on the basis of heredity alone, we should not go far astray in claiming that a child's environment after birth would serve to make him different from all other children. Even children brought up in the same family cannot be said to have the same home environment because home conditions are constantly changing. The first child, for example, has a different environment from that of the second, if only through the difference in the size of the family. Birth and death, marriage and divorce, fluctuations in family income with their effect on living standards, moving from one street or community to another, visits of relatives and friends—these are only a few of the events that may profoundly influence one child and have little or no effect on another, because of difference in age or experience or temperament or some other factor at the time they occurred.

The Child Himself. In spite of the emphasis laid here on heredity and environment as determiners of personality, it would be a mistake to assume that its form and pattern are merely the passive result of the child's physical and mental inheritance and the imprints made upon him by everything coming into his body or acting on it from without. It must be remembered that his body is equipped at every point with sensitive nerve endings that supply him with information about the external world, and with a skeletomuscular system that enables him to bring himself into active contact with a wide variety of objects and events. Even as a tiny baby he is capable of the purposeful activity

[2] SCHEINFELD, AMRAM, "You and Heredity," p. 29, Stokes, Philadelphia, 1939.

required to modify the impressions made upon him by his environment. By his cries in protest against discomforts caused by unpleasant sensations, for example, he gets needed attention—his diaper changed, his hunger satisfied, a pricking pin removed, or an extra blanket supplied.

As time goes on, the internal changes incident to his own growth and development and the accumulation of new experiences enable him to bring even greater pressure to bear on the unending series of external forces with which he is continually bombarded. As a result, the child, already roughhewn by heredity, gradually acquires attitudes, tastes, and behavior patterns that are peculiarly his own. He himself then will have the last word about how he shall be modified. Within the limits set by his inborn constitution and by the raw materials in his environment, he will become the architect of his own body, of his own character. If this were not so, there would be no point in trying to give children the incentives and the knowledge that will help them to take advantage of their opportunities for the best possible growth and development.

Physiological Sameness

Although the personality of every human being is unique, the bodies of all healthy human beings are built and work pretty much alike within normal variations. It is of great importance to keep this fact in mind in observing children. Upon it are based everything we know and teach about the human body and its care and everything that tells us whether a child is healthy or needs medical attention.

What would be the sense of telling children what they need in the way of food and what foods supply these needs if each body differed from every other body in its food requirements? And how could any doctor examining a child find "something wrong" if there were no universal right—if it were natural for each child to possess a stomach or a heart or any organ that was constructed and worked differently from every other child's?

The many different signs and symptoms that may indicate that something is wrong physically all have a background of physiological sameness. Even when the trouble is primarily due to some form of emotional or social maladjustment, characteristic physiological signs may appear.

DO YOU KNOW?

1. Several subjects for a speech or group discussion are given below. Following each subject are listed four talking points. Select the right one to use or emphasize. For example: The Art of Diagnosis: parental

interest, a medical responsibility, teacher observation, nursing skill. "A medical responsibility" is the most important talking point, because only the physician is trained in the art of diagnosis.

a. The Leading Cause of School Absences: accidents, respiratory infections, skin diseases, digestive disorders
b. The Conquest of Diphtheria: antibiotics, isolation of cases, diphtheria immunization, sulfa drugs
c. Decline in the Pneumonia Death Rate: pneumonia immunization, use of sulfa drugs and antibiotics in prevention and treatment, decrease in the prevalence of colds, improved community sanitation
d. Typhoid Fever as a Disappearing Disease: the safeguarding of community water and milk supplies by public health sanitarians, typhoid fever immunization, isolation of cases, improved methods of diagnosis

2. Suppose you are on the affirmative side in a debate on the following question: Resolved that it is safer to have certain contagious diseases in childhood than in adult life. Select from the following list the diseases you would cite: scarlet fever, smallpox, mumps, diphtheria, typhoid fever, German measles, rheumatic fever.
3. Suppose you are on the negative side in a debate on the following question: Resolved that heredity is the sole determining factor in personality development. What arguments would you use in refutation?

SUGGESTED ACTIVITIES

1. Unobtrusively observe for 5 minutes a group of children or fellow students assembled in a classroom. Then write the answers to the following questions:

a. How many students have straight hair? curly hair? light hair? dark hair? blue eyes? brown eyes?
b. How many are left-handed?
c. How many wear glasses?
d. How many are pale? tanned? freckled? rosy-cheeked?
e. What are the names of the girls in the front row?

Check your answers in another more leisurely period of observation. Practice with different groups until you are able to make a perfect score.

2. Unobtrusively observe a strange child in a bus, streetcar, or train. Afterward write a description of the child's appearance and behavior.

Then observe and describe in writing a child you know well—a member of your family or a child in a class you are teaching. Which is the fuller description? Why?

3. As a group activity appoint a committee to stage a dramatic episode in the classroom or lecture room—an accident, a fire, a fight, for example. Afterward, have each witness write down what he saw and heard. Compare the descriptions. Then have the actors describe exactly what they did and said. Who was the best observer?

✓ 4. As a class activity have the members of the class make reports on the school-health-service set-up in the high schools they attended. In the opinion of each reporter, how could the health examinations, health counseling, and other services have been made more effective in improving his or her own living habits and attitude toward health?

5. Arrange with the nurse serving your laboratory or practice school (or the school in which you teach) to have a teacher-nurse conference on a child with a health problem who is scheduled for medical examination by the physician serving the school. Talk over with the nurse things you have observed which in your opinion should be brought to the physician's attention. Arrange to attend the examination. Afterward talk with the nurse and the parents (if present) about the physician's recommendations and how they can best be carried out at home and in school.

6. As a class activity make a survey of the community in which your college or training school is located in order to find out what facilities are available for getting needed medical, dental, or other specialized services, without charge or at low cost, for school children who would not otherwise obtain them. Things to look for include a community or neighborhood health council; clinics (hospital out-patient, cardiac, dental, child guidance, etc.); health centers operated by the official public health unit serving the community; facilities made available by voluntary health agencies (local tuberculosis association, local chapter of the National Foundation for Infantile Paralysis, local Red Cross Chapter, etc.) and by clubs or organizations interested in child welfare (Lions Club, Kiwanis Club, church clubs, American Legion post, etc.).

7. Obtain from the public health unit in your college town (or county) or your home town (or county), the community's mortality rates for typhoid fever, tuberculosis, and the "big four" communicable diseases of childhood (measles, scarlet fever, whooping cough, and diphtheria) at 5-year intervals from 1925 to 1955. Construct graphs showing the decline in mortality from these diseases. Discuss these questions in class:

a. How has the discovery that infectious diseases are caused by micro-organisms made possible the control of many such diseases?

b. What once common infectious diseases are now comparatively rare?

c. What measures are currently being used to combat each disease mentioned?

SELECTED REFERENCES

The School Health Program

AMERICAN ASSOCIATION OF SCHOOL ADMINISTRATORS (a department of the National Education Association): *Health in Schools; Twentieth Yearbook,* rev. ed. Washington, D.C., 1951.

BROWNELL, CLIFFORD LEE: *Principles of Health Education Applied,* New York, McGraw-Hill Book Company, Inc., 1949.

COOPS, HELEN LESLIE: *Health Education in Elementary Schools: Activities—Materials—Methods,* New York, A. S. Barnes and Company, 1950.

DENVER (Colorado) PUBLIC SCHOOLS: *Health Interests of Children,* 2d impression, 1949.

DEPARTMENT OF ELEMENTARY SCHOOL PRINCIPALS (of the National Education Association): *Health in the Elementary School, Twenty-ninth Yearbook,* Vol. XXX, No. 1 (September), 1950. (A bulletin of the Department.)

DEPARTMENT OF ELEMENTARY SCHOOL PRINCIPALS (of the National Education Association): *Science for Today's Children, Thirty-second Yearbook,* Vol. XXXIII, No. 1, 1953. (A bulletin of the Department.)

GROUT, RUTH E.: *Health Teaching in Schools,* 2d ed. Philadelphia, W. B. Saunders Company, 1953.

METROPOLITAN LIFE INSURANCE COMPANY, HEALTH AND WELFARE DIVISION: *The School Health Program,* New York, 1950.

METROPOLITAN LIFE INSURANCE COMPANY, HEALTH AND WELFARE DIVISION: *What Teachers See,* New York, 1954.

METROPOLITAN LIFE INSURANCE COMPANY, HEALTH AND WELFARE DIVISION: *The School Administrator, Physician, and Nurse in the School Health Program,* School Health Monograph No. 13, New York, 1949. (A report sponsored by the National Conference for Cooperation in Health Education.)

METROPOLITAN LIFE INSURANCE COMPANY, HEALTH AND WELFARE DIVISION: *Absent from School Today,* New York, 1949.

NATIONAL COMMITTEE ON SCHOOL HEALTH POLICIES (of the National Conference for Cooperation in Health Education): *Suggested School Health Policies: A Charter for School Health,* New York and Minneapolis, Health Education Council, 1945. (Revision in process.)

NATIONAL EDUCATION ASSOCIATION AND AMERICAN MEDICAL ASSOCIATION, JOINT COMMITTEE ON HEALTH PROBLEMS IN EDUCATION: *Health Education,* 4th ed. Washington, D.C., National Education Association, 1948.

NATIONAL EDUCATION ASSOCIATION AND AMERICAN MEDICAL ASSOCIATION, JOINT COMMITTEE ON HEALTH PROBLEMS IN EDUCATION: *School Health Services,* Washington, D.C., National Education Association, 1954.

OBERTEUFFER, DELBERT: *School Health Education,* rev. ed. New York, Harper & Brothers, 1954.

OVERSTREET, HARRY, and BONARO W. OVERSTREET: *Where Children Come First—A Study of the Parent Teacher Association Idea,* Chicago, National Congress of Parents and Teachers, 1949.

ROGERS, JAMES FREDERICK: *What Every Teacher Should Know about the Physical Condition of Her Pupils,* Pamphlet No. 68 (revised), Washington, D.C., U.S. Office of Education, 1945.

STRANG, RUTH M., and DEAN F. SMILEY: *The Role of the Teacher in Health Education,* New York, The Macmillan Company, 1951 (reissue).

TURNER, CLAIR E.: *School Health and Health Education,* 2d ed. St. Louis, The C. V. Mosby Company, 1952.

U.S. OFFICE OF EDUCATION: *Teachers Contribute to Child Health,* Bulletin No. 8, Washington, D.C., 1951.

Excellent manuals or guides on the school health program have been developed in many states by the state department of health or the state department (or board) of education or by joint committees or councils of both departments. Copies may be obtained through the department of health or department of education of the state.

The Human Body and Healthful Living [3]

BEST, CHARLES HERBERT, and NORMAN BURKE TAYLOR: *Living Body; A Text in Human Physiology,* 3d ed. New York, Henry Holt and Company, Inc., 1952.

[3] The books and pamphlets listed in this and the following category include several references which in many instances can be read to supplement the specific references given at the end of other units. This note applies particularly to books on the human body and the control of disease.

CLENDENING, LOGAN: *The Human Body,* 4th ed. New York, Alfred A. Knopf, Inc., 1945.

DAVIS, ARTHUR F., and WARREN H. SOUTHWORTH: *Meredith's Hygiene,* 5th ed. New York, Blakiston Division, McGraw-Hill Book Company, Inc., 1954. (A textbook for college students.)

DIEHL, HAROLD S., and ANITA D. LATON: *Health and Safety for You,* New York, McGraw-Hill Book Company, Inc., 1954.

JOHNS, EDWARD B., WILFRED C. SUTTON, and LLOYD E. WEBSTER (with Walter H. Brown as adviser and consultant, and foreword by Bernice Moss): *Health for Effective Living—A Basic Health Education Text for College Students,* New York, McGraw-Hill Book Company, Inc., 1954.

SCHIFFERES, JUSTUS: *Healthier Living,* New York, John Wiley & Sons, Inc., 1954. (A text in personal and community health.)

STACK, HERBERT J., ELMER B. SIEBRECHT, and J. DUKE ELKOW: *Education for Safe Living,* 2d ed. New York, Prentice-Hall, Inc., 1949.

STILES, WILLIAM W.: *Individual and Community Health,* New York, Blakiston Division, McGraw-Hill Book Company, Inc., 1953.

TURNER, CLAIR E.: *Personal and Community Health,* 9th ed. St. Louis, The C. V. Mosby Company, 1952.

WILLIAMS, JESSE FEIRING, and LLOYD GAGE WETHERILL: *Personal and Community Hygiene Applied,* Philadelphia, W. B. Saunders Company, 1950.

Medicine and Public Health

AMERICAN PUBLIC HEALTH ASSOCIATION: *Control of Communicable Diseases in Man,* 8th ed. New York, 1955. [A standard handbook listing diseases alphabetically and giving for each one the means of identification, causative agent (when known), source of infection, mode of transmission, incubation period, susceptibility and resistance, occurrence, and methods of control.]

FISHBEIN, MORRIS: *The Popular Medical Encyclopedia: The Standard Guide on Health and Disease,* rev. and enlarged ed. New York, Doubleday & Company, Inc., 1953.

KLEINSCHMIDT, H. E., and S. ZIMAND: *Public Health Education: Its Tools and Procedures,* New York, The Macmillan Company, 1953.

LEAVELL, H. R., and E. G. CLARK: *Textbook of Preventive Medicine,* New York, McGraw-Hill Book Company, Inc., 1953.

MOUNTIN, JOSEPH W., and EVELYN FLOOK: *Guide to Health Organizations in the United States,* rev. ed. U.S. Public Health Service, Publication No. 196, Government Printing Office, Washington, D.C., 1953.

MUSTARD, HARRY S.: *An Introduction to Public Health,* 3d ed. New York, The Macmillan Company, 1953.

PATTERSON, R. S., and B. J. ROBERTS: *Community Health Education in Action,* St. Louis, The C. V. Mosby Company, 1951.

SHEPARD, WILLIAM P.: *Essentials of Public Health,* 2d ed. Philadelphia, J. B. Lippincott Company, 1952.

SMILLIE, WILLIAM G.: *Public Health Administration in the United States,* 3d ed. New York, The Macmillan Company, 1947.

SMILLIE, WILLIAM G.: *Preventive Medicine and Public Health,* 2d ed. New York, The Macmillan Company, 1952.

SPENCER, STEVEN M.: *Wonders of Modern Medicine,* New York, McGraw-Hill Book Company, Inc., 1953.

SWANSON, MARIE E.: *School Nursing in the Community Program,* New York, The Macmillan Company, 1953.

Periodicals

Teachers who wish to keep abreast of developments in fields related to personal and community health and safety will find the following publications helpful:

Accident Facts. A valuable classified compilation of accident statistics, issued annually by the National Safety Council.

Canada's Health and Welfare. Issued monthly in English and French by Information Services Division, Canadian Department of National Health and Welfare.

Child Study. Child Study Association of America.

Children. Issued bimonthly by the U.S. Department of Health, Education and Welfare, Children's Bureau.

Health Bulletin for Teachers. Issued periodically during the school year, School Health Bureau, Health and Welfare Division, Metropolitan Life Insurance Company.

Journal of the American Association for Health, Physical Education, and Recreation. Issued monthly by the Association.

Journal of School Health. Issued monthly by the American School Health Association.

National Parent-Teacher. Issued monthly by Parent-Teacher, Inc.

Public Health Reports. Issued monthly by the U.S. Department of Health, Education and Welfare, Public Health Service.

Recreation. Issued monthly, except July and August, by the National Recreation Association.

Safety Education. National Safety Council.

School Life. U.S. Department of Health, Education and Welfare, Office of Education.

Science News Letter. "The Weekly Summary of Current Science," Science Service.

Statistical Bulletin. Issued monthly by the Metropolitan Life Insurance Company.

Today's Health. Issued monthly by the American Medical Association.

Understanding the Child. Issued four times a year by the National Association for Mental Health.

Government and National Voluntary Agencies

The agencies listed here have available educational material on a variety of subjects related to health. Organizations with special areas of interest are listed at the end of the units concerned with that area. For information regarding available materials, write to the organization. The addresses of these organizations, and of others mentioned in this book, are given at the end of the book.

American Council on Education
American Medical Association
American Public Health Association
Child Study Association of America
Metropolitan Life Insurance Company (Health and Welfare)
National Education Association
National Health Council
National Publicity Council for Health and Welfare Services, Inc.
National Safety Council
U.S. Department of Health, Education and Welfare: Children's Bureau, Office of Education, Public Health Service

Many state health and education departments also offer free or inexpensive material in the field of health.

Chapter 2   THE GROWING CHILD

Physical Growth and Development
Measuring Physical Growth and Development
Mental Growth and Its Measurement
Emotional and Social Development

PHYSICAL GROWTH AND DEVELOPMENT

There is no subject vaster and more complex than that of human growth and development. It can be discussed in this book only to the extent of giving teachers some idea of what should be kept in mind in observing the physical, mental, emotional, and social progress of school children toward maturity.

By strict definition, physical growth is limited to increase in size, and development to increase in complexity. Growth is an affair of time and space—children grow chronologically and dimensionally. Development also proceeds with age, but its relationship to increase in size varies greatly according to the process involved. A tremendous increase in complexity can take place with very little increase in size. There is, for example, a very close correlation between the head size (breadth and height from the ears up) of a three-month-old baby and a seventeen-year-old boy or girl, but there is a vast difference in the complexity of the brain at these two ages. On the other hand there can be considerable increase in size with very little or no increase in complexity. For example, the leg (from the knee to the floor) is nearly four times as long in a seventeen-year-old boy or girl as in a three-month-old baby, but practically no increase in the complexity of leg structure takes place between these two ages.

The Pattern of Growth

Growth is an expression of the tremendous power generated by the union of sperm and egg. A power belonging to life alone, it cannot be created and put to work in the laboratory, and so it can be studied only by observing how some of its results are achieved. Just so, without being able to duplicate the effects created by an artist, we can watch him at work and form some idea of his technique.

31

The process of physical growth has a beginning and an end. Beginning with the first mitosis, or division of the fertilized egg into two cells, it stops when full maturity has been achieved. The stoppage of increase in size is fully as important as its start. If we find it hard to think of ourselves as having once been microscopically small, our imaginations bog down completely at the idea of ever being infinitely large. Our only example of runaway growth—cancer—is a solemn reminder of the biologic necessity for keeping a tight rein on increase in size and for bringing it to a halt when maturity is reached.

If growth and development are defined in terms of progressive maturity, then it is evident that different parts of the body become adult —that is, mature—at different times. At birth or shortly after, an individual needs the services of almost all his body organs. Therefore we find that with a few exceptions—the sex glands, for example—an individual's organs are functionally mature even in early life. An organ must reach a certain size in order to function. After that it may keep on growing but usually does not grow a great deal. The internal ear is adult in size at birth. The olfactory apparatus in the nose reaches almost adult dimensions at the age of six months. The cranial cavity, which holds the brain, is nearly as large as it will ever be when a child is six years old. The eye, on the other hand, is usually not fully developed until age nine or ten.

The body framework, as a whole, is not fully mature until the third decade of life, but its various components have their own pattern of growth. In general these components, which together make up stature, consist of the head and neck, the trunk, and the lower limbs. The head and neck and the trunk are most fully developed at birth, because they contain all the organs upon which life depends; hence they need to grow less than the legs. At birth the legs make up only about 33 per cent of stature; at one year, 35 per cent; at six years, 45 per cent; and at seventeen years, 48 per cent. Of the three segments, the head grows at the slowest rate, because it is closest to adult proportions at birth and at two years of age is nine-tenths as big as it will ever be. Vertical growth in the arms and legs is comparatively greatest during grade school age, and in the trunk during high school age when the sex organs are reaching maturity.

So we see that, in growing, the body does not expand symmetrically as a bubble expands with an increase in the volume of its contents. It has a definite growth pattern, with different parts having their own time schedules for coming to maturity.

Influences on Growth and Development

Growth is motivated by forces contributed partly by heredity and partly by environment. In the germ cell, to which both parents contribute, is laid away each individual's growth pattern. But no matter what potentialities in the way of body build and physical stamina a child may have inherited, his actual size and shape and physical condition at any one time will show the marks left by any defects in structure that may have been present at birth (a congenital heart or blood-vessel defect, for example), the important illnesses and accidents he has suffered recently, the kinds and amounts of food he has eaten, the physical activities he has engaged in, and many other environmental factors.

Influences on Skeletal Growth. Hereditary influence is chiefly responsible for the so-called body types—the tall slender type at one extreme, the short and stocky type at the other, with an intermediate or "average" type in between. These variations in body build are largely determined by the size, shape, and density of the skeleton.

A newborn baby's skeleton is partly bone and partly cartilage. The shafts of the bones of the arms and legs, of the bones of the feet, and of the fingers and toes, for example, are well developed, but the ends are masses of cartilage which present in a general way the shape of the future bone. As the child grows older, ossification centers, called epiphyses, appear in the masses of cartilage as points of spongy bone. These juvenile pieces of bone, or epiphyses, gradually spread until at last they unite with the large, or parent, bone. With the fusion of the epiphyses, growth stops.

By taking x-ray pictures of the bones of large numbers of children at various ages, it has been possible to demonstrate with considerable accuracy not only the average time at which the various ossification centers make their appearance but also the average age when these centers (epiphyses) unite with the parent bone. The bone age of the child as revealed by the x-ray is therefore being used as an indicator of bodily maturity.

Many factors besides hereditary influence leave their imprint upon the skeleton as it matures.

Diet. In forming bone, the bone cells are dependent upon the bone-building materials supplied in food. These materials are the salts of calcium and phosphorus, which are combined to form calcium phosphate. Vitamin D is required for the utilization of calcium and phosphorus by the bone cells, and ascorbic acid (vitamin C) is necessary for the composition of intercellular cement, which affects the structure and the strength of bones as well as those of other tissues.

If babies and children fail to obtain adequate and balanced supplies of calcium, phosphorus, and vitamin D, the bones do not calcify normally and rickets (see Rickets, in Chap. 9) is the result. The typical rickety child—bowlegged, knock-kneed, or pigeon-breasted—is a dramatic reminder of the important part played by diet in skeletal growth.

Posture. Continual faulty posture during the growth years affects skeletal growth by changing the normal stresses in the architecture of the bones, and such deformities as lateral spinal curvature (see Posture and Its Appraisal, in Chap. 9) may possibly result.

Physical Defects and Illnesses. Congenital defects, chronic illness, and even acute attacks of common childhood diseases, such as severe diarrhea, measles, whooping cough, and mumps, sometimes delay the formation of various ossification centers beyond the time at which they usually appear. In most cases such delays are only temporary. In any event children in whom ossification centers fail to appear in the proper time sequence are not to be considered immature for their years, but merely delayed in their progress toward skeletal maturity.

Hormonal Influences. The force immediately responsible for the wide differences in body build and the many variants in body type and rate of skeletal growth that are readily observed in any large group of children consists of hormones produced by several different endocrine glands.[1] These hormones activate and control skeletal growth and, through their influence on sex maturation, bring it to a stop after adolescence. Variability in the functioning of the endocrine glands concerned results in variable amounts of the hormones they produce and consequently in variations in body build and rate of growth.

The known hormones that control the growth of the skeleton are secreted by the anterior pituitary, the thyroid, the gonads, and the cortex, or outer portion, of the adrenals.

During infancy and early childhood the spread of ossification centers in the bones is activated directly by the growth-promoting hormone of the front (anterior) portion of the pituitary. As the time of puberty approaches, another anterior-pituitary hormone works indirectly against the first by stirring up the gonads. The gonadal secretion speeds up bone growth, with the result that the epiphyses unite in a relatively short time and growth stops. The thyroid enters the picture through the influence of its hormone, thyroxine, upon energy metabolism, that is, all the chemical processes by which food and oxygen are transformed into heat and energy.

[1] See Observations Related to Endocrine Activity, in Chap. 3, for an account of the endocrine glands and how they work.

Table 1. VARIATIONS IN BODY BUILD AND APPEARANCE ASSOCIATED WITH HYPERFUNCTION AND HYPOFUNCTION OF ENDOCRINE GLANDS CONTROLLING GROWTH

	Anterior pituitary	Thyroid	Adrenal cortex
Hyperfunction (overactivity)	Relatively tall in stature, with greatest length in the arms and legs, owing to accelerated growth of the long bones, with rugged development of the face, hands, and feet *Gigantism*, when excessive hyperfunction occurs in youth, before the fusion of the epiphyses (This condition is marked by speedy lengthening of the long bones and a height far above average) *Acromegaly*, when excessive hyperfunction occurs after the fusion of the epiphyses (This condition is characterized by vigorous growth of the diameters of the bones, causing marked enlargement of the face, hands, and feet)	Relatively tall and slender in stature, with slender hands and feet and delicately formed facial features, owing to an acceleration of linear skeletal growth and a slowing down of lateral skeletal growth	Accentuated masculine appearance in both the male and female sex (The boy or man tends to be extremely masculine in build—the so-called "he-man" type; the girl or woman usually has a somewhat masculine build, masculine voice, much body hair, and frequently an excess of facial hair) *Virilism*, in a girl or woman, when hyperfunction is excessive (This condition is marked by the development of masculine physical and mental traits in the female)
Hypofunction (underactivity)	Relatively slight in stature, reflecting comparative delicacy of the skeleton and slower skeletal growth, especially in the long bones *Dwarfism*, when hypofunction is excessive	*Cretinism*, when complete absence or extreme deficiency of thyroid secretion is present in infancy (The cretin is a misshapen little creature with greatly retarded mental development) *Myxedema*, when thyroid deficiency develops after puberty (This condition is characterized by sluggish mentality, obesity, and puffy, rough, dry skin)	Underdeveloped and thin in appearance, with poor chest development and breathing capacity

In Table 1 are listed some of the possible variations in body build and appearance which may be produced by the overactivity or underactivity of the anterior pituitary, the thyroid, and the adrenal cortex. Hormonal influences on the puberal growth curve will be discussed in the section on stages and rates of growth.

Influences on Muscular Development. Both the structural pattern of the body and the pace of physical growth are set by the forces that bring the skeleton to maturity. But the bulk and modeling of the tissues that cover the bony framework also influence body dimensions and estimates of nutritional status. Height—from the top of the head to the soles of the feet—is practically skeletal height, but the width and girth of various parts of the body reflect the bulk of the muscles and the relative fullness or emptiness of the fat deposits just beneath the skin (subcutaneous fat). Normally muscle tissue constitutes approximately 40 per cent of body weight.

The type of skeletal build with which a child is endowed appears to be related in some measure to the amount of fatty and muscular tissue with which his bones are padded and operated. The two healthy six-year-old girls shown in Plate 3 illustrate this point. Jean is a tall child with big bones, and Frances is a delicate-looking child with small bones. Jean's large bony framework requires large muscles for its operation, while Frances' lighter framework requires smaller muscles. Also Jean is well equipped, skeletally speaking, to carry a relatively large amount of subcutaneous fat, whereas Frances is built for light loads.

Aside from constitutional factors, food and activity are the most important factors in muscular growth and development. Food supplies the raw materials, and activity leads to the building of extra material into the system. Hence the kinds and amounts of food a child eats and the extent to which he uses his skeletal muscles in work and play will have a great deal to do with the comparative heaviness or lightness and the comparative strength or weakness of his musculature.

Influences on Fat Deposits. The amount of subcutaneous fat is the most variable factor affecting the proportions and weight of the body. Unlike skeletal and muscular tissue, which are required for support and motion, adipose tissue plays a more or less passive role in body economy. Fat is found in every cell, tissue, and organ, but in certain regions great numbers of specific fat-containing cells are normally packed closely together to form adipose tissue. These groups of fat cells are the storehouses of fat, or fat depots, of the body (see How the Body Uses Food Materials, in Chap. 6).

A certain amount of fat (from 10 to 15 per cent of body weight) is found in all children who are reasonably well nourished. Excessive thinness or excessive fatness, no matter what may be its origin or nature, is not normal. The body in its wisdom would never on its own initiative reduce its store of fat below the danger point or hamper its movements and run the risk of shortening its life because of an excess of fat.

Some thin children who look as if they needed to be fattened up rapidly gain very slowly, while some roly-polies who look as if they needed to reduce may continue to gain rapidly. A history of leanness or obesity in the family seems in many cases to accompany a tendency to remain thin or to put on weight at every twist and turn in life's journey. Constitutional type and make-up and the degree of activity of different children seem to go hand in hand. The high-strung, strenuous child tends to be wiry and thin. He seems to burn up (metabolize) his food at a faster pace than does the more placid, easygoing type of child.

Usually there is nothing to worry about in these constitutional variations. This is especially true when they are brought about by differences in individual timetables of development. The little fat boy with well-padded hips may have an unawakened or sluggish endocrine system, which later on will become functionally mature, with the result that at seventeen or eighteen he has become as streamlined as his peers. The thin wiry child may begin to fill out during the puberal cycle. Whether medical intervention is necessary in cases of this kind or whether a policy of watchful waiting is indicated is, of course, for the physician to decide. Increased knowledge of the individual differences in growth and development has helped pediatricians to be a little more casual, a little less concerned, about some of the constitutional variations in degrees of fatness and rates of development.

On the other hand, more than a moderate degree of overweight in children and young people interferes with exercise and play, limits participation in the normal activities of the group, and may result in personality difficulties. And more than a moderate degree of underweight may be responsible for chronic fatigue, poor physical endurance, and lowered resistance to infection.

Sudden loss of weight or marked change in an established rate of growth may be a sign of some physical disturbance, for example, diabetes, rheumatic fever, or tuberculosis. Sudden gain in weight, in a very few cases, may accompany a glandular disorder. By and large, however, eating too much or too little is the direct cause of excessive fatness or excessive leanness.

Why May Some Children Eat Too Much or Too Little? There are many different reasons why children may eat more or less than they need to meet their energy requirements. In some families children may acquire the habit of overeating because good food and plenty of it is a family tradition. Children in other families may show little interest in food because eating is not considered to be important enough to have meals properly prepared and served at regular times.

Emotions often play a part both in overeating and in undereating. A child who feels unwanted or unloved, for example, may turn to food for comfort. Another child with unhappy feelings may react in just the opposite way and show an exasperating indifference toward food. Emotional conflicts also may interfere with normal digestion or metabolism.

Any child who is excessively fat or excessively thin should have a thorough medical examination to determine the cause. The physician will then evaluate any physical or emotional factors or individual living habits involved and work out the proper diet.

Teachers can help older children on weight-reducing or weight-gaining diets to understand that taking off or putting on extra pounds is largely a matter of decreasing or increasing their calorie intake. Less exercise in addition to more food may help the underweight child to gain. But more exercise cannot counterbalance the excessive storage of fat resulting from overeating. For example, a person would have to walk about five miles to use up the calories in one chocolate sundae and about one mile to work off two graham crackers.

Girls in their teens who are anxious to take off weight or to remain slender are likely to go in for drastic reducing programs without making provision for all the essential food elements required for growth and good health. They should understand that only a physician has the necessary skill and equipment to decide how much weight they can safely lose, how fast they can lose it, and with what diet.

Stages and Rates of Growth

Very roughly the stages of growth are divided into four periods: prenatal, preadolescent, adolescent, and postadolescent. By far the most rapid growth takes place in the prenatal period. During these 9 months, the biologic forces that motivate growth and development work at tremendous speed, adding inches to stature and pounds to weight and bringing about rapid increases in complexity of structure, for example, forming the four-chambered heart of the infant from the simple pulsating tube of the embryo. At birth the individual has grown from an imponderable zygote, or fertilized egg, into a ponderable infant weighing seven or eight pounds, more or less, and measuring about twenty inches from top to toe. And from a single dependent cell he has developed into an exceedingly complex multicelled organism with all his equipment for living an independent existence either actually or potentially present.

Following birth the biologic workmen slow down. Their remaining task is to put on the finishing touches—to bring their masterpiece to the perfection of maturity. But there is no hurry about this. For a number of years the rate of growth gradually slows down before speeding up again in preparation for puberty. Yet the biologic workmen do not lie down on the job altogether. Indeed, according to the yardstick and the scale, they seem to be putting on a very creditable performance.

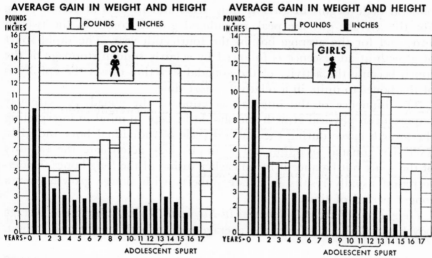

FIGS. 4 and 5. Yearly gains in pounds and inches of the average boy and girl from birth to seventeen years. (*From "How Old Are You?" Metropolitan Life Insurance Company.*)

Rates of Gain in Height and Weight. In Figures 4 and 5 are shown the yearly gains in weight and height of the average boy and girl for each year from birth to seventeen years of age. They indicate that gain in height progresses at a rapidly decelerating rate from birth to age two, and at a slowly decelerating rate from two to nine in girls and from two to eleven in boys. The rate of gain in weight during these childhood years, before the start of the puberal cycle, decelerates rapidly to age two years, decelerates very slowly from age two to age three, and thereafter picks up speed. From nine years to twelve years, in girls, and from eleven to fourteen in boys, gain in both height and weight progresses at an accelerating rate and then begins to decelerate until terminal size is reached. This happens at age sixteen in the average girl and age seventeen in the average boy, but there are many individual variations.

The Puberal Cycle. The anterior pituitary ushers in the onset of puberty by stimulating the production of the internal secretion of the gonads, or sex glands. The gonadal hormones are responsible for the emergence during puberty of the characteristic differences in body structure (secondary sex characteristics) which distinguish members of the male sex from those of the female. At the beginning of the puberal cycle there is a spurt in growth because the gonadal secretion speeds up skeletal growth, particularly in the long bones. On the average the puberal cycle begins in girls at nine years and in boys at eleven years. For the average girl the peak in puberal growth comes in the twelfth year, and for the average boy in the fourteenth year. The rapid spurt of growth at adolescence is followed by a fairly sudden stoppage of the spurt, because the activity of the gonadal secretion causes the epiphyses of the bones to unite in a relatively short time.

The influence of the internal secretion of the gonads is extremely important in physical growth and should be kept in mind in interpreting the growth curve during the puberal cycle of individual boys and girls. Excessive gonadal secretion, for example, may accentuate the rapidity of the spurt but balance it by an earlier fusion of the long bones. Undersecretion usually results in a late puberty with slower growth over a longer period of time.

Height and Weight Differences in Boys and Girls. At birth the average boy has a slight edge over the average girl in both height and weight.

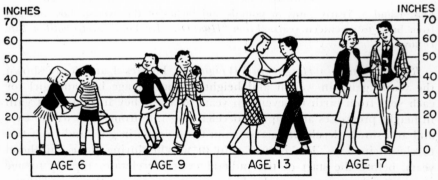

FIG. 6. Differences in height of boys and girls at various ages. (*From "How Old Are You?" Metropolitan Life Insurance Company.*)

The superiority of boys amounts to only about ¼ pound and ¼ inch. This tendency for boys to be a little taller than girls persists through the tenth year, but in the eleventh year the girls overtake the boys, and their stature continues to exceed that of boys up to age fourteen. The boys then pass the girls and in the end top them by more than 4½ inches.

Sex differences in weight are negligible or nonexistent from birth up through ten years, although the boys tend to be slightly heavier than the girls. At eleven years the average girl overtakes the average boy and continues to put on weight more rapidly until the end of the fourteenth year, when she begins to drop behind. On the average the boys at maturity are about 19 pounds heavier than the girls.

Since the average girl starts her adolescent spurt 2 years earlier than the average boy, it is natural to find many girls in junior high school who are taller than boys of their age. In some cases this may constitute a social or emotional problem, which can usually be solved by giving boys and girls an understanding of the principles of growth. It will be comforting to the boys to learn that their slight inferiority in height is almost certain to be temporary. And the girls will be glad to know that there is great likelihood that the "boy-taller-than-girl" ideal will eventually be realized.

Overlappings of Age and Size. In computing an average, or mean, for body dimensions at various ages, we find that the majority of children at each age are within a few inches or pounds above or below the average. However, the range of height and weight for the whole group will be wide. For example, the average height for a large group of healthy fourteen-year-old boys may be 65 inches, with most of them ranging from 3½ inches above to 3½ inches below. But the actual range in height for the whole group may be from 56 to 73 inches. In the same way, the average weight for a group of 100 healthy thirteen-year-old girls may be 100 pounds, with 50 of them weighing between 90 and 110, but the range of weight for the whole group will be much wider than this.

Physical growth takes place at such widely different rates in different individuals that two healthy young persons, separated in chronological age by several years, may measure the same in any one or more body dimensions. For example, it is not unusual to find a boy of ten and a boy of fifteen weighing the same, or a girl of eleven and a girl of sixteen being equally tall. Every teacher is familiar with these overlappings of age and size. She has only to look around her classroom to note that the variations in stature of the majority of the children of approximately the same age are not great, but that a few children will be noticeably shorter or taller than the average.

When "Outsize" Is a Problem. The physical measurements of boys and girls have little or no relationship with their mental measurements.

As a child passes from infancy to maturity, mental ability increases progressively with age but not with size. It has been found that the correlations between I.Q. and stature and I.Q. and weight are far too low to have much if any significance. Since this is so, in one grade there may be a few little chaps, several big huskies, and a great many in-betweens, all falling close to one another in chronological age and mental age. It sometimes happens that the exceptionally big husky boy at one extreme or the little runt at the other seems to himself and others to be "out of his class." This is only one of the many psychological problems that may arise as a result of being "outsize" as regards physical size or shape.

The physician may find that the hereditary pattern of growth or some other unchangeable constitutional factor appears to explain exceptionally small or large size for age or exceptionally slow or rapid progress in growth. In this case the most useful observation the teacher can make is to note whether being outsize—small or large—is having an unfavorable influence on the child's total development. If the physician's findings indicate that marked deviations from the average are likely to be permanent, the child's problem may be solved by helping him to organize his life on the basis of a frank acceptance of his physical characteristics.

In many cases, however, outsize, especially during adolescence, is temporary. Boys ignorant of the wide range of onset of puberty may develop a sense of inferiority when playmates mature more rapidly than themselves. The short boy whose schoolmates are enviably tall also goes through his period of depression. The very tall boy or girl, on the other hand, may be painfully conscious of overgrowth. Worries of this kind affect mental poise, and, indirectly, posture and other factors. Since the teen age is one in which mental and emotional reactions are closely knit with physical processes, the teacher may be able to find a way to improve the adolescent's emotional attitude toward himself by providing the thrill of accomplishment to offset unfavorable comparisons with others.

MEASURING PHYSICAL GROWTH AND DEVELOPMENT

Extensive studies during recent years have added greatly to our knowledge of how children grow and how the individual members of any group may be expected to deviate from the average, or mean, at various ages in body size, build, relative amounts of different tissues, nutritional state, and rates of growth. Body measurements are useful in appraising the physical status of a child at the time they are taken and in evaluating the progress made in the intervals between successive measurements. Much attention has been given to the selection of a system of body measurements for use in spotting children in need of medical investigation because of considerable deviation from normal growth patterns.

Height and Weight

The two measurements which are easiest to make and which have been made most consistently in checking up on a child's nutritional status and rate of growth are height and weight. Height is a measure of length —up-and-down size—and weight is a measure of mass. Since growth means an increase in size and bulk, and all healthy children grow, we expect a healthy child to become progressively taller and heavier as the years pass.

Height-weight-age Tables. The most common use to which measurements of height and weight in school have been put is to determine the appropriateness of mass (weight) to length (height) at successive ages. When school weighing and measuring first became popular a generation ago, it was considered desirable to have some standard of comparison for the individual child. For that reason, tables were devised showing average weight for height and age. In constructing such tables the average, or mean, weight for height at various ages of very large numbers of children were computed, and the average weight for a particular height, age, and sex were then set up as the standard of comparison for any boy or girl of that height and age.

It would be rare indeed for the weight of an individual child to be exactly the same as that arrived at by averaging the weights of thousands of children. All that can be expected is that his weight will fall within the weight range of a substantial fraction of the total number of children of his age and height measured. Hence, in using height-weight-age tables a child is considered to be overweight or underweight only if his weight is from 10 to 15 per cent above or below the mean weight reported for each height at different ages.

The use of tables of this kind has several disadvantages. One is the tendency to accept the average as the ideal or normal. After the anatomical dimensions of large groups of children have been tabulated and averaged, we have simply a collection of mathematical averages of weights for height at various ages. Because a child is within the weight range of the majority of those who were measured to arrive at the averages does not mean that he is "normal" or that his weight is optimum. He is only average. He represents what *is,* not necessarily what ought to be.

Another disadvantage in the use of average weight for height and age tables is the impossibility of determining which of the groups of tissues are involved in marked deviations from the average. Is it the relative lightness or stockiness of the skeleton? the relative bulkiness or thinness of the muscles? or the relative leanness or fatness of subcutaneous tissue? It is easy to see that mistakes may be made in appraising a child's health status if these factors are not taken into consideration in deciding whether or not a child is excessively thin or excessively fat. If the weights of the two six-year-old girls shown in Plate 3, for example, were compared with the average weight for their height, big-boned Jean might be classified as overweight and small-boned Frances as underweight. Yet both girls have been given a clean bill of health by the physician who examined them, because his physical examination was supplemented by a knowledge of their inherited body build and health history.

Height–weight–age–body-build Tables. In an attempt to allow for body build in comparing a child's weight with average weight for height and age, tables of weight in relation to age, height, and body type have also been worked out. Classifications of body build fall into three main groups: "tall, slender type," "average (medium) type," and "short, stocky type." It must be remembered, however, that there are many gradations in body build, or physique. The classification into which a child falls will depend upon the characteristics that are predominant. Without other measurements besides height and weight, it is often difficult to guess to which group a child belongs.

The trunk, with its powerful bone structure and tightly packed organs, contributes more to weight than do the head and limbs. Hence, a child with a long and roomy trunk, with broad shoulders and wide pelvis, would be classified as having a heavy frame irrespective of total height. And a child with a medium or short trunk would be classified as medium or slight in build, depending upon the ruggedness or delicacy of his skeleton.

Height-age and Weight-age Curves. By calculating the average, or mean, height and weight at various ages of very large numbers of children, and plotting average height and average weight separately against age, it is possible to construct charts showing average, or mean, height-age and weight-age curves for boys and girls together with normal variations from these averages. Examples of such charts prepared by Howard V. Meredith from data collected at the Iowa Child Welfare Research Station, State University of Iowa,[2] are shown in Figures 7 and 8. You

[2] See "A 'Physical Growth Record' for Use in Elementary and High Schools" by Howard V. Meredith in *Am. J. Pub. Health,* Vol. 39, No. 7 (July), 1949, for a detailed explanation of these charts. Reproductions of the charts are available in booklet form. Each booklet is designed for recording the growth in height and weight of a single child. The booklets may be obtained from the American Medical Association or the National Education Association. For addresses of these organizations, and of others mentioned in this book, see the list at the end of the book.

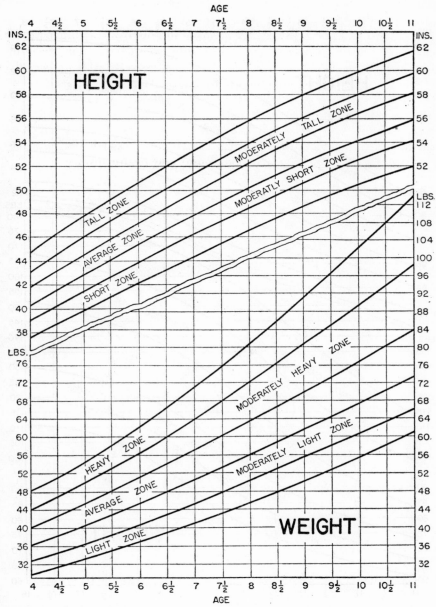

FIG. 7A. Physical growth record for boys, ages four to eleven. (*Howard V. Meredith, reproduced by courtesy of American Medical Association.*)

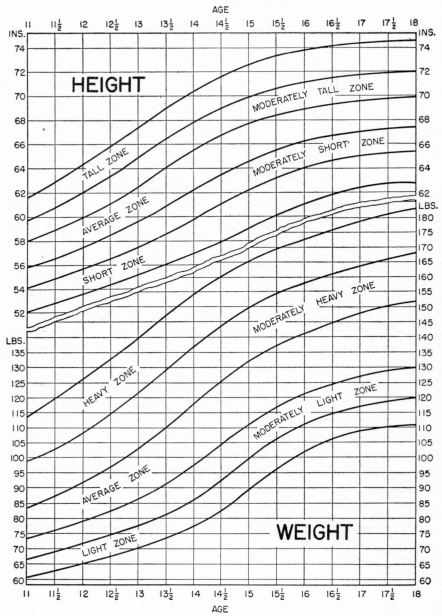

FIG. 7B. Physical growth record for boys, ages eleven to eighteen. (*Howard V. Meredith, reproduced by courtesy of American Medical Association.*)

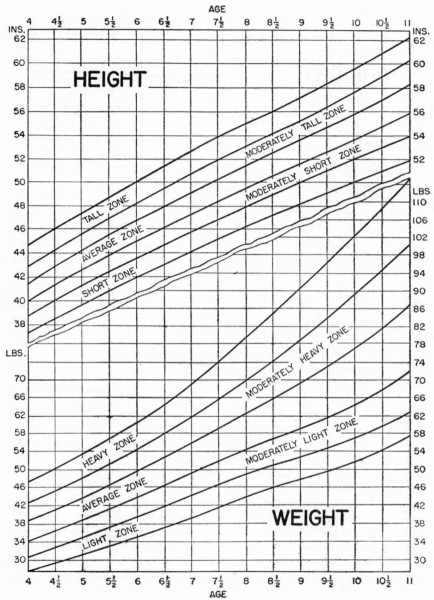

FIG. 8A. Physical growth record for girls, ages four to eleven. (*Howard V. Meredith, reproduced by courtesy of American Medical Association.*)

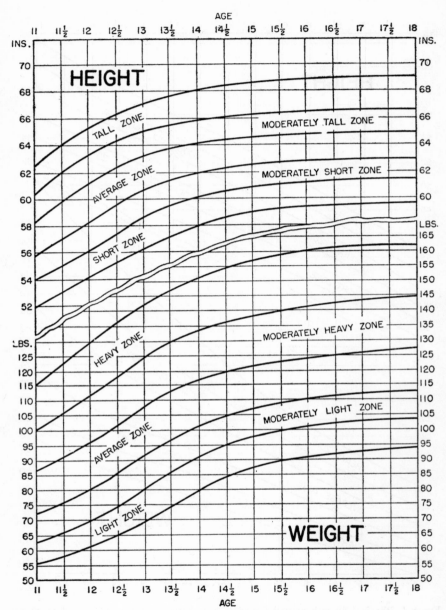

FIG. 8B. Physical growth record for girls, ages eleven to eighteen. (*Howard V. Meredith, reproduced by courtesy of American Medical Association.*)

will note that each of the graphs shows five "normative zones" for height: tall, moderately tall, average, moderately short, and short; and five "normative zones" for weight: heavy, moderately heavy, average, moderately light, and light. The normative zones in these charts furnish a pattern that may be used in checking up on the individual child's growth pattern. This is done by noticing the zone of location of the child's height and weight points as they are plotted on his individual chart. If a child's height and weight points do not fall in corresponding zones (as tall and heavy, or short and light), or if a child's height or weight jumps abruptly from one zone to another in the course of successive measurings, the child should be referred for medical investigation.

Wetzel's Grid. Another method of revealing trends in growth through the use of height and weight measurements is the grid developed by Norman C. Wetzel, known as Wetzel's grid [3] (Fig. 9*A*).

In the graph forming the first panel of this grid, the vertical scale is assigned to weight (pounds) and the horizontal scale to height (inches). When the child's weight is plotted against his height on this panel, a point is located which falls into one of several "physique channels" that traverse the graph obliquely from top to bottom. These channels are designated at the top by symbols. The more obese and stocky types are at the left of the channel system (A_4, A_3, A_2), the medium (A_1, M, B_1) in the center, and the thinner lighter types (B_2, B_3, B_4) at the right. The curve plotted from successive measurements represents the child's channel course. This curve tends to follow the particular physique channel that corresponds to the child's body build. The tendency to follow a particular channel is due to the tendency in health to preserve the same physique, or shape, at successive ages. Hence, if a child moves out of his established channel, a change in his nutritional or health status is indicated.

A second feature of the graph forming the first panel are numbered developmental-level lines which cross the channel lines at regular intervals. Each level represents a different size, that is, a different value of body surface. The numbered level at which a height-weight point is located measures the child's size (body surface area). The direction of the course taken by the child through the channel system is the result of change in size with respect to change in shape.

In summary, the channel system serves three purposes:

1. It identifies the child's physique, or body build, by the channel in which the various weight-height points fall.

[3] "Grid for Evaluating Physical Fitness in Terms of Physique (Body Build) Development Level and Basal Metabolism," published by NEA SERVICE, Inc.

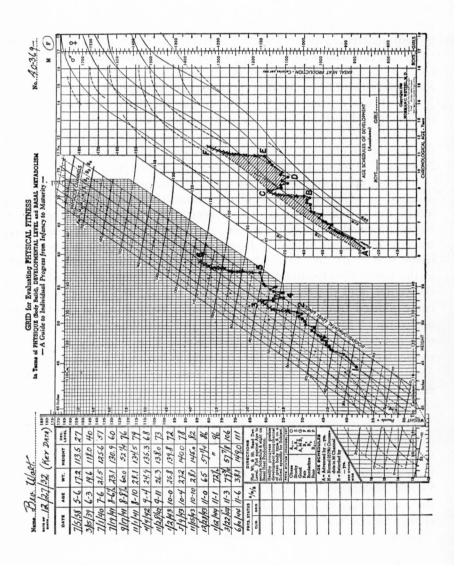

GRID for Evaluating PHYSICAL FITNESS
In Terms of PHYSIQUE (Body Build), DEVELOPMENTAL LEVEL and BASAL METABOLISM
— A Guide to Individual Progress from Infancy to Maturity —

Name: Bill Wolf.
No. A-0369

DATE	AGE	WT.	HEIGHT	DEVL. LEVEL
7/5/38	5-6	17.2	113.5	27
3/15/39	6-3	19.6	118.0	40
7/1/40	7-6	21.5	125.6	51
7/19/40	8-6½	23.1	130.9	60
9/17/41	8-8½	60.0	52¼	76
11/1/41	8-10	28.1	134.5	79
4/4/42	9-4	24.9	135.3	68
11/28/42	9-11	26.3	138.0	73
1/2/43	10-0	25.8	139.8	72
5/9/43	10-4	27.2	140.0	78
11/15/43	10-10	28.1	145.0	82
12/28/43	11-0	65	57¼	86
4/24/44	11-1	72½	"	96
3/22/44	11-3	77½	57½	106
6/6/44	11-6	38.1	149.0	111

Fig. 9A. Wetzel's-grid record showing two episodes of simple growth failure (malnutritional type), plotted from the data tabulated in centimeters (height) and kilograms (weight). (*Reproduced by courtesy of Norman C. Wetzel.*

Channel course: This child's normal body type, first observed at point 1, falls between physique channels B_1 and B_2. Segments 1–2 and 3–4–5 of her actual channel course represent moderate and severe departures from true channelwise direction (indicated at 1, 3, and 6) with corresponding losses of physique from her own B_1, B_2 body type. Segments 2–3 and 5–6 indicate recovery responses following treatment started at 2 and 5. Physique was completely restored at 3 and 6.

Auxodromic progress: The child's "own," or "expected," auxodrome (age schedule of development) is represented by the broken line *ACF*. The line *ABCDEF* is the child's actual auxodrome.

The slowing down, or lag, in speed of development, corresponding with the losses of physique shown in her channel course, is measured by the vertical difference between the expected auxodrome (*ACF*) and the actual auxodrome (*ABCDEF*). At *B*, for example, the level actually reached is 57, whereas according to the child's expected auxodrome it should be 74. Therefore, her lag in speed of development at *B* amounts to 17 levels. At *E* it amounts to 22 levels. Segments *B–C* and *E–F* of the actual auxodrome show speed-up during the first and second recovery phases, with complete return to her own schedule at *C* and *F*. Failure in both episodes continued to increase until definite action had been taken at 2 (in channel course), *B* (in auxodrome) and 5, *E* to investigate causes and to remedy them.

2. It measures the child's size by means of the developmental levels at which these points are located.
3. It acts as a direction finder for ascertaining the trend or direction of the child's own development.

In the second panel a field is provided for determining *speed* of development. On this graph, size (developmental level) is plotted from the

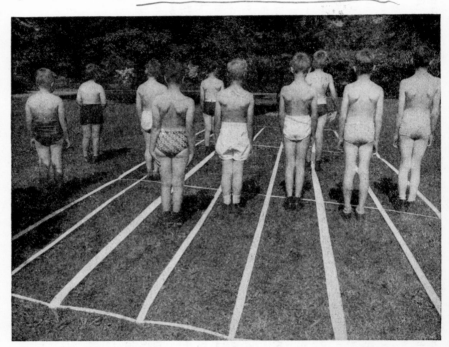

FIG. 9B. These boys are lined up in their respective physique channels (ranging from A_4 at the left to B_3 at the right) to illustrate the value of Wetzel's grid in determining body type. Observe the striking physical differences in the boys at approximately the same developmental level (level 95). (*Reproduced by courtesy of Norman C. Wetzel and* Science Illustrated.)

vertical scale, and age from the horizontal scale. The curve plotted for the individual child from successive points in this panel is called his "auxodrome," or age schedule of development. A set of standard auxodromes (blue curves for boys, red curves for girls) shows how many children at any given age (expressed as a fraction of the total number at that age in the general population) may be expected to have reached a given developmental level. Thus it is possible to recognize whether a child's developmental level is high or low in relation to the normal distribution of size for age and also to detect deviations from its expected course.

In a third panel the developmental-level lines are correlated with an energy scale which indicates the basal heat production in calories per day at each level. Daily fuel requirements of the child are approximately twice his basal heat production. These developmental-level–calorie relationships form the basis for planning additional dietary allowances in the medical treatment of malnutrition.

The principles upon which Wetzel's grid has been constructed lie in the realm of advanced mathematics, but the teacher or nurse making height-weight measurements can easily learn to plot them in the channel system, read the developmental level, and then plot developmental level against age in the second (right-hand) panel. The physician inspecting the grids of a number of children can readily select those which indicate deviations from the expected patterns of growth.

Wetzel's grid is of undoubted value to physicians in appraising the quality of growth in children. Also the American Association of Teachers Colleges is finding it helpful in laying new emphasis on the growth and development of school children in the teacher-training curriculum.[4]

Measurements of Skeletal Stockiness, Bulkiness of Musculature, and Subcutaneous Fat

The three tissues that have the greatest influence on body build, stature, and weight are the skeleton, the musculature, and the subcutaneous fat. Hence, in addition to measurements of length and mass (height and weight), measurements of the stockiness of the skeleton, the bulkiness of the musculature, and the quantity of subcutaneous tissue have been found helpful in the appraisal of a child's physical status.

Various measurements for determining the magnitude of these three attributes have been proposed by investigators who have carried on extensive studies relating to the appraisal of the physical status of children. One of the most recent sets of measurements to be recommended is that of Harold C. Stuart, Head of the Department of Maternal and Child Health, Harvard School of Public Health, Harvard University, and Howard V. Meredith, now professor in the School of Health and Physical Education, University of Oregon.[5]

[4] 1943–1944 Teachers College Collaborators, Lonzo Jones, chairman (1944), "Child Growth and Development Emphases in Teacher Education," American Association of Teachers Colleges.

[5] Table 2 and Figures 10, 11, and 12 are reproduced by special permission of the authors, from "Use of Body Measurements in the School Health Program," by Harold C. Stuart and Howard V. Meredith, in *Am. J. Pub. Health,* Vol. 36, No. 12 (December), 1946.

Table 2. SELECTED PERCENTILES FOR FIVE BODY MEASUREMENTS: * AGES 5 TO 7½ YEARS

Boys						Girls				
Percentiles							Percentiles			
10	25	50	75	90		10	25	50	75	90
					5 years					
36.6	39.6	42.8	46.5	49.7	Weight	36.1	38.6	41.4	44.2	48.2
105.3	108.3	111.3	114.2	116.7	Height	105.0	107.2	109.7	112.9	115.4
17.0	17.6	18.3	18.9	19.6	Hip width	17.0	17.4	18.0	18.7	19.4
51.6	52.8	54.5	56.2	57.5	Chest circ.	50.2	51.4	52.9	54.6	56.5
21.0	21.7	22.6	23.6	24.6	Leg girth	21.1	21.8	22.8	23.8	24.7
					5½ years					
38.8	42.0	45.6	49.3	53.1	Weight	38.0	40.8	44.0	47.2	51.2
108.3	111.2	114.4	117.5	120.1	Height	107.8	110.2	112.8	116.1	118.9
17.4	18.0	18.7	19.4	20.1	Hip width	17.4	17.8	18.4	19.1	20.0
52.4	53.6	55.3	57.1	58.5	Chest circ.	50.9	52.2	53.7	55.5	57.4
21.4	22.2	23.1	24.1	25.2	Leg girth	21.5	22.3	23.3	24.3	25.3
					6 years					
40.9	44.4	48.3	52.1	56.4	Weight	39.9	42.9	46.5	50.2	54.2
111.2	114.1	117.5	120.8	123.5	Height	110.6	113.2	115.9	119.3	122.3
17.7	18.4	19.1	19.8	20.5	Hip width	17.7	18.2	18.8	19.5	20.5
53.2	54.4	56.1	57.9	59.5	Chest circ.	51.5	52.9	54.5	56.3	58.2
21.8	22.6	23.6	24.6	25.7	Leg girth	21.9	22.7	23.8	24.8	25.8
					6½ years					
43.4	47.1	51.2	55.4	60.4	Weight	42.2	45.5	49.4	53.3	57.7
114.1	117.2	120.8	124.2	127.0	Height	113.7	116.2	119.1	122.6	125.6
18.1	18.8	19.5	20.2	21.0	Hip width	18.1	18.6	19.2	20.0	21.1
54.1	55.3	57.0	58.9	60.6	Chest circ.	52.2	53.7	55.3	57.2	59.2
22.2	23.1	24.1	25.2	26.3	Leg girth	22.3	23.2	24.3	25.4	26.4
					7 years					
45.8	49.7	54.1	58.7	64.4	Weight	44.5	48.1	52.2	56.3	61.2
116.9	120.3	124.1	127.6	130.5	Height	116.8	119.2	122.3	125.9	128.9
18.5	19.2	19.9	20.6	21.4	Hip width	18.4	18.9	19.6	20.4	21.6
54.9	56.1	57.8	59.8	61.6	Chest circ.	52.8	54.4	56.1	58.0	60.1
22.6	23.5	24.6	25.7	26.9	Leg girth	22.7	23.7	24.8	25.9	27.0
					7½ years					
48.5	52.6	57.1	62.1	68.7	Weight	46.6	50.6	55.2	59.8	65.6
120.0	123.5	127.1	130.9	133.9	Height	119.5	122.0	125.2	128.8	131.8
18.9	19.6	20.3	21.0	21.9	Hip width	18.8	19.3	20.1	20.9	22.1
55.8	57.1	58.8	61.0	62.9	Chest circ.	53.5	55.1	57.0	59.0	61.2
23.1	24.1	25.2	26.3	27.6	Leg girth	23.1	24.2	25.3	26.4	27.7

Source: The basic data were collected 1930–1945 on Iowa City children of northwest European ancestry attending University of Iowa experimental schools.

    * In this table and in Figures 11 and 12 length is recorded in centimeters. To find height in inches, for example, divide each measurement of height by 2.54 (i.e., 1 inch equals 2.54 centimeters).

Table 2 (Cont.). SELECTED PERCENTILES FOR FIVE BODY MEASUREMENTS: AGES 8 TO 11 YEARS

		Boys						Girls		
		Percentiles						Percentiles		
10	25	50	75	90		10	25	50	75	90
					8 years					
51.2	55.5	60.1	65.5	73.0	Weight	48.6	53.1	58.1	63.3	69.9
123.1	126.6	130.0	134.2	137.3	Height	122.1	124.8	128.0	131.6	134.6
19.2	19.9	20.7	21.4	22.3	Hip width	19.1	19.7	20.5	21.3	22.6
56.7	58.0	59.8	62.1	64.1	Chest circ.	54.2	55.8	57.8	59.9	62.3
23.6	24.6	25.7	26.8	28.2	Leg girth	23.5	24.6	25.8	26.9	28.3
					8½ years					
53.8	58.3	63.1	68.9	77.0	Weight	50.6	55.5	61.0	66.9	74.5
125.7	129.1	132.8	137.0	140.0	Height	124.6	127.3	130.5	134.4	137.5
19.6	20.3	21.1	21.8	22.7	Hip width	19.4	20.1	20.9	21.8	23.1
57.6	59.0	60.8	63.3	65.4	Chest circ.	54.9	56.5	58.7	60.9	63.5
24.1	25.1	26.3	27.4	28.9	Leg girth	23.9	25.0	26.3	27.5	28.9
					9 years					
56.3	61.1	66.0	72.3	81.0	Weight	52.6	57.9	63.8	70.5	79.1
128.3	131.6	135.5	139.8	142.6	Height	127.0	129.7	132.9	137.1	140.4
19.9	20.6	21.4	22.2	23.0	Hip width	19.7	20.5	21.3	22.2	23.5
58.4	59.9	61.8	64.4	66.7	Chest circ.	55.5	57.2	59.6	61.9	64.7
24.5	25.6	26.8	28.0	29.5	Leg girth	24.2	25.4	26.8	28.1	29.5
					9½ years					
58.7	63.7	69.0	76.0	85.5	Weight	54.9	60.4	67.1	74.8	84.4
130.6	134.0	137.9	142.1	145.1	Height	129.4	132.2	135.8	139.9	143.2
20.2	21.0	21.7	22.6	23.5	Hip width	20.1	20.9	21.8	22.8	24.1
59.3	60.9	62.9	65.5	68.1	Chest circ.	56.2	58.0	60.5	63.2	66.1
24.9	26.0	27.3	28.5	30.1	Leg girth	24.7	25.9	27.3	28.6	30.2
					10 years					
61.1	66.3	71.9	79.6	89.9	Weight	57.1	62.8	70.3	79.1	89.7
132.8	136.3	140.3	144.4	147.5	Height	131.7	134.6	138.6	142.6	146.0
20.4	21.3	22.0	22.9	23.9	Hip width	20.5	21.2	22.2	23.3	24.6
60.1	61.8	63.9	66.6	69.4	Chest circ.	56.9	58.7	61.4	64.4	67.4
25.3	26.4	27.7	29.0	30.7	Leg girth	25.1	26.3	27.7	29.1	30.9
					10½ years					
63.7	69.0	74.8	83.4	94.6	Weight	59.9	66.4	74.6	84.1	95.1
135.1	138.4	142.3	146.8	149.7	Height	134.4	137.5	141.7	145.9	149.7
20.8	21.6	22.3	23.2	24.4	Hip width	21.0	21.7	22.9	24.0	25.3
60.9	62.8	64.9	67.7	70.7	Chest circ.	57.8	59.9	62.8	65.8	69.0
25.7	26.8	28.1	29.5	31.4	Leg girth	25.6	26.8	28.3	29.9	31.8
					11 years					
66.3	71.6	77.6	87.2	99.3	Weight	62.6	69.9	78.8	89.1	100.4
137.3	140.5	144.2	149.2	151.8	Height	137.0	140.3	144.7	149.2	153.4
21.1	21.8	22.6	23.5	24.8	Hip width	21.4	22.2	23.5	24.6	26.0
61.7	63.7	65.9	68.8	71.9	Chest circ.	58.6	61.1	64.2	67.2	70.5
26.0	27.1	28.5	30.0	32.0	Leg girth	26.0	27.3	28.9	30.6	32.6

Table 2 (Cont.). SELECTED PERCENTILES FOR FIVE BODY MEASUREMENTS: AGES 11½ TO 14½ YEARS

	Boys					Girls				
	Percentiles						Percentiles			
10	25	50	75	90		10	25	50	75	90
					11½ years					
69.2	74.6	81.0	91.6	104.5	Weight	66.1	74.0	83.2	94.0	106.0
139.8	142.9	146.9	151.4	154.8	Height	139.8	143.1	148.1	152.9	157.0
21.5	22.2	23.1	24.0	25.3	Hip width	21.9	22.8	24.2	25.4	26.8
62.5	64.6	66.9	69.9	73.1	Chest circ.	59.6	62.5	65.5	68.5	72.2
26.4	27.6	29.0	30.6	32.8	Leg girth	26.6	27.9	29.5	31.2	33.2
					12 years					
72.0	77.5	84.4	96.0	109.6	Weight	69.5	78.0	87.6	98.8	111.5
142.4	145.2	149.6	153.5	157.9	Height	142.6	145.9	151.5	156.6	160.6
21.9	22.6	23.5	24.5	25.8	Hip width	22.4	23.4	24.9	26.2	27.6
63.3	65.5	67.8	70.9	74.2	Chest circ.	60.6	63.8	66.7	69.7	73.8
26.8	28.0	29.5	31.2	33.5	Leg girth	27.1	28.5	30.1	31.8	33.8
					12½ years					
74.6	80.6	88.7	102.0	116.4	Weight	74.7	83.7	93.4	104.9	118.0
144.5	147.5	152.3	157.2	161.6	Height	145.9	149.3	154.3	159.1	162.7
22.3	23.1	24.1	25.1	26.5	Hip width	23.0	24.0	25.5	26.8	28.3
64.2	66.5	69.1	72.4	75.8	Chest circ.	61.8	64.9	67.7	70.9	75.3
27.3	28.6	30.1	32.0	34.2	Leg girth	27.7	29.1	30.7	32.4	34.3
					13 years					
77.1	83.7	93.0	107.9	123.2	Weight	79.9	89.4	99.1	111.0	124.5
146.6	149.7	155.0	160.8	165.3	Height	149.1	152.6	157.1	161.5	164.8
22.7	23.6	24.6	25.6	27.2	Hip width	23.6	24.6	26.0	27.4	29.0
65.0	67.4	70.3	73.8	77.4	Chest circ.	62.9	65.9	68.6	72.0	76.7
27.8	29.2	30.8	32.7	34.8	Leg girth	28.2	29.7	31.2	32.9	34.8
					13½ years					
82.2	89.6	100.3	115.5	130.1	Weight	85.5	94.6	103.7	115.4	128.9
149.4	153.1	158.9	164.6	168.9	Height	151.1	154.4	158.4	162.6	165.9
23.2	24.1	25.2	26.4	27.8	Hip width	24.2	25.2	26.5	27.8	29.5
66.3	68.8	72.4	75.8	79.4	Chest circ.	63.8	66.6	69.3	72.9	77.7
28.5	29.9	31.6	33.4	35.3	Leg girth	28.7	30.2	31.6	33.4	35.1
					14 years					
87.2	95.5	107.6	123.1	136.9	Weight	91.0	99.8	108.4	119.7	133.3
152.1	156.5	162.7	168.4	172.4	Height	153.0	156.1	159.6	163.7	167.0
23.6	24.6	25.8	27.1	28.3	Hip width	24.8	25.8	26.9	28.1	29.9
67.6	70.2	74.5	77.8	81.4	Chest circ.	64.6	67.2	69.9	73.7	78.6
29.1	30.6	32.3	34.1	35.8	Leg girth	29.2	30.6	32.0	33.8	35.4
					14½ years					
93.3	101.9	113.9	129.1	142.4	Weight	94.2	102.5	111.0	121.8	135.7
155.0	159.4	165.3	170.7	174.6	Height	154.1	156.9	160.4	164.3	167.6
24.1	25.1	26.3	27.5	28.7	Hip width	25.2	26.2	27.2	28.4	30.3
69.4	72.3	76.3	79.6	83.1	Chest circ.	65.1	67.7	70.4	74.2	79.2
29.8	31.3	32.9	34.6	36.2	Leg girth	29.6	30.9	32.3	34.1	35.7

Table 2 (Cont.). SELECTED PERCENTILES FOR FIVE BODY MEASUREMENTS: AGES 15 TO 18 YEARS

	Boys						Girls			
	Percentiles						Percentiles			
10	25	50	75	90		10	25	50	75	90
					15 years					
99.4	108.2	120.1	135.0	147.8	Weight	97.4	105.1	113.5	123.9	138.1
157.8	162.3	167.8	173.0	176.7	Height	155.2	157.7	161.1	164.9	168.1
24.6	25.6	26.7	27.9	29.1	Hip width	25.6	26.5	27.5	28.7	30.6
71.1	74.4	78.0	81.3	84.8	Chest circ.	65.5	68.1	70.9	74.7	79.8
30.4	31.9	33.4	35.1	36.6	Leg girth	29.9	31.1	32.6	34.3	35.9
					15½ years					
105.2	113.5	124.9	139.7	152.6	Weight	99.2	106.8	115.3	125.6	139.6
160.3	164.7	169.7	174.8	178.2	Height	155.7	158.2	161.7	165.3	168.6
25.1	26.0	27.1	28.2	29.4	Hip width	25.9	26.7	27.8	29.0	30.8
72.8	75.8	79.4	82.9	86.3	Chest circ.	65.8	68.4	71.3	75.1	80.2
30.9	32.3	33.8	35.5	37.0	Leg girth	30.1	31.4	32.9	34.5	36.1
					16 years					
111.0	118.7	129.7	144.4	157.3	Weight	100.9	108.4	117.0	127.2	141.1
162.8	167.1	171.6	176.6	179.7	Height	156.1	158.6	162.2	165.7	169.0
25.6	26.4	27.4	28.4	29.6	Hip width	26.1	26.9	28.0	29.2	31.0
74.4	77.2	80.7	84.5	87.8	Chest circ.	66.1	68.7	71.6	75.4	80.5
31.3	32.7	34.2	35.8	37.3	Leg girth	30.3	31.6	33.1	34.6	36.3
					16½ years					
114.3	121.6	133.0	147.9	161.0	Weight	101.9	109.4	118.1	128.4	142.2
164.2	168.4	172.7	177.4	180.7	Height	156.2	158.8	162.4	165.9	169.2
25.9	26.7	27.6	28.6	29.8	Hip width	26.2	27.0	28.2	29.3	31.1
75.4	78.1	81.6	85.4	88.8	Chest circ.	66.3	69.0	71.9	75.7	80.7
31.5	32.9	34.4	36.1	37.6	Leg girth	30.5	31.8	33.3	34.8	36.5
					17 years					
117.5	124.5	136.2	151.4	164.6	Weight	102.8	110.4	119.1	129.6	143.3
165.5	169.7	173.7	178.1	181.6	Height	156.3	159.0	162.5	166.1	169.4
26.1	26.9	27.8	28.7	29.9	Hip width	26.3	27.1	28.3	29.4	31.2
76.4	78.9	82.5	86.2	89.7	Chest circ.	66.4	69.2	72.1	75.9	80.9
31.7	33.1	34.6	36.3	37.8	Leg girth	30.6	31.9	33.4	34.9	36.6
					17½ years					
118.8	125.8	137.6	153.6	166.8	Weight	103.2	110.8	119.5	130.2	143.9
165.9	170.1	174.1	178.5	182.0	Height	156.3	159.0	162.5	166.1	169.4
26.3	27.0	27.9	28.8	30.0	Hip width	26.4	27.2	28.4	29.5	31.3
77.0	79.4	83.0	86.7	90.2	Chest circ.	66.5	69.3	72.2	76.0	81.0
31.8	33.3	34.8	36.5	38.0	Leg girth	30.7	32.0	33.5	35.0	36.7
					18 years					
120.0	127.1	139.0	155.7	169.0	Weight	103.5	111.2	119.9	130.8	144.5
166.3	170.5	174.5	178.9	182.4	Height	156.3	159.0	162.5	166.1	169.4
26.5	27.1	28.0	28.9	30.1	Hip width	26.4	27.2	28.4	29.5	31.3
77.5	79.8	83.4	87.1	90.7	Chest circ.	66.6	69.4	72.3	76.1	81.1
31.9	33.4	34.9	36.6	38.1	Leg girth	30.8	32.1	33.6	35.1	36.8

In addition to body weight and standing height, the measurements selected by these authorities are chest circumference and hip width (pelvic breadth at the crests of the ilia, that is, the upper edges of the hipbones)

NAME   **BIRTH DATE**

AGE	WEIGHT		HEIGHT		HIP WIDTH		CHEST CIRC.		LEG GIRTH		THICKNESS SKIN & FAT	
YRS.-MOS.	M	P	M	P	M	P	M	P	M	P	CHEST	ILIAC

Fig. 10. Form suggested for use in the individual health records of school children. This allows for recording the measurements taken and their respective percentile positions at each of 20 ages. Reading the percentiles across a single age line reveals at a glance the interrelationships between all the measurements taken and the effect upon them of subcutaneous fat. Reading down each percentile column shows how the child's position within the range has changed with age in respect to each measurement. This form should follow the child to all schools attended throughout his school life.

Age. Give to nearest month, checking with birth date.
M. Measurement as taken.
P. Percentile rank in normal distribution from appropriate age and sex table.
Skin and fat. Clinical ratings on 5-plus scale. See directions for use.

to indicate the degree of skeletal stockiness, and leg girth (the greatest circumference of the calf) to indicate the bulkiness of the musculature. The method suggested for estimating subjectively the thickness of the skin and subcutaneous tissue is to draw together and elevate between the thumb and index finger a double layer of skin and subcutaneous tissue

(a) in the region slightly below and a little to the side of the left shoulder blade, and (b) in the region immediately above the top of the left hipbone. Ratings of the thickness of subcutaneous tissue are made according to a scale extending from 1 plus (+) at the lower end to 5 plus (+++++) at the upper end. To make these ratings, Stuart and Meredith point out, familiarity with the range of individual differences in given sex-age groups is required, as well as considerable experience in making judgments of subcutaneous tissue in the regions specified.

On the basis of measurements of large numbers of healthy American boys and girls in the school ages, Stuart and Meredith have constructed a table giving selected percentiles [6] (10, 25, 50, 75, and 90) at each half-year interval from five to nineteen for each of their recommended body measurements (Table 2). After a child has been measured and his percentile rank with respect to each of the five body measurements determined from the table, the teacher or nurse enters the values obtained on a form sheet (Fig. 10). It is recommended that these values also be used to plot curves for the child on graphs showing average normal curves as working standards of comparison (Figs. 11 and 12).

The physician referring to the record (Fig. 10) and the graph (Fig. 11 or 12) can readily note if a marked change has occurred between the successive measurement periods. Also, he can tell not only whether a particular measurement is above or below the average for the normative group of children of the same sex and age (percentile 50) but also how unusual the measurement is. For example, a girl aged ten with a percentile rank of 10 in chest circumference would be smaller in this respect than 90 per cent of her group and larger than 10 per cent. Additional interpretative value is attached to this single measurement when its percentile rank is compared with those of the other measurements. For example, if the percentile rank of this girl in weight, height, hip width, and leg girth is also at or near 10 and her rating for thickness of subcutaneous tissue is 3 plus, the physician would expect to find a small, proportionally well-balanced girl.

On the other hand, if the percentile rank of a ten-year-old boy is 75 in height and hip width; 75— in chest circumference; 50+ in leg girth and 50— in weight, with 1-plus ratings in thickness of skin and sub-

[6] By "percentile" is meant the expression of values in terms of per cent. The percentile rank of a child in a group of children arranged in order of magnitude in respect to a certain attribute indicates that child's superiority over children in the group with a lower percentile rank and inferiority to children with a higher percentile rank. For example, a child with a percentile rank of 75 in respect to height is taller than 75 per cent of his group and shorter than 25 per cent. If his percentile rank is 50, he occupies the middle position; hence, his height is medium or average (the mean). If his percentile rank is 25, he is taller than 25 per cent of his group and shorter than 75 per cent.

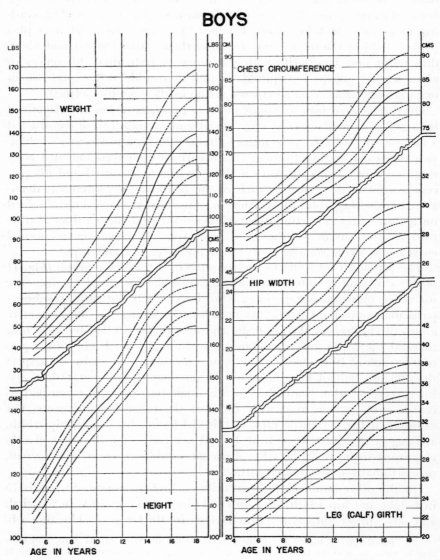

FIG. 11. Graphs for plotting measurements of boys. The trend lines shown—
proceeding from the highest to the lowest—represent the ninetieth, seventy-
fifth, fiftieth (mean), twenty-fifth, and tenth percentiles.

GIRLS

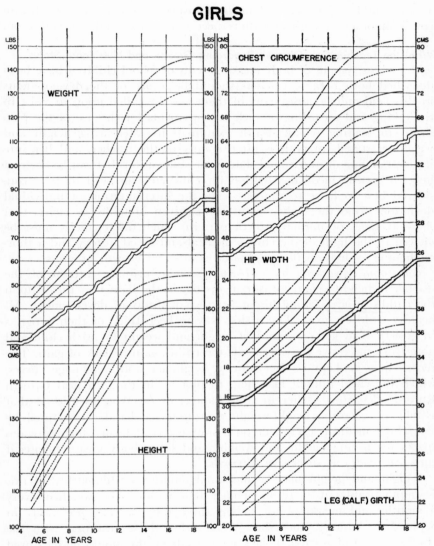

FIG. 12. Graphs for plotting measurements of girls. The trend lines shown—proceeding from the highest to the lowest—represent the ninetieth, seventy-fifth, fiftieth (mean), twenty-fifth, and tenth percentiles.

cutaneous tissue, the physician would expect to find a tall large-boned boy with underdeveloped musculature and too little fat padding. Such a boy would require careful medical inspection for a possible disease condition or a poor regimen with respect to diet, sleep and rest, and so on.

What the Teacher Can Observe Regarding Growth and Nutritional Status

The various systems of body measurements of school children have been described both because teachers should be aware of the developments in this field and because many of them may be called upon to assist in the taking and recording of such measurements for the use of the physician in making school health examinations. Measuring height and weight at stated intervals is often a duty of the teacher, and her subjective estimate of nutritional state is an observation that can be of great help in getting medical attention for children who need it. It is considered best to leave to the physician the interpretation of individual deviations from the body measurements given in tables or charts that show averages or normal growth patterns. Such discrepancies must be viewed in the light of the child's medical and social history and a thoroughgoing evaluation of his physical status and growth progress.

Classroom Weighing and Measuring. The primary interest of the teacher in height-weight measurements lies in the light they throw upon the child's progress along his or her own pathway of development. All healthy children grow. The easiest way to keep track of their progress in growth is to keep a record of height and weight for each child and note from successive measurements the child's gain or lack of gain. The record may be kept in the form of height-age and weight-age curves, which the child himself may help to plot, as in the "Physical Growth Record" described earlier in this chapter; or on Wetzel's grid, if that system of recording height-weight measurements has been adopted by the school medical service; or on a simple record form which provides spaces for noting height and weight (and other body measurements if they are made) at successive intervals.

Weight and height may be measured monthly or bimonthly. If this is impracticable, it is recommended that children be weighed every 3 months and measured for height three times a year—preferably in September, January, and May. Weight should be measured with the child's shoes and sweater or jacket removed; height should be measured with the shoes removed.

Failure to gain in weight over a period of one or two months may not have much significance, but a failure to make any gain for three successive months is nearly always a sign that something is wrong, either because of poor health habits or because of a disease or defect that needs medical attention. Studies made by C. E. Turner indicate that the majority of children fail to gain over a 1-month or 2-month period, but only 8 to 10 per cent of elementary school children fail to gain for three successive months between September and May. Such children and others who do not appear to be doing their best, and children who suddenly or persistently make excessive gains, should be called to the attention of the nurse or physician. At the time of making this referral a report should be given on the child's progress in school, the standard of living to which he is accustomed, and any other information that the physician may find significant in making a medical examination.

Continuous records of height and weight have specific value in several other ways:

1. They can be used to point out to the child the relation between growth and health. Thus, while they are not diagnostic in a clinical sense, they are a good educational device.

2. They can be used as an incentive to encourage the child to keep in good condition or to build up his health. His growth record is something the child can see and understand. In most cases it is a mirror revealing the relationship between growth on the one hand and nutrition, sleep, rest, and exercise on the other. By keeping track of his progress the child can see that his physical health is closely bound up with his health habits. This provides one way of appealing to the child to take some of the responsibility for his health.

3. The records are of interest to parents, who naturally like to have evidence of their child's progress. They may be helpful to the parents in arousing the child's pride in his health and in winning his cooperation in matters that affect his health.

Record keeping of this type in the classroom provides a valuable medium of health teaching. Through it the teacher, the parent, and the child collaborate regularly in a matter that is of importance to each one of them—the child's present and future well-being.

Subjective Estimates of Nutritional Status. The signs that indicate any departure from good health, like troubles, seldom come singly. Hence we should expect that a child who is not growing properly would show other abnormal variations besides a failure to gain, or an excessive gain, in pounds and inches. One of the principal factors that interfere with optimal growth is inadequate nutrition, whether it is due to faulty or insufficient food intake or whether there is some physical, emotional, or social condition that is interfering with the normal assimilation of food.

In Plate 4, ten-year-old Rosalie is shown with six-year-old Jean. Rosalie shows signs of being poorly nourished, not only because she is small and thin, but also because her face is pale, her hair dull, and her eyes ringed underneath with shadows. Her muscles, too, are very thin, and she has practically no fat between her skin and her bones.

The opinion of the teacher who referred Rosalie for a medical examination hardly differed from that of the physician. The teacher was going on her feeling for normality—her conviction that no healthy child should look the way Rosalie looked and get as tired as Rosalie got in the course of a school day. The physician based his opinion both on the teacher's observations and on his own findings during his examination of the child. Then he took the step the teacher could not take—he determined the cause of Rosalie's malnutrition and prescribed the measures necessary to correct it.

The story of Rosalie illustrates the fact that the observant teacher, because of her familiarity with healthy appearance in general and normal variations from it in particular, can hardly fail to be impressed by the signs which indicate that a child is ill nourished.

MENTAL GROWTH AND ITS MEASUREMENT

Exactly why one person should be better able or less able than another person to understand and deal with his environment in an adaptive fashion is not known. There is no doubt, however, that so far as functions of the central nervous system are concerned human beings are born with differences both in their ability to acquire and use facts and in their specific aptitudes. As they grow older, these individual variations in intelligence and power become far greater. At birth children's differences in intelligence and aptitude are only potentialities. They become real measurable differences through the opportunities for accomplishment provided in the environment.

Intelligence Tests

There is disagreement as to whether intelligence is a highly complex or a relatively simple function of the central nervous system. In any event, tests for measuring it have been devised. The norm of accomplishment in intelligence tests is determined by testing under similar conditions large groups of children of different ages so as to find out what tests the majority of children of a given age can do. Thus a mental age of twelve means that the child tested can do most or all of the tests that the majority of children of twelve can do. If a child of eight had a mental age of twelve and we wished to express his intellectual superiority in respect to his age group, we should say that he is older on the scale of mental growth than he is on the scale of chronological growth.

Speaking in terms of intelligence quotients,[7] we may think that an I.Q. of 100 represents the normal level of intelligence at a given age of childhood—that which the average child of that age possesses. However, intelligence cannot be measured accurately enough to spot it exactly at a single point, and so we say that normal intelligence ranges from an I.Q. of 90 to an I.Q. of 110.

Going up the scale of intelligence from an I.Q. of 110, we come to very bright children with I.Q.'s of 120 and above. The lower limit of exceptional brightness, or giftedness, is usually placed at an I.Q. of 125 to 130. In any mixed group of 100 children, five or six are likely to be found with I.Q.'s of 120 or above, three with an I.Q. of 125 or above, and only one with an I.Q. of 130 or above.

Going down the scale of intelligence from an I.Q. of 90, we come to the very dull children. The lower limit of mental backwardness at which these children can profit by education in regular school classes is placed at an I.Q. of 70 to 75.

Teachers are likely to encounter mentally backward children more frequently than intellectually gifted children because—on a percentage basis—the gifted are rarer than the backward. In schools of less than 100 students, an exceptionally bright child (I.Q. of 130 or above) may only occasionally be found.

Achievement Tests

Intelligence tests are not designed to find out how much is stored in the mind but rather how well the mind works. Achievement tests, on the other hand, measure what a child *has done* rather than what he *can do* in various subjects, such as reading or spelling or arithmetic. Standard achievement tests often pick out gifted children very much better than school marks. In one study, for example, it was found that in almost every school grade there were children whose achievement in one or more subjects was rated by the teacher as average or *below* for the grade but

---

[7] A child's intelligence quotient (I.Q.) is expressed as the ratio between mental age (M.A.) and chronological age (C.A.), multiplied by 100 to eliminate decimals. For example, suppose three children aged fourteen, twelve, and ten respectively all do equally well on an intelligence test that the majority of twelve-year-old children can do. Then all three children are said to have a mental age of twelve. The I.Q. of the fourteen-year-old child is:

$$\frac{12 \text{ (M.A.)}}{14 \text{ (C.A.)}} = .86 \times 100 = 86$$

By the same computation, the I.Q. of the twelve-year-old is 100 and that of the ten-year-old is 120.

whose achievement test scores showed them to be as much as two years *above* their grade norms in those same subjects.[8] One possible reason for this surprising finding is that few gifted children are as educationally advanced as their ability would warrant. In many cases boredom with school tasks develops when the mental nuts the child is called upon to crack are not tough enough for him. As a result the child falls into sloppy habits of work, which adversely affect his ability to achieve good marks.

Aptitude Tests

In addition to differences in general intelligence, children show differences in special gifts or aptitudes. Even among children of so-called normal intelligence, some are "good" at music or art, for example, and others at working with tools or working with people. Children of high intelligence are seldom equally good in all school subjects and sometimes show definite specialization in their interests and abilities.

Numerous tests have been devised to distinguish children who exhibit special gifts or skills regardless of what their intelligence quotients may be. Such tests are important not only for the detection of creative abilities in science, mechanics, music, art, literature, leadership, and social relations, but also for helping all children to develop along the lines of their major strengths.

Factors Influencing Mental Growth

Many different influences help or hinder a person in using the intelligence or the special abilities with which he is endowed. One person with an I.Q. below normal may function smoothly and efficiently. Another person with a high I.Q. may function so poorly that he might as well not have a "good brain."

Sometimes a child's physical condition may be to blame for his failure to use his intelligence to good advantage. That is why a physical factor like poor eyesight or poor hearing or a chronic infection or an endocrine disturbance is the first thing a physician looks for when a teacher reports that a child is obviously not using the intelligence he possesses. Frequently an emotional block of one kind or another profoundly influences the functioning of intelligence.

Environmental influences often wield the power to make or break the child of unusual promise. It is true that the history of genius is punctuated with tales of men and women who suffered cruel and bitter hardships in childhood either through poverty or through lack of social

---

[8] TERMAN, LEWIS M., and M. H. ODEN, "The Gifted Child Grows Up," p. 26, Stanford University Press, Stanford University, Calif., 1947.

or spiritual understanding. Such individuals possessed a drive to accomplish so forceful that they were able to overcome early adverse conditions. Less familiar because they are obscure are those with a high potentiality of giftedness which was never realized because there was no one at hand to give friendly guidance and suitable materials with which to work. Practically every study of giftedness has revealed the great waste caused by the failure to identify and encourage individuals who might have made significant contributions to society if they had been provided with opportunities to develop and use their gifts.

Even a child who is known to be intellectually superior through either intelligence testing or classroom performance often fails to come up to expectations because the mental tasks he has been given to do furnish no challenge to his intelligence. Like the children in Kenneth Grahame's "Dream Days," he has scorned to excel in subjects "held to be necessary even for him whose ambitions soared no higher than to crack a whip in a circus ring. . . ." Or he may be interested in his work but may finish it quickly and then be left to twiddle his thumbs because there is nothing else to do.

Identifying Superior Children

In general what may be called the best culture medium for the emergence of giftedness is an environment in which *all* children can reach the highest level of learning and accomplishment of which they are capable at each stage of their development. All children, no matter what their potentialities, are first of all children, each one setting his own pace and reacting in his own way to a variety of situations. As the teacher observes the day-to-day performance of all children in the classroom, a child here or there may astonish her with his keen insight and reasoning ability. Perhaps he is the youngest child in the class, because studies have shown that usually the youngest children in a grade are the brightest. Some very bright children, however, move along from grade to grade at the regular pace. In such cases general excellence in school work or consistently superior performance in areas of special interest may point to accelerated mental growth. The gifted child is the one who is most often able to supply the answers. He is eager to think things through and to extend his interests beyond the range of his immediate school tasks. Often the gifted child acquires an amount of special knowledge that seems "simply uncanny" in some subject that has caught his fancy or fired his imagination.

Whenever possible, the delightful discovery of unusual mental ability in one or more children should be verified by the results of performance on standardized tests of general intelligence. In many school systems such tests have long been an important factor in classifying students for schoolwork. Although current tests of general intelligence will not pick out all the mentally gifted, they are probably the most effective single *objective* measure for use in corroborating or casting doubt on the observer's judgment.

Administering standardized tests of general intelligence requires thorough training and experience. Teachers who have not had this preparation may call upon the services of a child-guidance or child-psychology clinic in the community if such services are not available through the school.[9] Standard tests of achievement can be administered by untrained teachers if directions are studied carefully and followed explicitly.

As for aptitude tests, there is a difference of opinion among psychologists as to the nature of special abilities and their relation to general intelligence. The question as to the best ways of measuring aptitude awaits to a considerable degree the settlement of such disagreements. Special abilities or talents are usually recognized through active performance, but sometimes a child expresses an interest which if encouraged leads to performance. Aptitude tests have been developed with a fair amount of success for identifying several abilities, for example, in music, mechanics, science, clerical work, and art. The value of these tests depends largely upon the background and training of those who interpret them.

Problems of Gifted Children

The possession of intellectual superiority is in itself a powerful drive. The mentally gifted child may have an unhappy childhood unless his dilemma is understood by his parents and teachers and an effort is made to help him solve it. It is natural to seek companionship on one's own intellectual level. Yet the children who are equal in mental age to the intellectually superior child are chronologically older—and hence physically bigger and stronger and socially more mature. These older children may not like to be tagged around by a "smart-aleck kid." Even parents and teachers may be goaded into irritability by his exhibitions of superiority. If the superior child tries to associate with children who are his chronological equals, he is likely to be bored by them and they are likely to be antagonized by him. As a result the child is caught in a situation in which he feels that he is not wanted anywhere. And like all people who feel unwanted, he will develop emotional difficulties. Unless the situation is corrected in time, he may be driven further and

[9] Teachers may write to the United States Office of Education for special help or advice regarding the use of standardized intelligence tests if such help is not available in their school systems.

further into himself and become a definitely asocial or even antisocial individual.

Great are the rewards of helping emotionally upset children of superior intelligence to solve their problems. Often the rapidity with which emotional difficulties disappear when adequate outlets are supplied is quite surprising. These children will grow up into the leaders we so sadly need "*if* their emotional problems do not constitute a barrier for the full exercise of their intelligence." [10]

Providing Educational Opportunities for Gifted Children

Whatever may be the methods of identifying gifted children, the school has the responsibility of planning an educational program that will give them adequate means of expression and satisfactory outlets for their drive to accomplish. Various plans are being tried in different school systems.

One of the most common methods used is acceleration. Acceleration means advancing an exceptionally bright child ahead of his group from one grade to the next after he has mastered the work in the grade from which he is moving. It does not mean "skipping grades," as is sometimes supposed.

At present, the wisdom of too-rapid acceleration, especially in the elementary school, is questioned by educators, largely because of the danger of social maladjustment. Bright children who are well developed physically, socially, and emotionally may get along well in a group in which the other members are one or two years older, but beyond that point social complications may arise. If acceleration seems to be the only answer to the problem, moderation is recommended, with special planning to make sure that there are no gaps in the child's experiences.

Many large school systems have organized special groups or schools in which superior children can find companionship and free play for their capacities. There is a difference of opinion among educators on this method also. Some believe that gifted children should learn to work and play with children of all levels of intelligence so that later on they will be able to adjust socially and emotionally to an adult world consisting of individuals of widely varying intellectual and cultural status. Others believe that it is not fair to the intellectually gifted to penalize them for the stereotyped education often made necessary by lack of funds or overcrowding or overworked teachers of varying qualifications. Until the argument regarding the organization of special groups for gifted

[10] THORNER, MELVIN W., "Psychiatry in General Practice," p. 36, Saunders, Philadelphia, 1949.

children is settled, each community is responsible for seeking the solution that best conserves and develops its human resources.

A third method, which occupies the middle ground between acceleration and the organization of special groups, is curriculum enrichment. The enrichment for children of unusual promise differs only in degree and variety—not in kind—from that which all school children need. The dominant factor is the provision of a flexible program of challenging experiences and large areas of interest in which gifted children are encouraged to seek higher levels of creative expression and a greater appreciation of problems than is attainable by less able children in the group. In some schools, gifted children are formed into special groups for activities in line with their special interests and into mixed groups of all levels of ability for subjects that are considered fundamental for all.

Backward Children

From the human point of view it is as important to spot the mentally backward child in a group as it is to spot the superior child and the "intellectually average-minded." Nothing can be done to improve the basic ability to acquire and use facts in mentally retarded children unless their low intellectual capacity is due to some reversible change in the central nervous system, like that caused by an infection or an endocrine disturbance. However, a great deal can be done to help such children use their basic intelligence to the utmost by removing as many adverse physical and emotional factors as possible.

Only teachers of young children are likely to come in contact with youngsters who reach their mental ceiling anywhere from kindergarten to third grade. Once having reached that ceiling they can go no further. When their low intellectual status is discovered through intelligence testing or through failure to progress at a normal rate in their schoolwork, their future education is usually placed in the hands of teachers who have specialized in the training of mentally retarded children.

Educational authorities agree that children who have been given individual tests by competent testers and are found to have I.Q.'s between approximately 50 and 70 should be enrolled in special classes. The so-called slow learners with I.Q.'s of 70 to 90 will do well in regular classes if their teachers recognize their mental handicap "and sympathetically give them opportunities for success and adjustment within their range of achievement." [11]

[11] "Suggested School Health Policies," National Committee on School Health Policies of the National Conference for Cooperation in Health Education, Health Education Council, New York, 1945.

Dull or backward children often have emotional difficulties that they are incapable of solving by themselves. The services of the physician and the teacher are required to help them make the best possible compromises with life. Many children whose mental deficiency is not too severe may be trained to take a useful place in the world if they are given the education suited to their needs. There are many routine tasks in industry and business that call for individuals who are easily satisfied with simple work that would irk the intellectually average or superior person. However, it is important to protect such individuals from being unfairly treated or exploited and to help them realize that their work is important in the organization.

EMOTIONAL AND SOCIAL DEVELOPMENT

Children when they first come to school—even the three- to six-year-olds dealt with in the nursery school and kindergarten—are already "complex miniature personalities whom it is by no means easy to influence." [12] Their emotional and social development, intimately linked with their physical and intellectual growth, has been a continuing process since birth. It was Sigmund Freud (1856–1939) who first turned our attention to the early life of the individual as the period in which the infinite complexities and peculiarities of personality may be traced to their origins.

The Drama of Personality Development

Before describing the phases of personality development through which the child passes before physical maturity is reached, it may be helpful to review the forces that operate in the formation of personality. First comes the biologic, intellectual, and emotional constitution of the newborn baby. Constitution is what is born into the tissues and remains with the individual throughout his life. However, it is subject to an infinite variety of modifying influences springing from the environment.

Within the newborn baby are powerful instinctual drives or forces (technically called the Id) which seek for expression. Not only do these inner forces war among themselves, but also they come eventually into conflict with forces in the outside world. These outer forces seek to mold the child into an acceptable member of the family and the society into which he was born. The child's Ego, the part of his personality that he knows as "I, myself," emerges during this process. An essential part of Ego formation is identification with the wishes and ideas of the parents. The parents are always giving, the child always taking and putting

[12] FREUD, ANNA, "Psycho-analysis for Teachers and Parents," p. 16, Emerson, New York, 1935.

together in his own mind, the various pieces of the picture of what is expected of him as a responsible member of society. Naturally the Ego is weaker than it will be later when the child is able to think and function independently and when his own ideal of what he wants to be becomes firmly established.

As the child grows older the parents cannot always be with him to remind him that some things are wrong and must not be done, and some things are right and must be done. To overcome the feeling of insecurity that arises from not being able to remember what is right and what is wrong, the child erects a mechanism that operates automatically to keep him on the right track. This mechanism is called the conscience, or Superego. At first, the child's conscience is the reflection of his parents' consciences. But as the child gains more knowledge of the moral concepts and behavior ideals of the society in which he lives, his conscience takes on substance and becomes an integral part of his personality.

With the arrival on the scene of the Superego, the stage is set for the lifelong drama of personality development. The central figure in the struggle—the hero—is the Ego. The self must defend itself from the machinations of both the Id and the Superego. The instinctual impulses of aggression and sexuality arising from the Id threaten individuality by urging the Ego to be too independent and grasping—too self-centered and selfish. The cultivated impulses arising from the Superego threaten individuality by urging the Ego to be too dependent upon social dictates, too self-effacing and submissive. The happy denouement of this struggle is the development of a well-balanced and mature personality— an individual with a profound sense of personal worth combined with a lively sense of responsibility toward others.

Phases and Aspects of Personality Development

The child's emotional and social life from birth onward follows as precise a pattern as the stages of his physical development. Indeed, most of the phases of emotional and social growth have been given names that indicate the closeness of their tie-ups with the physical aspects of personality development. Their chief characteristics are summarized in Table 3.

Introduction to the Requirements of Social Living. The baby's chief source of satisfaction comes through sucking—being fed—and the feeling of close warm contact with his mother that goes with it. If he is loved and properly cared for, he is not denied the reasonably prompt gratification of his instinctual needs and drives. He does not have to wait for the relief of tension caused by discomforts, such as hunger, cold, and pain.

Table 3. PHASES OF EMOTIONAL AND SOCIAL GROWTH

Period	Age	Zone of preoccupation	Characteristic interests and events
Oral........	First year	The mouth and everything connected with it	Pleasure in nursing (being fed)
			Finger sucking
			Weaning
Anal........	From first through third year	The anus (outer end and outlet of rectum) and the surrounding area	Pleasure in bowel and bladder functions
			Playing with feces (transferred to playing with mud, water, finger paints, etc.)
			Toilet training
Phallic (or genital)	From third through sixth year	The genital organs	Romantic attachment to parent of opposite sex
			Pleasure in playing with genital organs
Latency.....	From sixth year to onset of puberty (about 11th, 12th, or 13th year)	No special area	Pleasure in companionship with children of same sex
			Curiosity about sex
			Overflow of hostile impulses (naughtiness, aggressiveness)
			Interests outside of home (going to school)
Early adolescence	From puberty to age 16 or 17	Physical and psychic phenomena connected with maturation of the sex glands at puberty	Interest in children of opposite sex
			Menstruation (in girls)
			Nocturnal emissions (in boys)
			Increased frequency of masturbation
			Emergence of secondary sex characteristics
			Awkwardness in body movements and in social relationships
Late adolescence	From age 16 or 17 to age 20 or 21	No special area	Preparation for assumption of adult responsibilities
			Emancipation from home and parents
			Deciding on a career
			Working out a satisfactory love life

A little later, however, he does have to learn to wait. Little by little he finds that the pleasure of relieving the inner tensions set up by his instinctual needs and urges must be postponed for the attainment of some greater or more distant good. The acquirement of toilet habits, which usually begins toward the end of the first year, is emblematic of the child's introduction to the training that grooms the human being for social acceptance. Giving up the satisfaction of wetting and having a bowel movement when and where he pleases wins for the child his parents' approval, which eventually gives him more satisfaction than the immediate relief of tension.

Learning to Meet Reality. Every child at each stage of his development has pleasures, desires, and purposes upon which he wants to act "right here and now." Taking action, however, may conflict with what is considered right and proper by his own developing Ego or by outside authorities. In postponing action, or in directing his energies into more acceptable channels, or in repressing unworthy impulses for the sake of the more solid lasting satisfaction represented by his own or outside approval, he gains practice in dealing realistically with the forces that influence him. In this process, however, he is bound to experience the pangs of frustration.

The easier and pleasanter dealing with reality is made, the quicker the child will learn, and the fewer will be his feelings of frustration and resentment against authority. Each success in learning new skills in living strengthens his Ego and makes him better able to take the next step forward in his development.

Many of the things required of the child are in line with his own needs and desires. He overcomes his feelings of frustration fairly quickly because of his pleasure in finding that the new patterns of behavior are preferable to the old. For example, the child must learn eventually to feed, wash, and dress himself. At first he may feel disappointed or hurt when his mother does not give him all her attention. But he finds that being able to do things for himself gives him a pleasant feeling of independence. Even though it may take him two or three times longer than it would take his mother to button his coat or to tie his shoelaces, he insists upon doing it. Walking all by himself frees him from the restraining hand that often keeps him from going where *he* wants to go. And so the tremendous effort required in learning to walk alone is worth it—it is made gladly.

However, there are many requirements that seem to interfere with the child's freedom or threaten his Ego. The time comes when he must begin to give up the satisfaction of having his playthings all to himself. He learns that certain things and certain persons are inviolable. There are, for example, things which he may not take without permission or without paying for them, things which he may not touch or even go near. He learns that the penalty for kicking, biting, hitting, or otherwise assaulting grown-ups and younger children is much greater than for similar encounters with children of approximately his own age.

As the child grows older and his environment widens, he comes up against many other requirements that force him to give up his freedom to do as he pleases. To be socially acceptable he finds, for example, that in playing and working with others he must "take turns," obey the "rules of the game," refrain from crying even when hurt, go to school regularly although sometimes he'd much rather be somewhere else, be on time when he feels like loitering, walk in the school corridors when he'd rather run, keep still in the classroom when he wants to talk, and so on.

The child learns to meet many such requirements because he has been convinced that failure to do so will delay or block the coming of some greater good, or will seriously handicap his personal well-being. However, he seldom meets them with equanimity. We have all seen the prototype of Shakespeare's boy "creeping like snail unwillingly to school" because he has learned that the fruits of truancy are less appetizing than the fruits of attendance.

Also the child often experiences overwhelming emotions such as anger or fear when he is frustrated or confronted with the unknown. Experience gradually teaches him that it is safer or nicer or wiser to keep such feelings bottled up. So he learns to control overwhelming emotions—to be angry or afraid inside and not show it, to be frustrated and not sulk or weep. During the learning process, however, his feelings often spill over. This is natural, because it takes time to learn to repress strong feelings successfully or to divert them into channels of constructive activity (see Behavior Reactions to Frustration, in Chap. 3).

As the child grows up he is expected to put away such childish things as temper tantrums, or fits of sulkiness, or crying. On the surface, at any rate, he is expected to have worked out the adjustments that make possible what we label adult behavior. But the impulses that aroused childish behavior cannot be thrown away or given away. Like the dolls and the tin soldiers in the attic, they remain unclaimed in the lost-and-found department of his mind as reminders of the child he once was. More often than he realizes, they influence his conscious thoughts and actions.

Development of Sexuality. During the period of life that extends roughly from three to six years of age, the sexuality that is born in everyone begins to take shape. The sensual pleasure that children get in the oral stage from nursing and sucking their fingers and in the anal stage from their bowel and bladder functions is experienced in the genital stage through playing with the genital organs. This act is called masturbation.

Usually the child discovers that touching the genital area is pleasurable even before the end of the first year. However, the two phases in the normal child's life when masturbation tends to increase in intensity are in the genital period, when children go through a period of emotional attachment toward the parent of the opposite sex, and in the adolescent period, when the maturation of the sex glands gives impetus to sexual development.

Masturbation becomes a problem when it is indulged in excessively or under circumstances that make it embarrassing. As with finger sucking and other immature ways of getting satisfaction, this is not likely to happen in happy contented children who have interesting, wholesome activities and congenial playmates. Above all, an abiding assurance of the love of both parents will help the child to curtail his indulgence in order to follow the pattern of behavior that wins his parents' approval. In children of school age, this manifestation of emotional or social immaturity is not uncommon. Usually, it is symptomatic of a complex problem of maladjustment which requires for its solution the understanding of school authorities as well as parents, and perhaps professional medical or religious guidance.

The Oedipus Complex. It is generally agreed that sometime between the ages of three and six most children have their first romantic experience. The little girl "falls in love" with her father and resents the mother's claim on him. The little boy has the same romantic devotion to his mother and feels hostile toward the father. This is the famous Oedipus complex, named for the legendary Theban lad who grew up without being aware of the identity of his parents and fulfilled his tragic destiny by slaying his father and marrying his mother.

While the miniature love affair is going on with the parent of the opposite sex, the child is still dependent upon both parents and knows that he is supposed to love both. Hence, the resentment toward one parent aroused by the frustration of the possessive love for the other seems to threaten the child's security. The child fears the disapproval, anger, and possible punishment of the parent toward whom he feels hostile. At the same time, the harboring of such hostile feelings toward one whom he is expected to love, honor, and obey fills him with a sense of guilt.

Of course, the child does not consciously think this through. Without knowing why, he simply feels uncomfortable and anxious. To relieve the tension he may draw on his own body for comfort. That is why masturbation is more frequent at this time in some children.

Understanding parents who do not let themselves become upset by the outward manifestations of the inner struggle through which the child is going—sudden bursts of hostility and irritability, for example —can be of great help in steering the child safely through this emotionally stormy period. If the child is made to feel that he amounts to something in his own right and that his parents cannot be divided in their affection for each other and for him, his progress toward sexual maturity is likely to be healthy. On the other hand, if the child is encouraged in his love for one parent at the expense of his love for the other, or if his parents are "at outs" with each other and the child is forced to take sides, it may be difficult, and perhaps impossible, for him to express the sexual side of his nature in a normal, mature way later in life.

Hostility and Guilt. There are innumerable life situations besides the Oedipus complex in which conflicts within the child give rise to feelings of hostility toward persons in the child's immediate surroundings. Instinctual impulses seeking gratification come up against many prohibitions and frustrations, emanating from the world outside. The hostile impulses arising when such brakes are applied on forceful instinctual drives come in conflict with the friendly impulses arising from the child's love and respect for those who show their love and respect for him. The inevitable outcome of this conflict is a feeling of guilt that is often a source of much anxiety.

The solution of the difficulty raised by hostile impulses which make the child feel guilty must be found in one of two ways. Either the child must repress them or he must redirect them into acceptable channels.

Unconscious Conflict. The most frequent way in which the child solves his emotional problems is repression. That is, he succeeds wholly or in part in banishing from consciousness those impulses which he has discovered to be condemned and forbidden. However, many of them continue to lead an active existence in the unconscious mind, where they constantly seek for expression. Opposing them are the Ego—the self— and the Superego—the conscience. As a result, there is continual conflict between repressed desires and impulses and the Ego ideals, social taboos, and standards of conduct derived from the interaction of the child and his environment. This inner conflict, together with the struggle between the personality and the outside world to which everyone must adjust, continues throughout life. It is important to remember that the battleground of this conflict is in the unconscious. The individual is not aware of what is going on. However, he does consciously experience the symptoms of anxiety generated by it.

Individuals vary greatly in their capacity to resist anxiety. One person may have a strong enough sense of personal worth and integrity to keep from being overwhelmed either by powerful instinctual drives and repressed impulses or by the "thousand several tongues" of conscience condemning him "for a villain." Such a person seems able to let off emotional steam in satisfactory, useful pursuits and to stand up under any or all of "the slings and arrows of outrageous fortune." Another with a less well integrated personality structure may be able to jog along comfortably even when the going is not too good, but breaks down in the face of extraordinary or greatly prolonged emotional stress. Still another may be so lacking in Ego strength that he is unable to make a satisfactory compromise even under reasonably favorable circumstances.

Latency. When the child enters the first grade in school, at about the age of six, he is just entering the phase of personality development known as the latent period. From its name we should expect it to be a fairly quiet time. So it is, compared with the stormy periods immediately preceding and following it. However, many of the symptoms of the emotional disturbances of adolescence may be present in mild unnoticed form.

Children in the latent period tend to seek the company of their own sex. The boys think of the girls and their games and other occupations as "silly." The girls look upon the boys and their activities as "too rough." The boys form gangs; the girls make chums. The residual resentment and hostile impulses repressed during earlier periods of development tend to break out of bounds, with the result that many children of this age are aggressive toward one another and toward their parents and teachers.

The teacher becomes an unusually important person in the child's life. For the time that the child is in school, his teacher stands in place of his parents, at least to the extent of occupying a position of authority in his life. An emotionally stable, impartially kind, and understanding teacher may go a long way toward effacing the stigma attached to authority in the minds of children who have suffered from abuses of this adult prerogative. The teacher who is really interested in making friends with her students, in inspiring and guiding them as well as in imparting knowledge, is a potent stabilizing force in the lives of children.

Adolescence. Puberty has been taken as a convenient landmark for the beginning of adolescence. With the maturing of the sex glands and the development of the reproductive function, the tide of childhood gradually recedes and the tide of maturity comes in. Puberty is not only a period of rapid growth in body (see The Puberal Cycle, earlier in this chapter) but also one of rapid changes in mental and emotional life. In respect to the latter, physiological age is more significant than chronological age, because mental and emotional attitudes depend more upon how far the body has progressed toward maturity than upon how old the child is in years. The fact that girls mature about two years earlier than boys accounts in part for the relative lack of understanding between boys and girls of the same age which is frequently noted in the late elementary and junior high school periods.

There is a marked change in the attitude of boys and girls toward each other as sex becomes a conscious urge. Children whose reactions to companions of the opposite sex have hitherto been sexless soon discover that there is an intriguing difference between boys and girls. This is as it should be, because adolescence is the time for working out satisfactory relations with the opposite sex in preparation for courtship and marriage.

Physical changes take place so rapidly during puberty that young people usually cannot make adjustments in the management of their bodies with enough speed to give the effect of a smooth performance. In boys the voice "cracks." Arms and legs may grow so fast that their owners do not quite know what to do with them. Masturbation may again increase in frequency as the endocrine secretion of the sex glands heightens tensions associated with sexual development. Boys and girls both may be troubled with poor complexions (see Acne, in Chap. 7).

The stormy emotional weather peculiar to this period is due partly to the fact that the adolescent is beginning to take his life into his own hands before he has acquired mature perspectives. It is not surprising that in the process of shifting from the thoughts and feelings of a child to the thoughts and feelings of an adult all sorts of puzzling problems should arise. The adolescent can no longer act childish, because he is no longer a child. On the other hand, he cannot do many of the things that adults do, because he is not yet grown up. Lack of understanding and inconsistencies in dealing with him aggravate his bewilderment. At the very time when he shows signs of "feeling his oats" his parents may tighten up on the reins. He may be told on one occasion, "You're as big as a man. Why don't you act like one?" and on another, "You're only a boy. What makes you think you can decide such an important matter?"

Many of the problems of adolescence can be solved satisfactorily when parents and teachers cooperate in giving young people every opportunity to achieve success in their progress toward maturity. The ability to manage one's own life with wisdom grows slowly, and boys and girls need experience that only life can give. Their Egos need to feel what it is like to be "on one's own"—to have only the self to congratulate when things go right, only the self to blame when things go wrong.

Emotional Needs of Children

Although children of different physiological ages differ in their interests, they are all alike in having certain basic emotional needs. Anything that prevents the satisfaction of these needs will have a harmful effect on the development of the child's personality. The basic emotional needs of children may be summarized briefly as follows:

1. *Every child needs the feeling of security that comes from being loved, being wanted, being understood.* This need must be met in the school as well as in the home. Children brought up in broken homes in which there has been no attempt to provide a satisfactory substitute for an absent parent, and unwanted (rejected) children deprived of the love of one or both parents, are those who are likely to live their early lives in the shadow of insecurity.

The personalities of parents and teachers also have a profound effect upon the developing personality of the child. Emotional instability is quite frequently mirrored in the behavior of children whose feelings of insecurity stem from not knowing where they stand with adults. In such cases, perhaps one or more adults in positions of authority may themselves be emotionally unstable and show their anxiety in their inconsistency in dealing with the child, for example, by punishing him for a certain misdemeanor on one occasion and overlooking it on another, or by adopting an attitude that differs from a previously expressed attitude, or by making promises or threats that cannot be carried out.

Most children are ready and willing to accept reasonable rules of conduct. An orderly, just code of rules, implemented with consistent rewards and punishments, helps to give them a sense of security. But they are bewildered or antagonized by too many rules, or by constantly changing rules, or by rules that seem to apply to them but not to others, or by impossibly high standards, or by too much disapproval and too little approval.

Children in school are bound to feel insecure—sometimes even humiliated and demeaned in their own eyes—if the methods of controlling them are determined by an arbitrary, rigid set of rules that does not take into account individual differences in family and cultural background, developmental level, physical and psychological make-up, and other factors.

2. *Every child needs to achieve enough success in dealing with the things and persons in his environment to build up a strong sense of personal worth.* The child begins to think of himself as a separate entity when he emerges from the complete dependence of infancy and realizes that certain things are expected of him. He finds that he cannot always be on the receiving line; he, too, must be a giver, and his success in giving helps to strengthen his Ego—himself. He acquires his feeling of personal worth—his self-respect—from doing things that win expressions of approval from others and from his own conscience. Every child every day should have opportunities to win approval from both sources.

Religious experience often plays an important part in strengthening the child's sense of personal worth and in giving authority to the dictates of his conscience. During the adolescent period, especially, there is likely to be a resurgence of interest in spiritual needs.

To give opportunities for success in school, the capacities and the inadequacies of each child in the group should be taken into account and appropriate situations should be taken advantage of or created in which all children can capitalize on their abilities. Whatever immediate goal the teacher wants the children to reach should be attainable by sharing the work rather than by starring those who can do it best.

If the emphasis is placed on cooperation rather than on competition, the children will have many opportunities to find satisfaction and success in their relationships with their contemporaries. In the good-natured give and take of working and playing together, feelings of failure may disappear as children learn that other children, in general, are fairly easy to get along with—that one needn't be athletic or beautiful or especially gifted or rich or clever, for example, to be acceptable to one's group.

3. *Every child needs to acquire the ability to make necessary compromises with life.* Gradually, as the lessons of experience are learned, children discover that they are limited in what they can do. As a result they are bound to have disappointments and failures. Some of the limitations are man-made—the forces of custom, policy, law, and order in family, school, and society. Others arise from the child's own physiological and psychological make-up. Some children have physical or mental handicaps with which they must learn to live. All children are good at some things, not so good at others. Learning to accept necessary limitations gracefully and to work effectively within them is an important part of the child's education.

DO YOU KNOW?

1. Match each word or term in Group A with the word or term in Group B which you associate with it.

Group A	Group B
Epiphyses	Growth-promoting hormone
Rickets	$\frac{M.A.}{C.A.} \times 100$
Anterior pituitary	
Puberty	Overactivity
I.Q.	Conscience
Latency	Vitamin-D deficiency
Superego	Activation of gonads
Ego	The self
Hyperfunction	Ossification centers
	Elementary school age

2. How would you help a youngster who

   a. Is painfully conscious of being much smaller or larger than others in the class?
   b. Is anxious to reduce in weight?
   c. Is embarrassed because the girl he likes best in junior high is taller than he?
   d. Has failed to gain in weight over a period of 3 months?
   e. Has an I.Q. of 75?
   f. Shows evidence of being much brighter than others in the class?
   g. Shows that he resents your authority?
   h. Is suffering from the physical and social awkwardness characteristic of early adolescence?

SUGGESTED ACTIVITIES

1. Obtain the latest record of the heights and weights of the children of approximately the same age in the class you are teaching. Compute both the average, or mean, height and weight of the group and the percentile rank of each child with respect to height and weight. Are there any children who are much above or below the average? Are there any with very low or very high percentile ranks? What conclusions do you draw regarding the individuality of physical growth?
2. Obtain copies of Meredith's "Physical Growth Record" issued in booklet form and Wetzel's "Grid for Evaluating Physical Fitness"

(see Measuring Physical Growth and Development). Divide the class of children for which you are responsible into two groups and arrange to assume the responsibility over a period of 6 months or more for making the measurements and keeping the records called for in these two methods of visualizing trends in growth. Discuss the records at appropriate intervals with the nurse or physician serving the school.

3. If possible, arrange to attend the administration of standard intelligence tests or achievement tests to a group of children. Are there any children in the class for whom you are responsible whose schoolwork or special interests give you grounds for believing, on the basis of observation alone, that they are intellectually superior or gifted in some way? intellectually backward? Give specific illustrations to back your opinions.

4. Select two or three children you now know well to whom you were attracted at first sight. From memory, list the personality traits (posture, facial expression, manners, etc.) which impressed you. Have these children come up to your expectations on better acquaintance? What characteristics, not at first obvious, have confirmed or changed your first impression?

5. Observe a child and make notes on his behavior in different situations. In what phase of emotional and social growth is the child (see Table 3)? How does his behavior differ from your own in ways of expressing joy, sorrow, and anger? ways of meeting frustration? ways of getting what he wants? the ability to cooperate with others in work or play? What signs of emotional and social maturity do you possess which the child does not possess?

6. Discuss these questions with your fellow students:

   a. Why is it important to help children understand that emotions like anger and fear are common to everyone in certain situations?

   b. How can we help children to acquire techniques for meeting difficulties ranging from minor disappointments to conditions that cannot be changed, such as irreversible mental retardation, intellectual superiority with its hazard of social maladjustment, and irremediable physical defects or handicaps?

SELECTED REFERENCES

BAKER, HARRY J.: *Introduction to Exceptional Children,* rev. ed. New York, The Macmillan Company, 1953. (A text for teachers on the characteristics and problems of all types of children, including such topics as physical handicaps and mental growth and development.)

BRECKENRIDGE, MARIAN E., and E. LEE VINCENT: *Child Development; Physical and Psychological Growth through the School Years,* 2d ed. Philadelphia, W. B. Saunders Company, 1949.

CHAMBERLAIN, N. H., and D. H. MOSS: *Three "R's" for the Retarded;* a program for training the retarded child at home, New York, National Association for Retarded Children, 1954.

CUTTS, N. E., and N. MOSELEY: *Bright Children;* a guide for parents, New York, G. P. Putnam's Sons, 1953.

EDUCATIONAL POLICIES COMMISSION, NATIONAL EDUCATION ASSOCIATION AND AMERICAN ASSOCIATION OF SCHOOL ADMINISTRATORS: *Education of the Gifted,* Washington, D.C., National Education Association, 1950.

FARNHAM, MARYNIA F.: *The Adolescent,* New York, Harper & Brothers, 1951.

GESELL, ARNOLD L., and FRANCES L. ILG: *The Child from Five to Ten,* New York, Harper & Brothers, 1946. (Observations on the development of children through the ages from five to ten.)

GESELL, ARNOLD L.: *Studies in Child Development,* New York, Harper & Brothers, 1948. (A collection of Dr. Gesell's papers on the characteristics and conditions of child development observed at the Yale Clinic of Child Development.)

HYMES, JAMES L., JR.: *Understanding Your Child,* New York, Prentice-Hall, Inc., 1952.

HYMES, JAMES L., JR.: *Behavior and Misbehavior;* a teacher's guide to action, New York, Prentice-Hall, Inc., 1955.

HYMES, JAMES L., JR.: *A Child Development Point of View,* New York, Prentice-Hall, Inc., 1955.

JENKINS, GLADYS GARDNER, HELEN SHACTER, and WILLIAM W. BAUER: *These Are Your Children,* expanded ed. Chicago, Scott, Foresman & Company, 1953. (Child guidance related to the physical, mental, and emotional development problems peculiar to each age group; for parents and teachers.)

JERSILD, A. T.: *Child Psychology,* 4th ed. New York, Prentice-Hall, Inc., 1954.

MARTIN, W. E., and C. B. STENDLER: *Child Development; the Process of Growing up in Society,* New York, Harcourt, Brace and Company, Inc., 1953.

Overstreet, Harry A.: *The Mature Mind,* New York, W. W. Norton & Company, Inc., 1949.

Overstreet, Harry A., and Bonaro W. Overstreet: *Mind Alive,* New York, W. W. Norton & Company, Inc., 1954.

Pollock, Morris P.: *New Hope for the Retarded;* enriching the lives of exceptional children, Boston, Porter Sargent, Publisher, 1953.

Rand, Winifred, and others: *Growth Development of the Young Child,* 5th ed., revised by Marian E. Breckenridge and Margaret N. Murphy. Philadelphia, W. B. Saunders Company, 1953.

Scheifele, M.: *Gifted Child in the Regular Classroom,* New York, Teachers College, 1953.

Simmons, Katherine: *The Brush Foundation Study of Child Growth and Development: II. Physical Growth and Development,* Washington, D.C., Society for Research in Child Development, National Research Council, 1944.

Strang, Ruth M.: *An Introduction to Child Study,* New York, The Macmillan Company, 1951.

Terman, Lewis M., and Melita H. Oden: *The Gifted Child Grows Up,* Stanford, Calif., Stanford University Press, 1947.

Tuddenham, R. D., and M. M. Snyder: *Physical Growth of California Boys and Girls from Birth to Eighteen Years,* Berkeley, Calif., University of California Press, 1954.

Witty, Paul, ed.: *The Gifted Child,* The American Association for Gifted Children. Boston, D. C. Heath and Company, 1951. (A nontechnical book giving practical suggestions for meeting some of the outstanding needs of gifted children.)

Organizations
National Association for Retarded Children
Public Affairs Committee
The American Association for Gifted Children

Chapter 3   THOUGHTS AND FEELINGS, ACTIONS AND REACTIONS

Ins and Outs of the Nervous System
Observations Related to Endocrine Activity
Defense Reactions of Physical Origin
Psychogenic Reactions
Organic Disorders of the Nervous System
Mental Illness of Psychogenic Origin
Identifying Children with Emotional and Social
Problems

INS AND OUTS OF THE NERVOUS SYSTEM

The child comes to school with a whole constellation of thoughts, feelings, and patterns of behavior that is uniquely his own. He also has a body that reacts to stimuli from both without and within, according to physiological laws that apply to every body. The forces that condition both uniqueness of personality and physiological sameness are lodged in the central nervous system (the brain and spinal cord). For that reason teachers will find it helpful to have some background knowledge of this system as a basis for the intelligent observation of children as individuals and as members of a group.

The Seat of Thought and Voluntary Action

The part of the brain known as the cerebral cortex makes it possible for each person to think, to remember, to learn, to act voluntarily—in short, to be himself in thought, word, and deed. It is a corrugated layer of gray matter composed of nerve cells, which covers the two hemispheres of the cerebrum, or upper part of the brain, as bark covers the trunk of a tree. *Cortex* is the Latin word for bark.

The cerebral cortex belongs to the division of the central nervous system which is sometimes called the outward-acting system because through it the individual governs his dealings with people and things in the world outside himself. Information received about the world from his special sense organs makes it possible for him to govern intelligently. And voluntary muscles supplied with motor nerves from the seat of government make it possible for him to act as he wills.

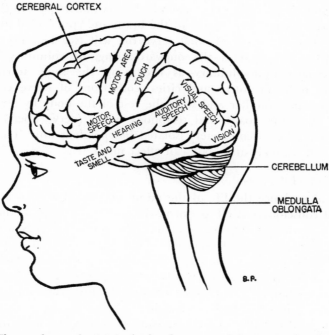

FIG. 13. The cerebrum (brain) is the headquarters of the outward-acting nervous system.

Department of Internal Affairs

That part of the central nervous system which manages the internal affairs of the body is the autonomic (self-controlling) nervous system. The inward-acting nervous system is another good name for it. It supplies nerves to the glands and to the involuntary muscles of the eyes, heart, lungs, digestive tract, kidneys, blood vessels, skin, and other organs. Autonomic impulses, which may be provoked by emotional as well as by physical stimuli, are responsible for the rate of the heartbeat; for the amount of digestive juices secreted by the stomach and small intestine and the amount of sweat secreted by the sweat glands; for the dilation and contraction of the pupils of the eyes and of the tiny blood vessels (arterioles) in the skin; and for a great many other actions. In short, the autonomic system takes the government of our bodies off our minds so that we do not need to bother about what goes on inside to regulate the work of the organs and to maintain the living conditions to which the cells are accustomed.

Two in One

The autonomic nerve centers from which nerve fibers pass to the organs they influence have their places in the brain and spinal cord along with the groups of nerve centers that serve the will (see Fig. 14). We may visualize the two systems—the outward-acting, or voluntary, and the inward-acting, or involuntary—as occupying the same territory but located in different towns and cities (collections of nerve cells), connected with one another and with the rest of the body by an intricate network of streets, roads, and telephone wires (nerve fibers). Neither system operates as a completely isolated independent unit. That is why mind can affect body and body can affect mind.

The Psyche and the Soma

In medical parlance the life of the mind—emotional as well as intellectual, and conscious as well as unconscious—is referred to as the psyche. In Greek mythology, Psyche, meaning the soul, was personified as a lovely, butterfly-winged maiden, emblematic of immortality. The body, in medical language, is known as the soma, which is the Greek word for "body." Putting the two words together, we get "psychosomatic," which designates body-mind relationships. Bodily symptoms and signs of psychic origin are called psychogenic.

Blushing with shame or embarrassment, turning white with joy or rage, having a sinking feeling at the pit of the stomach from fright, watering at the mouth when an appetizing food is smelled are all psychogenic manifestations. That is, they are physical changes brought about by the effect of the psyche on the autonomic and endocrine systems. Since such changes occur automatically—when the proper psychic button is pushed—it is easy to see why a person may have all sorts of physical signs and symptoms without having anything organically wrong. Although thoughts and emotions have their home in the brain, they are not confined to home. Their echoes reverberate in every cell and tissue of the body. The reverse is also true. Physical sensations, as we all know, have a profound effect on our thoughts and feelings.

What Sensations Are and Why We Have Them

Sensations are conscious impressions produced by the reaction of sensory nerve endings (receptors) to stimuli to which they are sensitive. The simplest way to represent our sensory mechanism is, first, to draw a circle and place on its circumference (representing the outer, or periph-

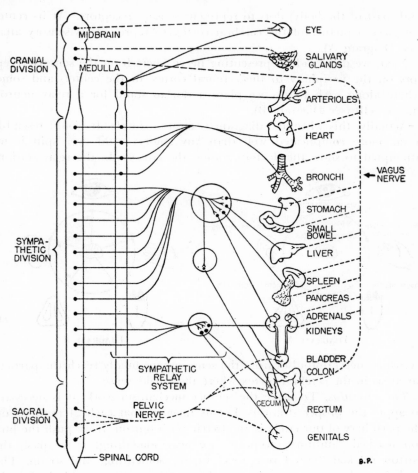

FIG. 14. The nerve fibers of the autonomic system pass out from the central nervous system in three regions: (a) the lowest portion of the brain (cranial division); (b) the lower end of the spinal cord (sacral division); and (c) the spinal cord between the cranial and sacral divisions (sympathetic division—solid lines in diagram). The two end divisions (cranial and sacral) together form what is called the parasympathetic division (broken lines in diagram). The vagus nerve and its branches carry the impulses from the cranial division to the organs of the trunk. In their influence upon any one organ, the parasympathetic division and the sympathetic division work against each other. For example, the sympathetic division supplies the nerve fibers over which impulses to contract the skin arterioles (vasoconstrictors) are transmitted, whereas the parasympathetic division supplies the nerve fibers that carry the impulses responsible for their dilation (vasodilators).

eral, part of the body) dots to represent sensory receptors.[1] At its center we place a picture of the cerebral cortex to represent its sensory areas (see Diagram A).

Next, we draw radii representing nerve fibers from the sensory receptors on the periphery to the cerebral cortex in the center, and somewhere along each radius we place a dot to stand for a relay neuron (nerve cell) (see Diagram B).

Actually, this wheellike diagram is far too simple. It would resemble a far more complicated web than any spider could ever spin if we attempted to show the devious routes, the crossroads, the relay stations

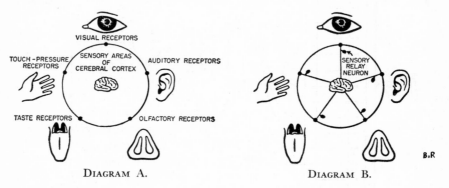

DIAGRAM A.   DIAGRAM B.

by which nerve impulses from the sense organs finally reach the particular areas in the cerebral cortex where they make sense.

The Stimulus. To make the sensory mechanism work, it is necessary to apply the proper stimulus. Let us imagine that each of the dots on the periphery of our circle is an electric push button. If we push the button marked "auditory receptors" we hear something; if we push the button marked "visual receptors" we see something; and so on. The push in each case is the stimulus. It must be a different kind of push, or stimulus, for each kind of receptor. For example, only light waves can stimulate visual receptors; only sound waves can stimulate auditory receptors; only odors can stimulate olfactory receptors. However, it does sometimes happen that a receptor is excited by an unusual stimulus. When that happens the sensation aroused is similar to that aroused by the usual stimulus. For example, we "see stars" (light) when hit between the eyes.

The Nerve Impulse. The force started along a nerve fiber when the proper stimulus is applied to its sensory ending, or receptor, is the nerve impulse. The impulses carried by sensory nerve fibers leading from one

[1] For the sake of simplicity only the receptors of the familiar five senses are represented here. There are other sensibilities, as will be explained later.

kind of receptors are practically the same as those carried by nerve fibers leading from other kinds of receptors. An electric current makes a bell ring or a light come on, according to the device to which it is connected by wires. Just so, the nerve impulse gives us the sensation of sight or hearing or some other sensation, according to the sensory area in the brain to which it is connected by nerve fibers. That is, the starting point of an impulse and its destination are what determine the character of a sensation, not the impulse itself. Although all impulses in themselves are more or less alike, no one has yet explained exactly *what* they are. The nearest we can come to defining a nerve impulse is to say that it is an excitation process associated with a series of electrical and chemical changes along its nerve-fiber route.

Somatic Sensibilities. So far we have been discussing the sensations which are so distinctive that they have been singled out and given special names. Four of these familiar quintuplets—sight, hearing, taste, and smell—still maintain their status as special senses. But in recent years touch and its refinements have been placed among the less distinct sensations designated as somatic, or body, sensibilities. These sensibilities make us aware, in varying degrees, of pressure, heat, cold, pain, and the movements and position of the limbs, trunk, and head. As their name implies, they are concerned with matters of vital interest to the body itself. When their receptors are stimulated, machinery is set in motion which brings about automatically the adjustments required, or calls our attention to conditions that only we, by thinking and acting voluntarily, can rectify.

Acting without Thinking

The adjustments that take place without our thinking about them are the simple, or unconditioned, reflexes. They are brought about by impulses that travel to nerve centers in the spinal cord or brain stem, and then out again over motor nerves to the gland or muscle that acts in response to them. They do not get to the boss—the cerebral cortex—because the personal attention of the boss is not necessary.

Ordinarily, we are not aware of the great majority of the simple reflexes that bring about desirable adjustments; for example, secretion of the digestive juices when food enters the mouth, and the widening or narrowing of the eye pupils according to the amount of light entering the eyes. But in the case of many reflexes we are aware of the action taken, even though we do not consciously initiate it. Often we think about it and, if necessary, take further conscious steps to remedy the situation. Without thinking, we snatch our hands from a hot stove. But some of the impulses started on their way by contact with the hot surface reach the cerebral cortex. As a result, we consciously feel the pain of the burn and go for the burn ointment. We may not be able to stop a sneeze. But we are aware of the premonitory tickle in the nose and reach for a handkerchief if we have learned regard for our fellow men. We cannot stop a blush, the mechanics of which are handled autonomically. However, we are conscious both of the blush and of the embarrassment responsible. On the other hand, we may be completely unconscious of some other emotion or inner tension and yet be all too well acquainted with the violent headache or upset stomach caused by it.

Habit Acts

There are other things, like walking, dressing, and bathing, which we do *almost* without thinking, as we say, but which once gave our brains a lot of work. When definite nerve tracks and switches had been established for the impulses that initiate every move in these complicated acts, we could then devote our minds to higher things like deciding where to walk, or what to wear, or when to take a bath.

It is only necessary to watch a little child learning to string colored wooden beads to get an idea of the tremendous concentration required to master a performance which the child who has already mastered it does with the greatest ease. And once it has been mastered, what delightful ways of expressing himself are opened up! Be it reading or skating or stringing beads or walking or what not, it is only when the basic operation has become a habit act, or series of conditioned reflexes, that the child can proceed to the fairy tales or the figure eights or the soul-satisfying patterns or the desired destinations.

Thinking before Acting

The kind of mental activity through which we express ourselves—our own unique personalities—is the highest function of the mind. It requires our constant and direct personal attention. Thinking things through to arrive at decisions and performing the voluntary acts required to deal with new situations as they arise require the association of vast numbers of neurons in the cerebral cortex and often involve widely separated regions of the body.

OBSERVATIONS RELATED TO ENDOCRINE ACTIVITY

"Their name is legion" is an expression that might well have been invented for the chemical products that influence body functions. Among them are the hormones—almost unbelievably powerful substances produced in minute quantities in one part of the body and carried in the blood stream to other organs or tissues. The term hormone is derived from a Greek word meaning "to excite."

Hormones exert a profound influence on the physical appearance, body processes, and mental and emotional manifestations of every individual. This influence is expressed in many of the variations in body build and personality which teachers observe in school children. Many organs carry on the manufacture of hormones as a sort of side line. Others are especially designed for the sole business of producing and secreting hormones. These organs are the endocrine glands. They have no ducts, like the salivary and tear glands, for example, but deliver their secretions directly into the blood stream. Hence another name for them is ductless glands.

Roll Call of the Endocrines

The known endocrine glands are (a) the pituitary, the master of them all, reposing snugly like one small pebble in a tiny ditch, or fossa, in the

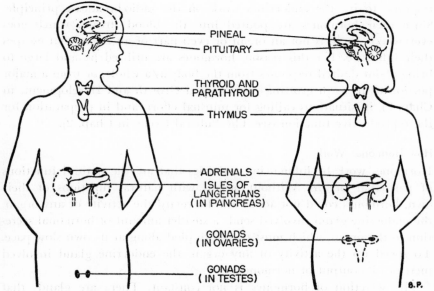

PINEAL
PITUITARY
THYROID AND PARATHYROID
THYMUS
ADRENALS
ISLES OF LANGERHANS (IN PANCREAS)
GONADS (IN OVARIES)
GONADS (IN TESTES)
B.P.

Fig. 15. Diagram showing the location of the endocrine glands.

base of the skull; (b) the thyroid, sprawling like the letter H across the front of the larynx and windpipe; (c) the adrenals, perched like triangular cocked hats over the rounded upper pole of each kidney; (d) the parathyroids, resembling minute reddish-brown beans marking the corners of an imaginary square on the back surface of the thyroid; (e) the islands of Langerhans, clusters of cells embedded in the connective tissue of the pancreas; (f) the ovaries, or female sex glands, and the testes, or male sex glands.

The tiny, reddish-gray pineal gland (in the middle of the substance of the brain), supposed by the French philosopher Descartes to be the seat of the rational soul, and the lymphatic thymus behind the breast-bone, waxing during infancy and waning after puberty, have not yet had their status as endocrine glands firmly established.

Why We Have Endocrines

The function of the endocrine glands is to secrete individual hormones at the proper time and in suitable quantities to regulate and coordinate the work of other organs and tissues. The autonomic nervous system cooperates with the endocrine system in this task. But whereas the nervous system in large measure exercises individual control (operating through a central switchboard to put through "person-to-person" calls from the receptor of a stimulus to the muscle or gland that acts in response to it), the endocrines work on the radio-broadcast principle. Since their hormones are poured into the blood stream, which goes everywhere, there is not an organ or even part of an organ that escapes their influence. For this reason, hormones are utilized by and large to bring about desired responses from the body as a whole, or from a major portion of it, as in growing (see Physical Growth and Development, in Chap. 2), in situations calling for unusual effort, and in preparation for the reproductive function (see The Puberal Cycle, in Chap. 2).

How Hormones Work

Hormones work by influencing activities that are the natural functions of particular organs. Without organs with natural functions of their own, hormones could not act at all. To retard the activity of any organ, the endocrine gland involved sends a smaller amount of hormonal secretion to the organ, which must therefore plod along at its own slow pace. To speed up the activity of any organ, the endocrine gland involved increases its output of hormones.

The secretion of hormones is not constant. There are glands that secrete more or less continuously, it is true—for example, the thyroid, the adrenal cortex, and the anterior (front) portion of the pituitary during skeletal growth—but the amounts secreted vary according to need. Other glands secrete cyclically—for example, the ovarian gonads, or female sex glands, and the gonad-controlling portion of the pituitary. Still others secrete intermittently—for example, the islands of Langer-hans after carbohydrate food has been eaten, and the adrenal medulla when there is urgent need for the release of sugar from the liver to meet some sudden demand for energy.

The Sympatheticoadrenal Team

The teamwork of the sympathetic division of the autonomic system and the adrenal medulla (inner portion of the adrenal glands) in preparing the body to cope with threatened dangers accounts for many psychosomatic signs and symptoms. When the sympathetic division gives the word "go" to the adrenal medulla, the latter starts secreting its hormone, adrenaline, into the blood stream. The effect of this chemical is to put the body in a state of preparedness to take appropriate action in response to strong emotions like fear and anger. Surface blood vessels are tightened up to make extra blood available for the muscles; the force and frequency of the heartbeat are increased; the bronchial tubes are relaxed to ensure the ventilation of the lungs; sugar stored in the liver is released into the blood to provide extra energy; the pupils of the eyes are dilated, intestinal movements stopped, and all sphincters in the digestive tract closed. The ship of the body, so to speak, is cleared for whatever action seems appropriate—fighting or running away as the case may be.

It is worth pointing out that the standards of civilized behavior which demand the suppression of motor responses to primitive emotions, like fear and anger, often have undesirable physical repercussions. Upset digestions and nervous exhaustion are part of the price paid for mobilizing the body's forces for fight or flight when no such action is called for or even possible. The secretion of adrenaline under emotional stress on signal from the sympathetic nervous system accounts for many of the signs and symptoms observed in persons known to be suffering from intense prolonged anxiety—for example, dilated pupils, cold wet hands, and excessive sweating in the armpits. These observations are the basis for interesting speculations regarding a possible tie-up between long-continued anxiety or worry and such conditions as high blood pressure, gastric ulcer, asthma, and certain skin disorders.

Elementary school children are in the period of emotional and social development in which strong motor reactions to anger, fear, and frustration are natural and proper. Many teachers know this through their knowledge of child psychology or through their intuitive understanding of children's behavior. Yet getting mad and fighting with one another in the classroom or showing by hyperactivity or fidgetiness that some sort of emotional conflict is going on is not conducive to good working conditions. On the other hand, it is desirable to encourage acceptable forms of muscular response to strong emotion. Ordinarily this is accomplished during the school day by allowing periods for games and other motor activities during which children can work off the effects of the bodily changes provoked by their aggressive impulses.

When Endocrine Glands Go Wrong

The effects of the hormones secreted by the endocrine glands are so inter-related that an almost hopelessly complicated sequence of events takes place when one gland does not function properly. Like the old woman's pig that would not get over the stile until it was nipped by a dog, which had to be activated by a stick, which was in turn threatened by fire, and so on, the adequate functioning of one endocrine gland depends on the adequate functioning of a series of others.

Even physicians who specialize in endocrinology are cautious about diagnosing and treating endocrine disturbances. Temporary imbalances may occur, especially in children, which clear up spontaneously, that is, without special treatment. On the other hand, the endocrines do produce decided deviations from the normal, and teachers should have at least a speaking acquaintance with some of the possible effects of endocrine imbalance.

The more important variations in body build caused by the hyper-function or hypofunction of the endocrine glands that influence growth are described in Table 1. Brief accounts of the two endocrine disturb-ances that are most likely to be encountered in young people—simple goiter and diabetes—are given here.

Simple Goiter. The thyroid depends upon an adequate amount of iodine in the diet for the manufacture of its secretion, thyroxine. If it does not get enough iodine, it may become large enough to be noticeable. This condition is known as simple goiter. It occurs chiefly in regions where the drinking water and the soil in which foodstuffs are grown are deficient in iodine. In our country the chief goiter belts are in the Great Lakes region. In places near the seacoast many common foods contain iodine in small quantities. Sea food is especially rich in it.

Adding iodine to the drinking water, using iodized salt instead of ordinary salt, and administering iodine to school children in chocolate candy at regular intervals are ways in which the development of simple goiter may be prevented in goiter regions.

In children, simple goiter usually first manifests itself during adoles-cence when there is an increased demand on the part of the body for thyroxine. For this reason it is sometimes called adolescent goiter. Simple goiter appears as a swelling in the neck just below the Adam's apple (Fig. 16). It affects children of both sexes but is especially common in girls. It has a tendency to disappear around age twenty-five. In simple goiter without symptoms other than the slight enlargement of the gland in the neck, the feeding of small amounts of iodine will often hasten the disappearance of the swelling.

A child with noticeable enlargement of the thyroid gland should be referred to a physician. No one should take iodine in any form for this condition without medical advice. If the enlargement is not due to simple goiter but to a more serious condition, iodine may make matters worse instead of better. In some cases, it may cover up the seriousness of the condition for a time, until it is too late for the doctor to treat it successfully.

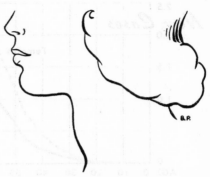

FIG. 16. A slight swelling of the neck may indicate simple goiter.

Diabetes. Diabetes is a disease of metabolism in which the body's power to use sugar is affected. Normally the body is able to oxidize (burn) and store sugar because of the presence in the blood of insulin, the secretion of the islands of Langerhans in the pancreas. Diabetes develops when the flow of insulin from these insulin-secreting cells is lessened or completely stopped.

What causes the islands of Langerhans to fall down on the job of producing insulin is not yet known with any certainty. These groups of cells are part of the whole endocrine system and are influenced by disturbances in other parts of the system. A hereditary factor is undoubtedly involved, because investigations have shown that diabetes runs in families. Overweight in middle age also seems to be an important predisposing factor.

When the tissues can neither use nor store sugar, signs and symptoms of diabetes appear. Sugar accumulates in the blood, and this causes thirst. Drinking large amounts of water to quench the thirst results in frequent urination. An excessive amount of sugar is present in the urine because that is the way in which the body gets rid of the sugar it cannot use. The inability to use sugar means that the body is robbed of this important source of energy. As a result there is constant hunger and a loss of weight and strength. Urinalyses made in connection with periodic school health examinations furnish the surest means of detecting diabetes in children in its earliest, most treatable stage (see The Kidneys, in Chap. 6).

In most cases the diabetic age "begins at forty." That is, diabetes is primarily a disease of middle and old age rather than of youth. Juvenile diabetes is not common, but when the disease does occur in children, it is usually severe and, if untreated, progresses rapidly. A diagnosis of diabetes in a child was equivalent to a sentence of early death in the days before 1922, when Sir Frederick Banting and his coworkers succeeded in extracting insulin from the pancreas of animals in a form that

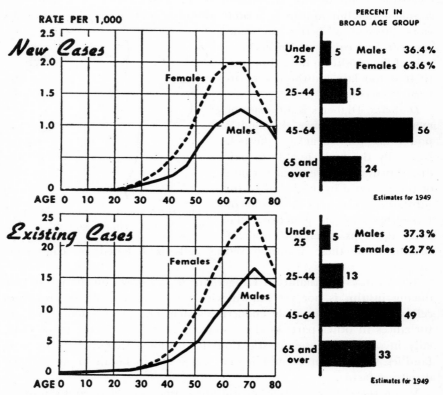

FIG. 17. The incidence of diabetes is low in the early ages. (*From "Progress in Diabetes," Metropolitan Life Insurance Company.*)

could be used in treating human beings. From the beginning of the insulin era to the present, the diabetes death rate at ages one to twenty-four has been reduced by about 75 per cent—that is, to an almost irreducible minimum.

If a child in the school has diabetes, his teacher should know it so that she can cooperate with him intelligently. To this end she should also know what the child has learned from the doctor and what he has been asked to put in practice. It is especially important to keep the child from thinking of himself as an invalid.

The diabetic child, as well as his parents, is told "all about diabetes" by his physician so that he may show the self-restraint and intelligence upon which his life depends. The "three R's" of the child's education in living with his diabetes are diet, insulin, and exercise. The kinds and amounts of insulin, food, and exercise that seem best are worked out by the doctor with the child's help.

The diabetic child is also given the information that will help him to keep out of trouble. The two chief dangers are diabetic coma and insulin reaction. These seldom occur in the child who conscientiously follows the program his doctor outlines for him.

Diabetic coma is due to poisons from acids formed in the body when sugar is not being burned. As coma may come on surreptitiously like a thief in the night, this is a condition that the diabetic child must understand thoroughly and learn how to avoid. *Even slight deviations from normal health,* such as a mild cold or other infection, while not a cause for alarm, should be treated with respect. This means that when the child has an acute illness the parents will want to keep him home for bed rest and medical care until he is fully recovered.

Insulin reaction takes place when there is too little sugar in the blood as a result of (*a*) too much insulin, (*b*) too little food or delay in eating after taking insulin, or (*c*) unaccustomed or unusual exercise. Hunger, trembling, sweating, and nervousness are the beginning signs when regular insulin is being used. If one of the long-acting forms of insulin is being taken, headache, nausea, drowsiness, a sick feeling, hunger, and sweating occur. The treatment is to take sugar immediately. Diabetic children who are taking insulin should always carry two lumps of sugar to be eaten in case symptoms of insulin reaction develop.

DEFENSE REACTIONS OF PHYSICAL ORIGIN

In our conscious efforts to defend the body from sickness and injury, we sometimes forget that the body itself has a great many arrangements for dealing with emergencies that arise very often without our knowledge. The remarkable power of the body to defend itself accounts for a wide variety of reflex actions which teachers constantly observe in healthy children. It also lies back of the mechanisms that operate to produce the outward manifestations of inward trouble of one kind or another. An understanding of these mechanisms cannot but give us a profound admiration for what Dr. Walter B. Cannon called "the wisdom of the body."

It is encouraging to learn that the body's power to deal with adverse conditions "is extraordinarily biased in favor of life as against death. . . . It does not win every time, and it still leaves plenty of work for us

doctors to do; but still it does about ten times as much as all that we
can do to keep life from being overcome by death." [2]

Signs and Symptoms

In most cases signs and symptoms are indications that the body is engaged
in a struggle to defend itself from harmful influences or to adjust itself
to adverse conditions that it cannot overcome. The signs and symptoms
of an infectious disease, for example, are the direct results of the interaction between living, multiplying germs and the defense forces of the
infected body.

Symptoms are unpleasant sensations felt by the person affected. Signs
are evidences of physical change that can be seen, heard, felt, or measured by someone else. A person whose signs and symptoms can be
traced to a definite physical cause is said to have an organic illness. A
person whose signs and symptoms have no detectable physical cause is
said to have a functional illness. Roughly, the proportion of organic
illness to functional illness is about half and half. In both types of
illness the autonomic nervous system has a leading part in the production of signs and symptoms.

In organic illness or physical injury the autonomic nervous system acts
upon impulses coming in from parts of the body that are in distress.
In most cases the action taken is the instigation of remedial measures.

In functional illness, the impulses calling for action go out from the
mind, or psyche, without prompting from outside. The action taken may
exactly simulate that taken when some organic irritation is the exciting
factor. To put it very simply indeed, a child may vomit because he has
eaten green apples or because he doesn't want to go to school. In the
first case the autonomic nervous system, acting in response to impulses
from the stomach, initiates the appropriate action to help the stomach
get rid of an irritating substance. In the other, the autonomic nervous
system, acting in response to forceful impulses from the mind itself,
helps the child to escape from a stressful situation.

Various Types of Defensive Arrangements That Give Rise to Signs and Symptoms

Protective Reflexes. Some defensive arrangements are the familiar protective reflexes that enable us to meet the emergencies of everyday living.
Sneezing, coughing, watering of the eyes, gagging, and vomiting, for
example, take place immediately, without an act of the will, to force
out irritating substances that might cause damage if they were not
expelled.

[2] Quoted from a speech given by Dr. Richard C. Cabot before the Massachusetts
Medical Society and printed in *New England J. Med.* for November 18, 1937.

Quick Adjustments. Many different kinds of adjustments enable us both to cope with the vicissitudes of daily life and to mobilize defense forces of one kind or another. Among such adjustments is the stepping up of the tempo of breathing and the rate of the heartbeat when more oxygen is needed in vigorous exercise and fever. Another is the formation of a clot over a break in the skin to prevent the escape of an excessive amount of blood.

Related to protective adjustments of this kind are reactions to infection, allergic reactions, reactions to overproduction and underproduction of heat within the body, and reactions to injurious stimuli. As such reactions account for many of the signs and symptoms that teachers are asked to observe in children and report to the nurse or doctor, some explanation of them is given here.

Reactions to Infection

Reactions to infection take place only when bacteria or viruses in sufficient number have managed to get by the outer barriers of the skin or the mucous membrane which lines all body openings, tubes, and cavities, or have escaped destruction by the antiseptic or flushing action of various secretions, such as tears (in the eyes), mucus (in the nose), saliva (in the mouth), and gastric juice (in the stomach).

Once the bacteria or viruses have succeeded in getting through these outer lines of defense into the blood and lymph streams and eventually into the tissues, they are confronted by a very powerful inner line of defense. This is the army of phagocytes (literally "cell-eaters") to which the white cells of the blood (see Blood and Its Composition, in Chap. 4) and many other cells widely distributed throughout the body belong. The main object of the phagocytes is to keep an infection localized. If this can be done, the whole body may be saved from bacterial invasion. The struggle between germs and phagocytes is marked by two signs that are familiar to us all. The first is inflammation, or the so-called inflammatory reaction, and the second is pus formation.

Inflammation. Inflammation is the typical first response of any part of the body attacked by bacteria.[3] The capillaries (see Circulation Survey, in Chap. 4) in the region become irritated and, as a result, their walls become more permeable. Thus fluid and white blood cells can escape from the blood stream into the tissue spaces.

The classic signs of inflammation are the four "-ors": *calor* (heat), *turgor* (swelling), *rubor* (redness), and *dolor* (pain). The heat and redness are caused by the rush of blood to the invaded area; the swelling,

[3] Inflammation also may be caused by physical or chemical forces, such as a blow or excessive heat or a strong acid or alkali.

by the excess fluid in the tissue spaces; and the pain, by pressure on nerve endings in the neighborhood.

The lay observer can see the objective signs of inflammation only if they are in an exposed region of the body, such as the eyes and the skin of the face, arms, and hands. Complaints of pain, of course, can be heard by all. Severe or extensive inflammation is also accompanied by fever, in most cases, and by other signs and symptoms of acute illness.

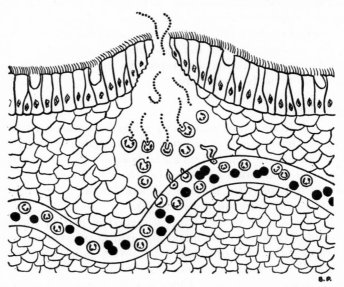

FIG. 18. The drama of phagocytosis. The invading army of bacteria (streptococci), entering through a beachhead in the skin, encounter the defending army of white blood cells passing through the capillary walls.

The noun ending "-itis" attached to the name of any part of the body denotes inflammation of that part. Appendicitis, otitis media, conjunctivitis, bronchitis, and neuritis, for example, mean respectively inflammation of the appendix, of the middle ear, of the conjunctiva of the eye, of the bronchial tubes, and of the nerves. Since inflammation is only a sign that *something is wrong*, the use of a term denoting inflammation of a part is not, strictly speaking, a diagnosis. Only the physician or surgeon is competent to tell what is causing the inflammation.

Pus Formation. Pus is simply a collection of the dead microbes and phagocytes that have lost their lives on the field of battle. It is white or yellowish white because that is the color of the phagocytes.

The phagocytes devour bacteria after the fashion of amebas by means of the extension and retraction of their cytoplasm (the part of a cell outside the nucleus). The meeting of a phagocyte with a germ is not a chance encounter, nor does the phagocyte wander about seeking what it may devour. Apparently the aimless movements of phagocytes are directed by chemical attraction toward bacteria or other substances foreign to the body. Probably this accounts for the migration of large numbers of wandering phagocytes to points of infection or injury.

Pus is a danger signal because it nearly always indicates that an infective process is going on. We see it in infected pimples and cuts, and in discharges from the nose, ears, and throat. Many of the conditions described later on in connection with what may be observed about different parts of the body are characterized or accompanied by pus formation.

Antigen-Antibody Reactions. When specific bacteria or viruses or the powerful poisonous substances (toxins) they manufacture come in con-

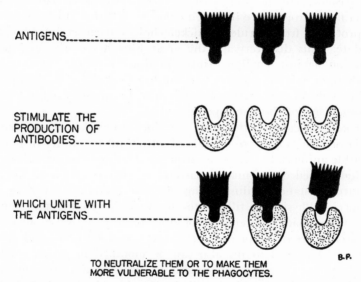

ANTIGENS

STIMULATE THE PRODUCTION OF ANTIBODIES

WHICH UNITE WITH THE ANTIGENS

TO NEUTRALIZE THEM OR TO MAKE THEM MORE VULNERABLE TO THE PHAGOCYTES.

B.P.

FIG. 19. A diagrammatic representation of the mechanism of antigen-antibody reactions.

tact with body tissues, another defense mechanism comes into action. This is antibody formation. Any substance taken into the body which gives rise to the development of antibodies is called an antigen. Each complete antigen stimulates the production of an antibody that reacts to it alone. Hence antibody formation is a specific line of defense.

The antigen may be either the germs themselves or a toxin produced by them. If the germs act as the antigen, the antibodies unite with the germs and help to dissolve them or make them more vulnerable to attack by the phagocytes. If a bacterial toxin is the antigen, the antibody substance produced is an antitoxin that neutralizes the toxin.

Immunity. The ability to form antibodies that help the regular defense forces of the body to fight invading bacteria or viruses explains why one attack of certain communicable diseases protects the body against sub sequent attacks. In many diseases—for example, typhoid fever, smallpox, scarlet fever, measles, chickenpox, mumps, and poliomyelitis—specific antibodies developed as the result of an attack stay in the blood plasma (see Blood and Its Composition, in Chap. 4) and in most instances give long-lasting protection from that disease.

Immunization

The foundations of the modern science of immunology were laid by Louis Pasteur. He discovered that doses of weakened chicken-cholera bacteria failed to produce illness in chickens, but that chickens so treated were protected from virulent chicken-cholera bacteria introduced at a later date. This discovery led the great French scientist to infer that vaccination against smallpox (introduced by Edward Jenner in 1796) works because microorganisms that are too weak to cause disease stimulate the body to set up specific resistance (immunity) against virulent microorganisms of the same species.

Vaccines. Pasteur gave the name "vaccines" to weakened, or attenuated, bacteria or viruses that are capable of setting up immunity in previously susceptible animals. Later, the meaning of the word vaccine was extended to include killed or attenuated bacteria or viruses that have the ability to induce resistance against living virulent bacteria or viruses of the same species. Physicians still use the term vaccine to designate immunizing substances made of attenuated or killed bacteria or viruses. Examples of such vaccines are those for whooping cough, typhoid fever, and smallpox.

Toxoids. Bacterial toxins also can be modified in such a way as to make them harmless and yet capable of arousing the body to produce antitoxin. A modified toxin is called a toxoid. The best known toxoids used in medical practice are diphtheria toxoid and tetanus toxoid.

Active Immunization. The injection of a vaccine or a toxoid stimulates the body to form antibodies which remain in the blood plasma for varying lengths of time. This process is called active immunization. Usually the protection given by active immunization does not last so long as the protection given by an actual attack of the disease. For that reason, reinforcing, or booster, doses of the immunizing substance are necessary from time to time.

Passive Immunization. Temporary immunity from certain communicable diseases can be given by injecting antibodies obtained from the

Table 4. IMMUNIZATION TIMETABLE *

Diseases	Ages and special times
Diphtheria Tetanus Whooping cough	At 3 months of age or earlier—the first of a series of injections with combined toxoid (diphtheria toxoid, tetanus toxoid, and whooping cough vaccine). At 4 and at 5 months of age injections are repeated to complete the series. One year after the first, or primary, immunization has been completed—a reinforcing, or booster, injection of combined toxoid. At about 3 or 4 years of age the booster injection should be repeated.
Diphtheria	On entering school and at 9 or 10 and at 12 to 14 years of age—a Schick test or a small booster dose of diphtheria toxoid. After exposure and during epidemics—a booster injection of diphtheria toxoid may be given to increase the protection of previously immunized children. An antibiotic can be used to give temporary protection to children not previously immunized. In some cases diphtheria antitoxin also may be given. In older children and adults the physician may make tests for susceptibility to diphtheria as well as sensitivity to the injection material before deciding what treatment to give.
Tetanus	On entering school (or at about 6 or 7 years of age) and about every 3 to 5 years throughout life—booster injections of tetanus toxoid. Following an injury from which there is danger of tetanus infection—a booster injection of tetanus toxoid may be given to those previously immunized. Tetanus antitoxin can be used to give temporary protection (lasting about 10 days) to those not previously immunized.
Whooping cough	On entering school (or at about 6 or 7 years of age)—a booster injection of whooping cough vaccine. After exposure and during epidemics—a booster injection of whooping cough vaccine may be given to previously immunized children. Several substances are available to give temporary protection to children not previously immunized.
Smallpox	At 6 months of age or earlier—the first vaccination with smallpox vaccine. On entering school—revaccination. Every 5 years and in epidemics or after exposure—revaccination. A successful vaccination usually protects from 5 to 7 years.
Typhoid fever	Periodically or when going on a vacation trip where there is danger of exposure to typhoid fever—an injection of typhoid vaccine (protection lasts for about 1 year).

* Adapted from recommendations of the American Academy of Pediatrics and the American Public Health Association.

If there is a poliomyelitis epidemic in the community, the physician may advise postponing immunizations to a later time.

blood plasma of an actively immunized animal or from the blood plasma of human beings who have had an attack of the disease. Examples of antibody substances which are used to give temporary, or passive, immunization from a communicable disease are diphtheria antitoxin, obtained from a horse actively immunized from diphtheria, and gamma globulin obtained from pooled adult blood plasma (see Passive Immunization under Poliomyelitis further on). Immunizing substances of this kind give only temporary protection because the body quickly eliminates as foreign substances any antibodies which it has had no part in producing.

In using the protection of vaccines, toxoids, antitoxins, and other immunizing substances, physicians make use of one of the most extraordinary and ingenious natural defenses of the body—the production of antibodies. The use of such substances has led to our present control of diphtheria, smallpox, tetanus, and other once dreaded diseases.

Allergic Reactions

It has been said that " 'allergy' is rapidly becoming a large wastepaper basket into which many diseases of unknown cause are being tossed—a catch-all phrase like 'eczema' or 'rheumatism.' " [4] "It must be an allergy" is a remark quite frequently made to explain the sudden appearance of some otherwise inexplicable skin rash or swelling. As a matter of fact, the skin and mucous membranes are the tissues most frequently involved in allergic reactions. The common manifestations of allergy are outlined in later chapters, but it may be helpful to get some idea of what is meant by allergy itself.

The word "allergy" comes from the Greek *allos* meaning "other," plus *ergon* meaning "work." It was proposed by C. von Pirquet in 1906 to designate the change that is produced in the body as a result of coming in contact with a specific substance that it has found to be harmful. As a result of that first encounter, the body's relation to the substance becomes permanently changed. We have this broad conception of allergy in mind when we say that we are "allergic" to something or someone who has once annoyed or irritated us. And just as we set up ways of protecting ourselves from sources of annoyance or irritation, so the body has defense mechanisms for dealing with various substances that have once irritated or harmed it.

We have learned that one of these defense mechanisms is antibody formation in response to stimulation by antigens. Antigens and antibodies also play a part in allergic reactions. In such reactions the antigen is called an allergen. Allergens stimulate the manufacture of specific allergic

[4] DOWNING, JOHN G., "Cutaneous Medicine," *New England J. Med.,* Vol. 217, No. 24 (Dec. 11), 1947.

antibodies, just as bacterial antigens stimulate the production of specific bacterial antibodies. Unlike disease-causing antigens, however, allergens are substances that are harmless for the majority of people. For the most part, they are protein substances which cause allergic reactions only in individuals who are sensitive to one or more particular proteins.

Shock Tissue. Allergic manifestations are usually localized. That is, a particular allergen sets off a reaction in one tissue or organ but not in others. The sensitive tissue is called the shock tissue. The shock tissue varies with each individual and may differ even in the same individual in response to different allergens. For example, in one person the shock tissue may be the mucous membrane of the nose (hay fever and allergic rhinitis); in another, the mucous membrane of the gastrointestinal tract (allergic stomach or intestinal upsets); in still another, the skin capillaries (hives and eczema).

Once allergic antibodies have been formed, the shock tissue becomes irritated every time they unite with the allergen that led to their creation. Instead of the silent combats that take place without our knowledge when the body is invaded by bacterial antigens against which it has developed antibodies, in allergic reactions the shock tissue—the field of battle, as it were—joins in the fray. And far from getting used to such encounters and ignoring them, the shock tissue, as if "remembering" former experiences, becomes much prompter and more violent in its expressions of resentment at each fresh meeting of the allergen and the allergic antibodies.

Types of Allergy. There are two principal types of allergy: (*a*) the familial type, and (*b*) the acquired or induced type.

In familial allergy, the shock tissue is inherited, that is, it "runs in the family." Examples of familial allergies are eczema, hay fever, bronchial asthma, allergic rhinitis, and some cases of urticaria (hives) and migraine (severe, one-sided headache). The allergens involved are usually those to which almost everyone is almost constantly exposed, such as common protein foods and plant pollens. Probably that is why allergy is most often defined as a condition of unusual or exaggerated sensitivity (hypersensitivity) to a substance harmless in similar amounts for most people.

Some forms of allergy are caused by substances with which most individuals seldom or never come in contact. Such uncommon substances include animal serums used in medical treatments, various drugs, products of bacterial growth, certain ingredients in cosmetics, and various materials used in industry. Allergy caused by some of these substances may be either familial or acquired, but usually it is acquired or induced. The defense mechanism involved is, in many instances, unknown; that is, no specific antibodies can be demonstrated. The reactions are so typical, however, that there is no doubt that they are allergies.

Sensitizing the Shock Tissue. Whether a predisposition to a certain form of allergy is inherited or hypersensitivity to a particular substance is acquired, *no form of allergy ever develops unless previous contact with the allergen has occurred.* That first contact results only in sensitizing the shock tissue. There is no sickness, no indication of what is going to happen the next time that particular allergen is encountered. A baby who has inherited a shock tissue sensitive to egg white, for example, will show no signs of distress when first given egg white. But after that first sensitizing dose, as it is called, all subsequent or exciting doses will result in allergic manifestations, the kind of manifestation depending upon the shock tissue inherited.

Finding the Offending Substance. Physicians now have various tests by which the offending substance, or substances, can be identified when some form of allergy is suspected.

Patch Tests. If the trouble seems to be a contact dermatitis, that is, a skin inflammation caused by sensitivity to one or more substances that come into contact with the skin (see Table 15, in Chap. 7), the tests given will be patch tests, because in contact dermatitis the epidermis or surface layer of the skin is the shock tissue. In the patch test the suspected material is placed on the skin, covered with a small square of cellophane, and held down with a strip of adhesive, Scotch tape, or collodion. The reaction is read by the physician in 2 to 4 days.

Scratch Tests. If suspicion lights on a food or foods or some other allergen that is brought to the shock tissue by the blood, the tests given will be scratch tests or intradermal tests. These tests are based on the fact that the allergic antibodies in the familial type of allergy (reagins) are skin-sensitizing antibodies. That is, when they are present in the blood they are also found attached to the skin. When the corresponding allergen is injected into the skin, fluid collects between the cells, giving rise to a wheal (see Observing Cutaneous Deviations from Normal, in Chap. 7). In giving a scratch test, a specially prepared extract of the suspected substance is put into scratches made through the upper layers of the epidermis without drawing blood. In the intradermal test, a small amount of a liquid extract of the suspected substance is injected between the layers of the skin. The appearance of a wheal and a surrounding area of redness indicates a positive reaction.

The Mechanism of Allergy. Although different individuals react to different substances in skin tests to find the allergens responsible for allergic conditions, the skin reactions themselves are alike. The lump or wheal raised on the skin after the injection of an extract of wheat in a person allergic to wheat, for example, will be no different from the wheal raised after the injection of a pollen extract in a person sensitive to that pollen. For this reason, scientists have long believed that there must be some substance released in the tissues which is common to all allergic reactions. It is now believed that histamine, which is a normal component of many tissues, is such a substance. According to the newest and most plausible theory of allergy, the irritation of the shock tissue, which takes place when the allergen unites with its sensitizing antibody,

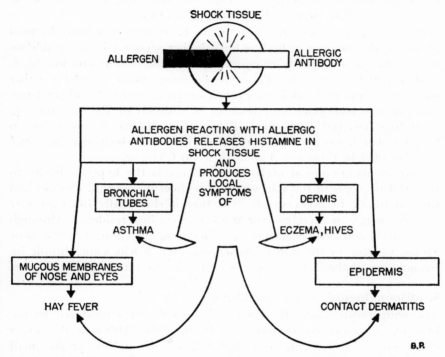

FIG. 20. A diagrammatic representation of the mechanism of allergic reactions.

results in the setting free of histamine (or a histaminelike substance). It is the liberated histamine that produces the manifestations of allergy.

The discovery of the role of histamine in allergic reactions naturally led to a search for substances that would neutralize or act as an antidote to histamine. A large number of drugs that act as histamine antagonists have been found. These drugs do not cure any form of allergy but merely relieve its distressing symptoms—the intense itching of hives, for example, or the sneezing in hay fever.

Permanent cure of any allergic condition depends upon finding the offending allergen and then avoiding it or being protected from it. The means used to confer protection is to give the offending substance in very small amounts, which are gradually increased until the patient is able to tolerate it nearly as well as persons who are not allergic to it.

Emotional Influences. The emotions exert a strong influence on allergic disorders. Under the stress of worry, fear, anger, resentment, or excitement, an allergic attack may flare up in a susceptible person or an existing condition may become worse. Or persons not known to be allergic may develop symptoms of a severe physical allergy when emotionally disturbed. Sometimes the physical condition does not improve until the person is helped to iron out his emotional conflicts.

Bacterial Allergy. Several skin tests that have an allergic basis are used as aids in diagnosis or in finding out whether a person is susceptible to, or immune from, a specific communicable disease. The reason for this is that certain bacteria bring about the development of an allergy either to the protein in their bodies or to their secretions or toxins. This allergic reaction may take place instead of, or in addition to, the formation of protective bacterial antibodies. Tubercle bacilli are the best known bacteria that bring about a changed response in a body that has once been invaded by them (see Tuberculosis, in Chap. 5).

Another manifestation of bacterial allergy is the hypersensitivity to bacterial residents of the skin which sometimes develops in chronic skin inflammations. In other words, skin that is chronically inflamed may become allergic to alien bacteria that it receives into residence. Although the bacteria may not produce open evidences of infection, they may slow up the progress of the skin to normality. That is why some chronic inflammations of the skin, eczema, for example, are often difficult to cure.

Reactions to Internal Temperature Changes

The temperature inside the body is due to the heat produced by the burning, or oxidation, of foodstuffs by the cells. Although there is a daily swing of a few tenths of a degree from a normal low in the small hours of the morning to a normal high in the afternoon, 98.6°F. is generally accepted as normal mouth temperature.

How Body Temperature Is Regulated. A "thermostat" in the lower brain regulates body temperature. When too much heat is being produced in the body, as in strenuous exercise, the blood flowing through this thermostat is hotter than usual. This is a signal for sending the autonomic impulses to the small blood vessels in the skin which cause them to open up. As a result, the warmer blood of deeper regions is diverted through them and in its passage loses its excess heat through radiation, conduction, and convection.[5]

However, the air surrounding the body may already be so warm that not much heat from the skin can flow into it (conduction). Or the air

---

[5] Radiation is the giving off of heat in all directions; conduction, the flow of heat from a warmer surface to a cooler one; convection, the transmission of heat by means of currents of air or water.

may be so still that the heated air cannot be shifted away from the skin by means of air currents (convection). In these cases autonomic nerve impulses cause the sweat glands to pour out perspiration on the surface of the skin. The evaporation of the sweat aids in the removal of heat from the body.

In cold weather the temperature of the surrounding air is considerably lower than that of the skin. Then autonomic nerve impulses from the surface of the body cause the thermostat to send orders to shut down (constrict) the skin blood vessels. As a result, little or no blood can flow through them. Instead of being "red" with heat, the skin may become "blue" with cold and covered with goose flesh (see Chilling, in Chap. 5). Also, the sweat glands are inhibited to prevent the flow of perspiration to the skin. Thus heat loss is reduced to a minimum. At the same time, body metabolism is speeded up so that additional heat is produced. If the amount of heat thus made available is still not enough, shivering sets in and perhaps the teeth chatter. Shivering is really forced exercise induced to increase muscular activity and thereby the production of additional heat.

Fever. Fever is a sign that the body is producing more heat than usual because of some unusual or abnormal stimulus. In the great majority of cases, the stimulus is the toxin produced by the germs or virus responsible for an infection. Yet a person coming down with an infectious fever usually feels chilly and looks pale. This is explained by the fact that the toxin of the infecting organism at first touches off the same mechanism which in health prevents a fall in temperature when the body is exposed to cold. That is, the surface blood vessels are constricted and the heat production of the body is increased by shivering.

We all know that the fire in a furnace may be blazing merrily, but the building will be cold if the radiators in the different rooms are turned off. Just so, a person may have a high fever and yet shiver and complain of feeling cold because his skin radiators (surface blood vessels) are closed to the warm blood which in health keeps him comfortably warm by stimulating the heat receptors in his skin. Later on, in fever, heat impulses from the deeper structures of the body result in the opening up of the surface blood vessels, the blood flow through the skin increases, the skin becomes flushed, and the sick person feels hot. This is a sign that the balance between heat production and heat loss has been restored but has been set at a higher level than in health. In other words, "the body's 'thermostat' has been turned up a point or so."

Although fever rightly alarms us and we are glad when it starts to go down during an acute illness, it is actually a protective device. There is good reason to believe that its occurrence is an important aid to the body in fighting disease. The very fact of its presence, however, is an indication that the body is engaging in such a fight and needs the aid that only the physician is prepared to give.

Indications of Fever. The quickest and surest way of telling whether a child has a fever is to take his temperature with a clinical thermometer. In schools that have nursing service, the nurse usually does this when the teacher suspects that a child is feverish. Indications of fever may be pallor, chilliness, and shivering; or flushed skin and languor, drowsiness, or restlessness. Such signs and symptoms may or may not be accompanied by others, such as nausea or vomiting; headache, earache, or aching in the limbs and back; running nose, sore throat, sneezing, red watery eyes, or tight dry cough.

Some slowly developing infections may be accompanied by low-grade fever and other mild warnings before more alarming signs and symptoms develop. Rheumatic fever (see Chap. 4) and tuberculosis (see Chap. 5) are illnesses of this type.

The Mechanism of Pain

The stimulation of specific receptors called "pain receptors" arouses the sensation of pain. These end organs of pain are free nerve endings located in the skin, in blood vessels, in muscles and joints, in nerve sheaths, and in many other body organs. They are the most widely distributed receptors in the body.

It is generally agreed that a physical stimulus adequate to excite pain is one that threatens damage to the tissues. In other words, "where there is pain, there is injury." For this reason pain has been classified as a protective sensation, as opposed to sensations like sight and hearing which convey information. Pain gives warning of the injurious nature of a stimulus. It provokes reflex actions that are defensive or protective or result in withdrawal of the part from the stimulus. The classic example is the rapid withdrawal of a hand from a hot stove. Pain, if it is severe enough, inhibits all other reflexes and is imperative in its demand for attention. It is not protective, in the usual sense, because some injury is already done before it is felt. Indeed it may actually be harmful, for example, in preventing full function of a part, as in a sprain, or in setting up a reflex that makes pain continue long after its original cause has disappeared. Under ordinary circumstances, however, pain is highly useful in calling attention to many conditions that might cause serious illness or death if allowed to progress.

Pain receptors do not respond to any one kind of stimulus as the other sensory receptors do. To produce the sensation of pain any type of stimulus—mechanical, chemical, or thermal (heat and cold)—will do, provided it is intense enough. No definite sensory centers for pain like those for sight and hearing have been located in the brain. Nevertheless, the brain interprets the sensation as coming from the part of the body which it associates with the particular nerve fibers affected. That is, it is trained to localize pain. This ability of the brain permits us to know that we have a pain in the stomach, or the foot, or the head, and so on. But what actually is causing the pain, unless it has a perfectly obvious cause, like a nail in the sole of a shoe, or a bee sting, or a burn is beyond us. Of course, this does not keep us from making guesses, which may or may not be correct.

Referred Pain. The ramifications of the nervous system are so complex that pain impulses originating at one point are often felt at some other point. Any area from which pain originates has been called a "trigger point." The trigger point becomes a "miniature sending station" when stimulated by an anatomical or physiological change. Just as a man in California may tune in through a local hookup on music broadcast over a radio network from New York, so one area of the body may tune in through a local hookup with pain impulses broadcast over a nerve network from some other area. In whatever area pain impulses are aroused, either directly by contact with the stimulus or indirectly by referral from some other area, pain is felt.

The phenomenon of referred pain, as it is called, explains why any one organ, like the heart, or one part of the body, like the head, may be innocent of causing many feelings of discomfort blamed on it. For example, the cavity of the chest and the upper part of the abdomen, which is separated from the chest by only a thin sheet of muscle, are packed tightly with organs. Any extra pressure, such as gas in the stomach or small intestine, may give rise to pain in the region of the heart with which the heart has nothing whatever to do.

Psychogenic Pain. Pain may be caused by psychic influences as well as by physical stimuli. If it seems strange to think that such an unpleasant symptom may in some cases have no physical basis, we have only to remember that emotion, when strong enough, can raise up many objective signs of distress—goose flesh, sweating, pallor, and so on. When pain occurs without any discoverable physical stimulus, then it is ascribed to the influence of the psyche on the autonomic nervous system.

"Nervous headache" and "nervous indigestion" are two well-known terms which show that practically everyone has at least a vague understanding of the influence of emotional tension or worry in the causation of pain. The school child who persistently has "nine o'clock headache" has a pain no less real than has the child suffering from eye fatigue. And in both cases there is need to find the reason why.

Dealing with Complaints of Pain. In dealing with children it may be difficult to decide what complaints of pain warrant immediate medical investigation. As with many different signs and symptoms, pain as an indication of illness seldom occurs alone. It is so often associated with other indications of trouble that it is a common component of a symptom complex, that is, a combination of two or more signs and symptoms. That, in itself, may serve as a guide in deciding whether a child who complains of headache or stomach-ache or leg ache, and so on, is in immediate need of medical attention. But whether other symptoms and signs are present or not, it is good sense to send children to the nurse or physician for any puzzling, unusual, severe, or persistent ache or pain. Only a physician has the training and experience required to detect signs hidden from a layman which help to supplement the evidence of pain and so point the way to a discovery of its cause.

Itching

The sensation of itching is caused by irritation of the touch-pressure or pain receptors in the skin. It has been called a low-grade form of pain. It draws attention to skin irritants and sets up the scratch reflex. The scratch reflex was designed to serve a useful purpose as a means of getting rid of causes of irritation. However, it has turned out to be something of a nuisance. Whenever intense itching impels us to scratch we remember that it is not good to scratch, since that act increases irritation of the skin and, in some conditions, leads to the spread of infectious material.

Itching is a common annoyance in a great many different varieties of skin irritations as well as in some systemic diseases. Children who complain frequently of itching, or show scratch marks, should be referred for medical attention (see also Chap. 7).

PSYCHOGENIC REACTIONS

Reference has already been made to some of the ways in which children may show by bodily signs and symptoms (pain, for example) that they are emotionally disturbed. Patterns of behavior also may be profoundly influenced by repressed feelings of hostility or frustration.

Psychosomatic Mechanisms

Sometimes somatic manifestations are mechanisms used by the child to get satisfaction for some need inadequately met during earlier periods of his life, or to express resentment against his parents, or to punish himself for harboring hostile feelings. Many of them are connected with the mouth or the function of eating, for example, lack of appetite (see Loss of Appetite, in Chap. 6), vomiting (see Vomiting, in Chap. 6), finger sucking, nail biting, overeating, and speech disorders (see Speech Difficulties, in Chap. 5). Others are related to bowel and bladder functions, for example, constipation (see Signs and Symptoms of Gastrointestinal Disorders, in Chap. 6) and urinary frequency (see The Kidneys, in Chap. 6).

Disturbances of vision and hearing in the great majority of cases are due to some physical defect or condition (Chap. 8). Sometimes, however, they may arise because of a desire to close the eyes or the ears to some distasteful idea or unpleasant feeling associated with seeing or hearing. A child may have a reading difficulty, for example, because he associates his personal difficulties with his teacher with the subject matter of what he is required to read or because he wants to annoy his parents who have shown that they are anxious for him to learn to read. A child may fail to come when he is called or to answer when spoken to simply because he hears only what he wants to hear. If he doesn't hear, then he cannot blame himself or be blamed for his willfulness.

Restlessness is natural in children. They cannot be expected to sit still for any length of time. But there are some children who are extremely fidgety and "nervous." Excess motor activity when not due to some physical cause (chorea, for example) is, in most cases, a sign of frustration. Perhaps a child has had a long illness during which he has had to repress his desire to be active. After his recovery, his parents or teacher may try to restrict his activities unnecessarily. As a result the child feels frustrated and angry. Verbal expressions of his pent-up active impulses are objected to, and so he lets off steam by unpurposeful continual muscular movements. Children may be placed in many other situations in which they cannot express their anger or jealousy or resentment against too-exacting requirements in acceptable ways and so fall back on "the fidgets" as the solution.

In some children fidgetiness may be localized—that is, they may spasmodically blink their eyes or make queer grimaces with their mouths or twitch their noses. Such localized motions are called habit tics, or spasms, when no physical cause can be found. Their origin usually lies in some forgotten emotional experience in which the child was actually punished or feared punishment for something about which he felt guilty. If no notice is taken of a habit tic, it may clear up spontaneously. Usually, however, the child is ridiculed or urged to control it, with the result that he may begin to feel pleasure in possessing a trick so attention-attracting. It may then be hard for him to give it up.

Behavior Reactions to Hostile Feelings

As we have seen, guilt arises when the child's Ego and conscience tell him that he ought to be ashamed of himself for harboring hostile feelings toward those upon whom he is dependent for security and love. When he does things like lying, stealing, or other acts, of which he knows his parents disapprove, he feels guilty because parental disapproval has tagged them in his mind as hostile acts. When he is punished for his wrongdoing, the punishment becomes associated with the sense of guilt he already harbors. Hence, there is built up in his mind the idea that punishment—suffering—atones for guilt.

The idea that there must be punishment for every misdeed is deeply ingrained in our society. Even when acts or thoughts that are considered wrong remain undiscovered, practically everyone is bothered with the vague guilty feeling that punishment is merited.

In childhood, naughtiness brings concrete retribution like a spanking or the withholding of some pleasure or privilege. The suffering caused by the punishment brings with it the satisfaction of making up for the naughtiness. With the pangs of his guilty conscience relieved, the child can once more feel at peace with his parents.

Gradually the child learns to accept the rules of conduct of his social code. If they are reasonable and fair and opportunities are given to express his hostilities and antagonisms constructively, he learns how to deal efficiently with his hostile impulses.

However, if he is made to feel insecure because of a rigid or erratic system of discipline or a lack of true love and understanding in the home, or because of differences between the standards of behavior required at home and in school, or for some other reason, he may develop the guilty feeling that almost everything he does will meet with disapproval if it is found out. Hostile impulses seem as wicked to him as bad behavior would be. That is, he feels as guilty for harboring such impulses as if he had actually done the things that would bring punishment. The anxiety generated in this conflict, of which the child is completely unaware, is almost sure to lead to neurotic trends unless its cause is discovered and removed. Perhaps the child may be oversubmissive or overdependent or unusually demonstrative to atone for the guilt he unconsciously feels. Or he may behave badly in order to get the punishment that will relieve his guilty feelings. Or he may frequently show symptoms of illness to get the sympathy and attention he craves or to make himself suffer for his hostile impulses.

Accident-proneness. It has been found that suppressed rebellion against authority may result in some adults in a curious condition called accident-proneness. Such adults tend to have accidents when strong hostility against authoritative restrictions or external coercion is aroused. The subconscious motivation seems to be a desire to atone for the guilt they feel for their rebellion against authority and at the same time to punish those responsible for their frustration. A too strict bringing up is regarded as the source of this authority-hostility conflict in accident-prone adults.

There has been a tendency to attribute to children who have frequent accidents the personality characteristics and motivations seen in adult accident-repeaters. In order to explore methods for identifying and determining the significance of personality characteristics, parent-child relationships, and other factors in relation to the incidence of child accidents, a pilot study was begun in the fall of 1951 by the staff of the Pediatric Psychiatric Clinic of the Babies Hospital, Columbia-Presbyterian Medical Center, New York. In this study two groups of nine children from the same neighborhood—one consisting of children who had had repeated accidents and the other of children who had had no accident history—were compared by means of thorough physical examinations, a battery of psychological tests, and investigations of personal relationships and physical environment.

In the preliminary report [6] of this pilot study it is emphasized that the groups studied were too small to reach any conclusions which can be applied to accident-repeater children in general. Some of the findings, however, provide interesting leads for further investigations with larger numbers of children.

The physical findings and the scores on intelligence tests did not yield significant differences between the two groups in the pilot study. But the psychological findings [7] strongly suggest that the children in the accident group on the whole are more active and independent in doing and in thinking than those in the nonaccident group. They tend to overextend themselves in their activities in trying to keep up with their ambitions or to seek acceptance by the group. As they lead bolder, more daring lives than the nonaccident children, they have more opportunity for getting into difficulties. Some of them have a poor reaction to stress. They become more impulsive and disorganized than children in the control group in stressful situations and do not recognize or heed danger signals.

The studies of child-parent relationships seemed to indicate that the parents of the nonaccident children were closer to their children and supervised them more closely than did the parents of the accident children. But the accident group as compared with the nonaccident group showed no greater striving for parental attention and no greater need to be revengeful toward their parents or to atone for some misdeed with self-punishment.

[6] "Pilot Study of Childhood Accidents: Preliminary Report," by William S. Langford, Rodman Gilder, Jr., Virginia N. Wilking, Minnie Marder Genn, and Helen H. Sherrill, in *Pediatrics*, Vol. 11, No. 4 (April), 1953.

[7] "Report on the Psychological Test Findings in a Pilot Study of Accident Repeaters and a Comparison Group," by George Genn, Minnie Marder Genn, and William S. Langford; New York, Columbia Presbyterian Medical Center, 1954.

Behavior Reactions to Overdirection

Children as they grow older need freedom, within reasonable limits, to make their own decisions, and time in which to do what they want to do. Unfortunately, many solicitous or domineering or insecure parents try to limit the activities and conversation of their children long after the need for freedom to express themselves in their own ways has been established. As a result, difficulties arise which cause the child to be labeled a "problem child." Perhaps the child's feelings of resentment and frustration are expressed in a form of obstreperousness technically called "negativism." The child has received so much direction that he refuses to obey *any* commands whether they are reasonable or not. Or he may go to the other extreme and become abjectly submissive.

When overly aggressive, defiant, chronically disobedient children who are suffering from an overdose of protection or overdirection understand that they are free to act and speak or be silent as they choose, without penalty of any kind, in conference with a psychiatrist or guidance counselor, they often relax and pour out their troubles. This emotional catharsis not only is usually a great relief to the child but also may indicate the correct solution to the child's problems. Quite frequently, it is one or both parents who need treatment more than the child does. Children labeled as problem children are often essentially good children who are reacting in completely normal ways to overdirection or nagging.

Behavior Reactions to Frustration

All behavior patterns develop in the interactions of the child with his environment. Among the most important environmental influences are the requirements of the society in which he lives. No one—child or adult —is able to accept completely and gracefully all the frustrations and inconveniences imposed by these requirements. If a requirement is too severe, or interferes with his personal desires for no good reason that he can see or understand, it is perfectly natural to seek ways of circumventing it. Practically everyone does it, no matter how well adjusted he may seem to himself or others.

Psychologists tell us that there are two main forms of evasion—attack and withdrawal. By attacking a natural force or social regulation that frustrates his desires or by finding ways to escape from it, the individual may avoid the necessity for accepting it or adjusting himself to it. The motive for both attacking and withdrawing behavior is the same, and streaks of both are often found in the same individual. Some persons, however, learn to depend more upon one than upon the others.

Evasion by Attack. It is easy to see that evasion by attack may be a potent constructive force. Civilization could not have progressed if everyone had meekly accepted, or adjusted to, things as they were at any particular stage. A large part of human history is a record of circumventing natural restrictions like those of distance on going places and of unaided vision on seeing things. Social and economic change has its roots in discontent with the existing order. And practically every individual has some unfavorable conditions in his own life which he must attack in order to get ahead. However, evasion by attack may be destructive if it keeps a child from eventually making inner peace with himself, his parents, his teachers, and the forces of law and order.

In dealing with aggressiveness in children it is important to make distinctions both in degree and kind. "Being bad"—disorderly, disobedient, boastful, noisy, curious about sex, and so on—is natural in the period of child development characterized by the impulse to experiment, to investigate, to show off, to determine just how far it is possible to go before parental ire or pedagogical wrath is aroused. On the other hand, consistently defiant attitudes or extreme expressions of hostility or antagonism usually indicate some form of emotional or social maladjustment. Very often the pattern of aggressive behavior which the child presents to the world is a cover-up for feelings of inadequacy or guilt that he is afraid or ashamed of expressing.

The Teacher and the Aggressive Child. A teacher does not have to be an old-fashioned martinet to be annoyed by bullying, defiance, quarrelsomeness, truancy, failure to submit to school routine, and other forms of attacking behavior that interfere with her teaching and wreck her efforts to create a friendly, helpful classroom atmosphere. If she allows her annoyance to show, however, and responds to attack by counterattack—ridicules or punishes or penalizes the child in retaliation for the flouting of her authority—she simply drives in deeper the feelings of fear, or resentment, or insecurity, or guilt, which are making the child misbehave.

On the other hand, if she recognizes that the attacking behavior is not the tug-of-war between child and teacher that it appears to be, but is rather the outward sign of some unsatisfied emotional need or inner conflict, she will appreciate the importance of detecting and seeking help in correcting its underlying causes.

Evasion by Withdrawal. Evasion by withdrawal also has its constructive and its destructive aspects. There is no one who has not found ways of escaping at times from the troubles and cares of everyday life. Daydreams, sleep, literature, music, and drama, for example, provide natural and necessary channels of escape. In many cases, however, the retreat from reality becomes so pronounced that it interferes with the ability to meet the requirements and responsibilities of social living. Some individuals upon reaching maturity are able to make constructive use of their habits of withdrawal and escape. The ability to shut out the outer "working-day world" and labor undisturbed in the inner workshop of the mind has resulted in many great scientific discoveries and inventions and many great accomplishments in the fields of literature, art, and religion. Sometimes, however, the habit of withdrawing from active participation in normal social living because of some deep-seated anxiety leads to mental illnesses of varying degrees of severity.

It is just as important in dealing with shy, overdependent children as in dealing with the aggressive ones to make distinctions between what is normal and what, under the circumstances, may be a serious deviation from normality. In the adolescent period, for example, it is natural for boys and girls to have occasional spells of dreaminess. This is the spring of life, in which there is poetical license for being fanciful and starry-eyed. In younger children, however, aggressiveness and other forms of attacking behavior are more natural than dreaminess and other forms of withdrawing behavior.

Many different experiences may lead a child to develop overdependence. Perhaps the parents are overprotective or afraid of what might happen to their child in rough play with other children. Or they may be too anxious to hear good reports of their child—"He is such a little gentleman." "She is such a nice girl." Such parental attitudes may lead a child to shun physical competition with schoolmates, to withdraw more and more into himself, and to find compensation in daydreams or in a reputation for studiousness and excellence in schoolwork. As a result, the child may be unfitted to meet the hard facts of existence and deprived of the independence he needs to stand on his own feet.

Possibly, a child's views of the world or his manners or his ambitions may be radically different from those of one or both parents. The parents may be trying to make him conform to their conception of the ideal child, or taunting him for disappointing them, or disagreeing as to the best way of coping with him. In that case the child may be finding necessary solace in a dream world created by and for him, where he can be and think and do as he likes.

Another possibility is that unfortunate experiences of one kind or another in early childhood have given a child the feeling that he is weak or bad or that nobody loves him. To earn the affection and security he craves, he may have developed the pattern of behavior which he knows, from his own observation and experience, adults approve of. Yet without knowing it he may deeply resent this dependence. In that case, the conflict between his love for those who protect and discipline him and his desire to be free may make him feel fearful and guilty. And so the child forms the habit of retreating into a dream world or a storybook world where he can attain his desire with no strings of doubt or fear attached.

The Teacher and the Overdependent Child. The child who habitually resorts to withdrawing behavior in response to feelings of guilt or frustration or inadequacy may have a much easier time of it in childhood than the child who uses methods of attack, but he is more likely to develop pronounced neurotic tendencies later on. The submissive, shy, timid, solitary, dreamy child usually behaves well and gives his parents and teachers little trouble. His apparently inadequate equipment for dealing with life often arouses the sympathy and protective feelings of those in authority. If his respectful behavior and his diligence in school tasks win him the favor of his teachers, the habit of withdrawal tends to become entrenched, just as meeting attack with counterattack tends to entrench the habit of defiance.

The "teacher's pet" type of child may have heartburnings over his unpopularity with his schoolmates and secretly admire the "big bad boys," but he can take comfort in the snug warm feeling of being cherished and protected by those who matter most in the ordering of his life. His worst troubles come when he is thrown on his own—when there is no loving parent or sympathetic teacher to turn to in stressful life situations. The attacking type of child at least learns to depend on himself and, if he is properly handled, will more often than not outgrow his so-called naughtiness.

ORGANIC DISORDERS OF THE NERVOUS SYSTEM

The things that go wrong in body government as a result of disease or injury depend upon which part of the central nervous system is affected. When we remember that intelligence, thought, behavior, and all forms of voluntary and involuntary action are controlled by the central nervous system, we can readily understand that any disturbance at the seat of government is bound to be reflected in one or more deviations from normal in muscular action or in mental life or behavior.

Deviations of this kind include lack of nerve-muscle coordination, shown by such signs as dizziness, tremors, and twitching and spasm of the face and eyelids; rigidity or partial or complete paralyses of muscles; confused states, convulsions, drowsiness, and unlocalized headaches; and even changes in personality and character. Any one or more of such signs and symptoms may occur in infections or injuries of the brain or spinal cord or both, or in some disturbance of brain-cell activity.

Teachers may seldom have occasion to be the first to observe and call attention to the onset or aftereffects of conditions causing actual destruction of nervous tissue or erratic functioning of various groups of brain cells. However, they may find it useful to have some knowledge of the

more common disorders of the central nervous system which may affect
the school-age child.

Poliomyelitis

Poliomyelitis (commonly called *polio*), or infantile paralysis, is an infection caused by a virus of at least three distinct types. The paralytic

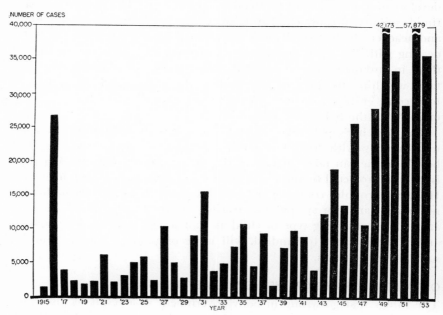

Fig. 21. Poliomyelitis cases reported in the United States, 1915 to 1953, inclusive.
(*Data from United States Public Health Service, furnished by the National
Foundation for Infantile Paralysis.*)

effects of polio occur in from 40 to 60 per cent of the cases in which the
virus invades the central nervous system (Fig. 22).

Inapparent and Abortive Polio. In the great majority of infections
with polio virus, the central nervous system is not involved. The
largest group of infections of this kind is made up of inapparent, or
"silent," infections. Available evidence indicates that these symptom-
less infections occur in most individuals at some time during life. Another group of polio infections in which the central nervous system is
apparently not involved occur mainly during epidemics and are classified
as abortive. Abortive infections are characterized by a brief febrile illness accompanied by lack of appetite, nausea and vomiting, headache,
sore throat, and vague abdominal pains. Recognition of abortive poliomyelitis is considered important, particularly during epidemic outbreaks,

because bed rest during the fever and for some days afterward may be a factor in preventing viral invasion of the central nervous system.

Paralytic and Nonparalytic Polio. In infections in which the central nervous system is involved, polio virus attacks motor neurons, that is

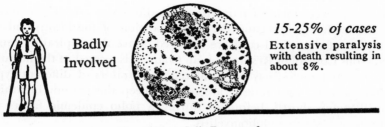

15-25% of cases
Extensive paralysis with death resulting in about 8%.

Many Nerve Cells Destroyed

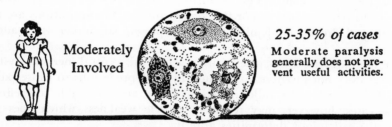

25-35% of cases
Moderate paralysis generally does not prevent useful activities.

Fewer Nerve Cells Destroyed

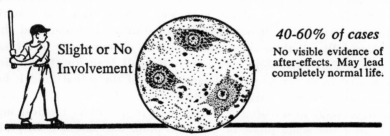

40-60% of cases
No visible evidence of after-effects. May lead completely normal life.

Very Few or No Nerve Cells Permanently Damaged

FIG. 22. The effects of infantile paralysis on the individual and his nerve cells. (*From "The Research Story of Infantile Paralysis," National Foundation for Infantile Paralysis.*)

nerve cells responsible for bringing about motion in the muscles to which their fibers run. In paralytic cases, destruction of motor neurons results in paralysis of the muscle fibers controlled by the destroyed neurons. Individual muscles or scattered groups of muscles are involved, according to the area in the central nervous system attacked by the virus. The destruction of motor cells in one area may result in the paralysis of fibers scattered throughout several muscles without affecting other fibers in the same muscles. In that case, there may be weakness rather than complete paralysis of certain muscles. Mild paralysis is often followed by complete recovery.

The most severe form of paralytic polio (bulbar poliomyelitis) results when the medulla oblongata (the lowest portion of the brain) and the neck region of the spinal cord are involved. Since the respiratory center (see Nervous Control of Respiration, in Chap. 5) is located in the medulla, the breathing muscles may be paralyzed. Respirators of different types, sometimes called "iron lungs," are used to keep the patient breathing. A tonsillectomy shortly before or during a polio epidemic favors the development of bulbar poliomyelitis.

There is some evidence to show that immunizations (see Immunization Timetable in this chapter) given during a polio epidemic may predispose a child to paralytic polio. For this reason routine immunizations are not encouraged during epidemics, as they represent an unnecessary added risk.

In nonparalytic cases, the virus reaches the central nervous system and yet does not progress far enough in its depredations to cause paralysis. In most of these mild infections there are no visible aftereffects. Some cases, however, may result in muscle weakness which goes unnoticed until minor deformities appear.

Early Signs and Symptoms. Among the signs and symptoms that may indicate the onset of polio are fever, drowsiness, headache, mild stiffness and pain in the muscles of the neck and back, nausea and vomiting, restlessness, irritability, diarrhea or constipation, sore throat, and chilliness. Naturally, all these signs and symptoms do not occur in the same individual. Early diagnosis is extremely difficult even for the physician experienced in detecting polio. Examination of the spinal fluid is helpful in reaching a diagnosis in doubtful cases.

Improvements in Treatment. Physical therapy [8] under medical supervision after the acute phase of paralytic polio has passed is helpful in aiding stricken muscles to regain their use through exercise, reeducation, and training. How successful this treatment will be depends upon the number of nerve cells destroyed or damaged by the virus (see Fig. 22). In recent years there has been great improvement in techniques and devices for restoring function to paralyzed muscles, for example, muscle transplants, early splinting of the extremities using rubber bands to assist

---

[8] Physical therapy, as defined by the American Physiotherapy Association, is "the treatment of disability, injury, and disease by nonmedical means, comprising the use of massage, exercise, and the physical, chemical, and other properties of heat, light, water, and electricity. . . ."

motion, and prosthetic devices to aid in moving paralyzed upper limbs. Great strides also have been taken in teaching patients whose breathing muscles have been affected to overcome dependence on iron lungs.

Mode of Infection. There is now almost complete agreement that entry of polio virus by way of the mouth is the usual mode of infection. As virus is present both in the throat and in the intestinal tract of persons harboring it, both the nose and throat discharges and the intestinal discharges of infected persons (frequently those not suffering from a recognized attack) are sources of infection. Infection takes place most frequently through intimate contact between a susceptible individual and a person harboring the virus. If one member of a family group has polio, the others often are infected. These "contacts" may have slight febrile illnesses or show no indication of illness whatever. Mildly ill or apparently healthy carriers of the virus are supposed to play a major part in the spread of the infection. That is why it is best during epidemics to keep children away from people with whom they have not been associated right along.

Apparently the period during which individuals stricken with polio can communicate the disease to others is covered by the latter part of the incubation period and the first week of the acute illness. The incubation period is from 7 to 21 days but commonly 12. The quarantine of family contacts of known cases during the period of communicability has not proved to be of practical benefit during epidemics because of the large number of unrecognized infections in the community.

How Polio Virus Reaches the Nervous System. Up to a few years ago polio virus had been isolated from the blood of only a few cases of paralytic polio. As it was known to be present in the alimentary canal even before the onset of symptoms, the most generally accepted idea was that it probably traveled directly from the alimentary canal along nerve fibers to the central nervous system.

Then in 1952, two investigators, Dr. Dorothy M. Horstmann and Dr. David Bodian, independently isolated virus from the blood of experimental animals (cynomolgus monkeys and chimpanzees) during the incubation period of polio. Further research revealed the presence of virus in the blood early in the course of human infections. It is assumed that previous failures to find virus in the blood of all but a very few recognized cases of polio were probably due to the fact that antibodies formed to combat the virus had cleared it out of the blood stream before symptoms of the disease developed. The weight of present evidence supports the idea that the virus invades the central nervous system primarily by way of the blood stream before enough antibodies have been formed to destroy it, rather than primarily along nerve pathways.

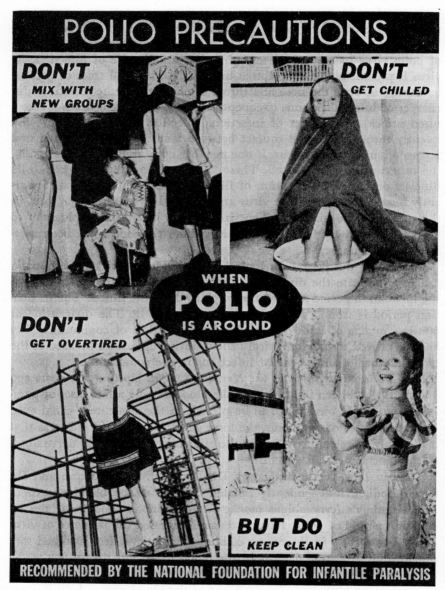

Fig. 23. A poster issued by the National Foundation for Infantile Paralysis to educate the public regarding polio precautions.

General Measures of Control. Probably no sanitary measures now practiced will prevent polio infection. The average age at which infection occurs seems to be higher in this country than in other areas where sanitary conditions are more primitive and children are naturally immunized early in life as a result of inapparent infections. Experience has proved, however, that certain precautions can be taken to lower the chances of having the disease in a severe form or of acquiring the infection at times when it is prevalent in the community. Such measures include (a) reducing contacts with individuals outside one's own immediate circle of family, schoolmates, and friends; (b) being extra careful to avoid *fatigue and chilling of the body;* (c) washing the hands carefully with soap and water before eating, after toilet, and when the hands are soiled with nasal or mouth discharges; (d) avoiding the use of common drinking cups and towels; (e) postponing, if possible, the removal of tonsils, the extraction of teeth, and other operations in or about the nose, throat, or mouth immediately before and during epidemic seasons; and (f) postponing routine protective immunizations except for polio vaccination.

Specific Control by Immunization. Protection from polio is conferred on the vast fortunate majority by infections so mild that they pass unnoticed. But a small unfortunate minority must pay the price of paralysis for immunity gained naturally. The target toward which research workers aimed for well over 40 years was the development of a practical and safe vaccine capable of producing artificially, and without incurring the risk of paralysis, the immunity which nature produces in the course of polio infection.

Typing Studies. One of the chief obstacles to the development of a vaccine was the complexity of polio virus. By 1949 three distinct immunological types of this virus had been identified. But did other types exist? The importance of this question lies in the fact that each immunological type stimulates the production of antibodies which work against it alone. An effective vaccine, therefore, must be capable of inducing antibody formation against all types of polio virus.

This problem was solved by 1951 through the cooperative efforts of investigators at four universities working under the sponsorship of the Committee on Typing of the National Foundation for Infantile Paralysis. The findings of these investigators indicated that all the many different strains of polio virus examined fall into the three immunological types already identified. That put the attempts to develop a vaccine on firm ground.

Studies on the Multiplication and Spread of Polio Virus within the Body. Up to a few years ago polio virus could be propagated only on nervous tissue in experimental animals. That seemed to indicate that polio virus had an affinity for nervous tissue alone. Then, late in 1949, came the dramatic announcement that Dr. John F. Enders (associate professor of bacteriology and immunology, Harvard Medical School), Dr. Thomas H. Weller, and Dr. Frederick C. Robbins had succeeded in growing polio virus in test tubes on nonnervous tissue. For this achievement Dr. Enders and his associates received the 1954 Nobel prize in medicine and physiology.

The discovery that polio virus could be grown in the laboratory on nonnervous tissue made it possible to grow large quantities of virus of all three types for immunological studies. It also supported the idea that polio virus may multiply in nonnervous tissue within the body and thereafter be carried in the blood to the central nervous system. If this proved to be the case, the paralytic effects of polio infection might be avoided by creating an antibody barrier in the blood stream to intercept the virus before it could invade the central nervous system.

There were two possible ways of doing this. The first approach was passive immunization, that is, the injection of polio antibodies which would destroy the virus before the body's own antibody-producing machinery was set in motion. This would give temporary protection only, because, as we have seen, the body eliminates antibodies which it has had no part in producing. The second approach was active immunization by the injection of a vaccine that would stimulate in the immunized person the formation of antibodies against all three types of polio virus. Both of these approaches were explored by investigators whose work was financed to a large extent by the National Foundation for Infantile Paralysis out of March of Dimes funds.

Passive Immunization. The first approach was tried on a large scale by Dr. William McD. Hammond (head of the Department of Epidemiology and Microbiology, Graduate School of Public Health, University of Pittsburgh) and his collaborators. In 1951–1952 these investigators made controlled field studies on the prevention of paralytic polio by gamma globulin.

Gamma globulin is the fraction of blood plasma which carries the antibodies developed by the body to fight disease-causing bacteria and viruses. When blood contributed by a thousand or more different adults is pooled, the gamma globulin obtained from the pool is sure to contain antibodies developed to combat the most common infectious diseases. Its protective effect in measles and infectious hepatitis has been known for many years. Whether it contains sufficient antibodies to confer protection against paralytic polio under conditions of natural exposure was the question Dr. Hammond and his collaborators set themselves to answer in their field trials of gamma globulin.

More than 25,000 children took part in these carefully controlled trials during the epidemic seasons of 1951–1952. Evaluation of the data collected indicates that gamma globulin is useful as a temporary protective measure against paralytic polio if the onset of infection occurs from one week through the fifth week after the injection of gamma globulin. In Dr. Hammond's words, however, gamma globulin, at best, "has an extremely limited application in the field of preventive medicine and will not produce dramatic results in general use."

Active Immunization. Dramatic results *are* expected of the vaccine for active immunization which was developed by Dr. Jonas E. Salk and his collaborators in the Virus Research Laboratory, Department of Bacteriology, University of Pittsburgh School of Medicine. This vaccine contains polio virus of all three types grown on minced monkey kidney and killed with a solution of formaldehyde, commonly referred to as Formalin. Every particle of the disease-producing property of the virus in the vaccine is destroyed without destroying completely its capacity to induce the formation of antibodies.

After exhaustive tests made in experimental animals to prove that the vaccine was safe and effective, it was cautiously tried on human volunteers. The success of these preliminary trials led to the famous large-scale field trial of the Salk vaccine in 1954. The study population was made up of more than 1,800,000 first, second, and third grade children in 217 study areas in 44 states. Nearly 624,000 children actively participated at the request of their parents by receiving the vaccine or a harmless inert substance called a placebo.

As all the world knows, the report on the safety and effectiveness of the vaccine was given on April 12, 1955, by Dr. Thomas Francis, Jr., Director of the Poliomyelitis Vaccine Evaluation Center at the University of Michigan. The report indicates that the vaccine used in the field trial was safe and 80 to 90 per cent effective in preventing paralytic polio.

Since the field trials of 1954 the vaccine has been improved and the schedule of inoculation has been changed, on Dr. Salk's recommendation, from 3 doses of vaccine within a period of 5 weeks to 2 doses for the primary immunization with a booster dose 7 months later. Dr. Salk's studies have shown that the booster dose induces a sharp rise in polio antibodies.

Authorities on polio believe that active immunization will be as effective in controlling paralytic polio as is this protective measure in controlling smallpox and diphtheria. A number of years may go by, however, before the grim story of paralytic polio arrives at this happy ending. There is much still to be done both in improving the vaccine and in working out ways of using it to the best advantage. Evidence shows, too, that no matter how successful a vaccine may be there are always individuals who do not avail themselves of its protection. Furthermore, the

National Foundation for Infantile Paralysis points out that there were tens of thousands of patients who were suffering from the aftereffects of paralytic polio at the beginning of what may be called the "vaccination era," and there will be many more victims before vaccination begins to have a marked effect in reducing the number of cases.

What the Teacher Can Do about Polio. With polio added to the ranks of the diseases from which children can be protected by vaccination, teachers can take an active part in the fight against this disease. In class discussions youngsters may have questions about vaccination which teachers can use to satisfy curiosity and allay fears. Some parents may need reassurance about the safety of the vaccine before they are willing to request vaccination for their children. Older boys and girls, especially high school students, will profit from the study of polio in their health and science classes. They will be interested in the story of the development of the Salk vaccine and in keeping abreast of the news in many areas of polio research, for example, the hunt for a drug that may be effective in the treatment or prevention of polio.

As the most optimistic estimates of the prospects for victory over polio by vaccination indicate that cases will undoubtedly occur for some time to come, teachers should continue to emphasize the precautions against infection that everyone should take during the season of highest incidence (summer and early fall). It is also important to keep on the lookout before school closes in the summer and after it opens in the fall for symptoms which may, or may not, indicate polio. Any child who seems ill in school should be taken home, and the parents should be impressed, without being unduly alarmed, with the importance of putting the child to bed, isolating him from others, and getting medical advice promptly.

Another important function of the teacher is the supervision of children who have returned to school after an attack. Often she can be very helpful in encouraging parents and children to return to the hospital or clinic for scheduled check-ups. Many children returning to school will have recovered completely. However, children who have had polio should be guarded for some time against fatigue and overexertion, as muscle weakness is a common aftereffect. It is recommended that they be watched carefully for at least two years for postural irregularities and speech defects.

Some children who return to school after a bout with paralytic polio may be severely or moderately crippled. It is generally agreed that "learning to help himself is the crippled child's salvation." The helpful sympathetic teacher will be able to find many ways of giving unobtrusive assistance to the disabled child and of guiding other children in giving him help and encouragement.

Other Infections of the Central Nervous System

Two other infections of the central nervous system—meningitis and encephalitis—may attack children. However, their incidence is rare. Brief accounts of them are given here for teachers who may be concerned about them because of the occurrence of cases in the school or community.

Meningitis. The outer covering of the brain and spinal cord consists of three layers of membrane called collectively the meninges. Meningitis is a general term for inflammation of these membranes. It occurs when bacteria of any one of several different families pass from the blood stream into the fluid that bathes the brain and spinal cord. By laboratory examination of a sample of cerebrospinal fluid, physicians can determine which form of meningitis—meningococcal, pneumococcal, or influenzal, for example—is causing the infection in suspected cases. Once the diagnosis is made, most patients can be cured with appropriate chemotherapeutic or antibiotic drugs if treatment is started early in the course of the disease. That is why prompt recognition of infections of the meninges is extremely important.

Meningococcal meningitis, which is caused by members of a genus of bacteria known as the meningococci, characteristically occurs in epidemics every 5 or 10 years. Since it attacks the meninges of both the brain and spinal cord, it is sometimes called epidemic cerebrospinal meningitis. The sulfa drugs and the antibiotics are now being used successfully to control outbreaks of this disease. In the epidemic waves, which last two or three years, the most severe infections occur among adults. In interepidemic periods sporadic attacks occur chiefly in children.

Susceptibility to clinical, or severe, meningococcal meningitis is very slight. That is, the attack rate among those who are exposed is low. However, there are many subclinical, or mild, cases. Slight attacks may be marked only by a mild sore throat with or without headache, malaise, low-grade fever, and pains in joints and muscles. Many people recover from a mild attack without knowing that they have had the infection.

Infection with meningococci takes place by way of the nasopharynx (see The Respiratory Passages, in Chap. 5). The microorganisms live in the throats of apparently healthy individuals and are present for weeks and sometimes even months after recovery from mild or severe infections. These carriers, as they are called, increase in the winter months, with increase in the attack rate, and are largely responsible for the spread of the disease during epidemic periods.

It is impossible to isolate carriers during epidemics because of their great number. Giving sulfadiazine in small doses for two or three days to all persons closely associated with one another (as in schools or camps) who have been exposed to a known case of epidemic cerebrospinal meningitis eliminates the meningococci from the noses and throats of carriers and usually stops the epidemic.[9]

Epidemic Encephalitis. There are several different types of the infection of the brain called encephalitis. The infecting agent in each form is a filtrable virus. Several species of mosquitoes are responsible for the spread of the virus of three of the types occurring in the United States (the St. Louis type and the Western and Eastern equine types). All types are serious diseases, but fortunately few people are attacked by them except in small localized outbreaks.

The form known as epidemic encephalitis has been recognized as a distinct disease only since 1917. Its popular name is "sleeping sickness" (not the same disease as African sleeping sickness, caused by trypanosomes which are spread by the bite of the tsetse fly). Modern studies of this serious disease began after the influenza epidemic of 1917–1918, when many cases of sleeping sickness were observed in different places. The specific virus causing it has not yet been identified.

Epidemic encephalitis begins usually with only a slight fever. Later, signs of brain or nerve involvement occur, such as sleepiness or insomnia, double vision, restlessness, twitching, and muscle spasm. Later still there may be psychic or behavior disturbances, amounting in some cases to alterations in personality. Often the disease takes a chronic course, waxing and waning over several years.

Epilepsy

Epilepsy comes from a Greek word meaning "seizure." It is not a rare disease. More than 700,000 persons in the United States are affected by it. This makes it nearly twice as common as tuberculosis.

The exact cause of the disarrangement of brain-cell activity which results in various forms of epilepsy is not known. However, as in some other diseases, the person who develops epilepsy has a tendency or predisposition to epileptic seizures which may or may not be inherited. Studies show that there is about one chance in 200 that the average person will have an epileptic child, while the chance is about one in 40 that an epileptic will have such a child.

A predisposition to epilepsy may be discovered by recording the electric currents that the brain, like the heart, gives off. These currents are recorded by an instrument called an electroencephalograph ("electro-," meaning "electric"; "encephalo-," meaning "brain"; and "-graph," meaning "writing"). The written record of the electric currents given off by

---

[9] Information concerning clinical meningococcus meningitis is given in Table 7.1. For general measures that should be taken in schools during epidemics of communicable disease spread by discharges from the respiratory tract, see The School and Respiratory-disease Control, in Chap. 5.

the brain is called an electroencephalogram (EEG for short). An EEG consists of a series of little waves, called brain waves. The waves form typical patterns known as brain-wave patterns.

In most persons predisposed to epilepsy the brain-wave patterns are different from those of most healthy persons. In analyzing the brain-wave patterns of thousands of individuals, it has been found that about one person in 10 has some irregularity that may indicate a predisposition to epileptic seizures or an allied disorder, such as migraine headache. However, only one person in every 200 actually does have seizures, so there must be something besides predisposition that brings them on. Among these influences are (a) damage to the brain caused by injury before or during birth, or by an infection, or by a severe head injury or brain tumor; (b) a disease in some other part of the body, kidney disease, for example, which may have a bad effect on the brain; and (c) emotional upsets or a sudden severe emotional shock. Persons who have epileptic seizures usually show the first symptoms before twenty years of age.

Whatever may be the disturbance in brain activity which causes epilepsy, each seizure is nearly always accompanied by a loss of consciousness. In the form of epilepsy known as petit mal, or "little illness," interruptions in consciousness lasting for a fraction of a second to several minutes often take place many times a day or when some critical situation arises. A child suffering from petit mal may "blank out" when a direction is being given by his parents or teacher, or during the playing of games with his playmates, or in the course of a conversation. As the child may only blink a few times, look blank, and then keep on with what he is doing at the time, these seizures are often overlooked. Not knowing what was said or done during his blank periods, the child may gain the reputation among adults of being inattentive or disobedient, and among his playmates of being stupid.

Teachers who have been especially tried by a child's inattentiveness or disobedience have, in some cases, been responsible for the discovery of hitherto unsuspected petit mal by reporting their observations to the school nurse or physician or to the child's parents. The confusion caused in the child's mind by frequent petit mal seizures usually clears up quickly when proper treatment is given.

The epileptiform seizure, characterized by convulsions as well as by loss of consciousness, is most commonly associated in the popular mind with epilepsy. This form of the disease is known as grand mal, or "great illness." Grand mal is a very ancient affliction. Many famous people including Julius Caesar, Napoleon Bonaparte, Algernon Charles Swinburne, the poet, and Niccolo Paganini, the violinist, suffered from it. In the popular mind it is often associated with mental defectiveness. Actually, the great majority of persons subject to epileptic seizures are in every other way perfectly normal human beings. Indeed, many of them are exceptionally talented or above average in intelligence.

An epileptic fit, as a grand mal seizure is often called, is frequently preceded by a warning called an "aura." The aura may consist of a feeling of unusual depression or exhilaration, smelling strange odors or seeing strange lights, pain in the limbs or stomach, trembling, or the impression that air is blowing on some part of the body and passing upward toward the head. A child subject to epileptic seizures should be watched for such premonitory symptoms. He may learn to report them immediately when he understands what they signify. When the aura occurs, the child should sit down or lie down in a safe place.

At the beginning of the actual attack, the epileptic becomes very pale, often cries or screams, and then loses consciousness. His body becomes stiff, and his arms, legs, and head contract spasmodically in a series of jerks, or convulsions. He ceases to breathe momentarily, and his face becomes blue. Often he froths at the mouth.

The convulsive stage usually lasts for only a few minutes and is followed by a return of breathing and of normal color. During the second stage, the person rolls his eyes and clamps his teeth shut. He may bite his tongue or cheeks, with the result that the froth on his lips becomes bloodstained. Urination and a bowel movement may occur involuntarily. This stage lasts for several minutes, after which the person slowly regains consciousness or falls into a deep sleep resembling unconsciousness.

An epileptic seizure seems very alarming to those who witness it. However, the person feels no pain and rarely hurts himself seriously unless he was in a precarious position at the beginning of the seizure. No attempt should be made to restrain the convulsive movements of a child in an epileptic fit. The most that should be done is to keep him from injuring himself. Placing a lead pencil wrapped in cloth between his teeth will keep him from biting or chewing his tongue. Putting something soft under him like a folded coat or a blanket will help to prevent injury which may be sustained in thrashing about during the convulsive stage.

In the third stage, or "afterstage," the child should be kept quiet until he has fully regained consciousness or has awakened from sleep. Usually he returns to normal within half an hour.

Medicines called anticonvulsants in combination with a special diet are proving to be very successful in controlling epileptic seizures of the grand mal type. Half the cases can be made completely free of seizures, and another 25 per cent can be benefited greatly. The treatment must, of course, be carried out under a physician's direction. It is important to remember that the epileptic child, like the diabetic child or the cardiac child, is in most cases no different from other children, except for his malady, and should be treated accordingly.

The Epileptic Child in School. Much consideration has been given to the question as to whether epileptic children should be allowed to attend regular school. It has been feared that an epileptic child may present a hazard either because the circumstances under which a fit occurs may result in injury to himself, or because other children may be thrown into a panic if a seizure takes place at the time of some school emergency such as a fire drill. However, the mathematical probability that a seizure might be a hazard either to the epileptic child or to his schoolmates is exceedingly slight. School authorities in most places agree that the occurrence of grand mal seizures without other physical or mental handicap does not justify the exclusion of the child from regular class attendance. The child should be taught at home or in special classes only if seizures are so frequent or so severe that their occurrence in the classroom seriously interrupts the work of the other children or are of such character that attendance in regular class is harmful for the child.

Like other handicapped children, the epileptic child should lead as normal a life as possible. Segregation in most cases is not necessary and is apt to be harmful. The good sense of the informed teacher will prevent fear in children who witness "fits" in a schoolmate suffering from epilepsy. Indeed, the teacher may profitably discuss the whole problem of epilepsy with her students and help them to understand that an epileptic needs sympathy and kindness. She may broaden the discussion to help her children develop proper attitudes toward all sick or handicapped individuals.

Cerebral Palsy

Cerebral palsy is a sign that certain areas of the brain which govern muscular action have been put out of commission. In the great majority of cases some developmental defect in the brain before birth, or an intracranial hemorrhage occurring at the time of birth (birth injury) is responsible for this condition. When the areas of the brain involved in the ability to acquire and use facts are not affected, the child's intelligence is not impaired.

One common type of cerebral palsy is characterized by tense, contracted muscles (spasticity). The muscles tend to react far more strongly to stimuli than is necessary to bring about desired movements of the limbs. Spasticity is caused by damage to the motor area of the cortex. Another common type of cerebral palsy is athetosis. This type is characterized by involuntary or unorganized muscular movements. Usually it is caused by damage to the brain stem (a cerebral area below the cortex).

There are several other less common varieties of cerebral palsy. In one variety the child may have trouble maintaining his equilibrium (ataxia). He walks uncertainly or staggers and has great trouble in climbing stairs. In another variety the child may have constant regular trembling of the extremities, and in still another, a special kind of muscle rigidity "in which the muscles feel like soft lead." In the last two varieties (tremor and rigidity) large areas of the brain may be involved, with the result that intelligence is affected. However, few children with cerebral palsy have these involvements.

There are more victims of cerebral palsy than is generally realized. The estimated number in the United States under the age of twenty-one is from 200,000 to 300,000.[10] According to Dr. Winthrop M. Phelps, an authority on cerebral palsy, six out of every seven children born with cerebral palsy survive. Of these, two are feeble-minded and require institutional care. Of the remaining four who are presumed to be mentally normal, one is so severely crippled that he is classified as "homebound," and one is handicapped to such a slight degree that he can compete on an equal basis with completely normal children. The remaining two are the ones "who present the greatest problems in physical and academic education."

With proper treatment and training, moderately disabled but mentally normal cerebral-palsy sufferers can be greatly improved. In many cases they can attend regular school after everything possible has been done for them in therapeutic nursing schools or in other treatment-training centers. The teacher who has one of these children in her class can do a great deal to make his school life successful and happy. She can help him to win acceptance in his relationships with the other children and can do everything possible to raise his general morale and strengthen his will to achieve, without seeming to give him undue attention.

MENTAL ILLNESS OF PSYCHOGENIC ORIGIN

Many of the bizarre, peculiar, often inexplicable, or annoying symptoms of the mentally ill are linked with lesions, injuries, or degenerative change in the brain or spinal cord. Also several infectious diseases—late syphilis, for example—are accompanied by or result in mental symptoms. There remains the stubborn fact, however, that it is at present impossible to find physical bases for more than half the illnesses characterized by mental disturbances.

Individuals who have failed to make a satisfactory adjustment between the needs and demands of their personalities and the requirements of

[10] "Impairments Among Young People," *Statistical Bulletin*, Metropolitan Life Insurance Company, Vol. 36, No. 8 (August), 1955. This range is based upon estimates made by Dr. Winthrop M. Phelps and confirmed by recent surveys of the incidence of cerebral palsy in a number of states and cities.

life as they must live it may develop the characteristic signs and symptoms of various forms of mental illness when exposed to environmental stress. The two best known forms are the functional psychoses and the neuroses. The functional psychoses, in general, involve marked disruption of personality. In some forms, particularly schizophrenia, there is abandonment of reality. Schizophrenics seem to live outside the world as we see it, in an inner world of their own. Neurotics are much closer to normal in their continuing awareness of reality, no matter how poor an adjustment they make to it. In spite of their basic anxiety, they are able to accept and react to explanations of the underlying causes of their illness.

Neurotic Patterns

A neurotic pattern often begins to develop in childhood when the Ego is weak and its ideals, largely a product of environmental prohibitions and demands, are threatened by strong instinctual drives or repressed impulses. A neurosis may be defined as a device used to bring about a compromise between irreconcilable drives which call for opposing courses of action. Since the mechanisms unconsciously used not only bring about the compromise but also disguise its purpose, the neurotic person does not know what is making him ill.

The mechanisms employed in a full-blown neurosis depend upon the pattern of behavior the individual has developed for dealing with anxiety. All of us as we go through life experience this emotion when we meet circumstances that make us feel afraid or guilty or frustrated or angry.

Even those of us who react adequately to most situations are familiar with many of the physical symptoms of anxiety which, as we have learned, are the result of the influence of emotions on the autonomic nervous system. We think of these symptoms as perfectly natural when the emotional stimulus is known. If it scares us to make a speech, for example, it does not surprise us to have the heart beat more rapidly and the mouth feel dry when we are called on for "a few words." The same mechanism operates when a bad headache or a spell of indigestion keeps a person from doing something he dreads doing, or expresses the outrage unconsciously felt when powerful impulses must be suppressed.

In childhood, physical responses to anxiety, such as an attack of nausea or vomiting or a headache or stomach-ache, or a reversion to some form of behavior that he has given up—for example, finger sucking or bed wetting or temper tantrums—are relatively common. These are neurotic manifestations which usually clear up as the child's Ego becomes stronger and he gains experience in handling the frustrations and instinctual drives which have produced his anxiety. However, if he fails to receive any real understanding or constructive help, he may use childish devices all his life long to escape from painful life situations.

In growing up there is always a tendency to regress to earlier patterns of behavior when faced with a situation that is difficult or painful. Even adults sometimes wish they could weep on mother's shoulder or throw a temper tantrum or have a convenient pain. When strong impulses to act childishly arise, some people have symptoms which indicate that the body is acting up as it did in childhood in periods of great emotional stress. This is called "conversion hysteria." The symptoms range all the way from complete or partial paralysis or blindness or deafness or amnesia to skin numbness, gastrointestinal upsets, fainting spells, or vague feelings of physical discomfort.

In another form of hysteria, called anxiety hysteria, the individual is troubled by fears that arise when instinctual forces pressing forward from the unconscious seem to threaten the Ego with danger from within. Never having learned as a child that aggressive and sexual impulses are normal and natural and can be successfully managed and directed, the individual threatened by such impulses falls into the same sort of helplessness that he felt as a child when confronted by the unknown. The symptoms are identical with those which arise when anyone is threatened by situations in the outside world that call for the mobilization of the body's forces for flight or fight (see The Sympatheticoadrenal Team, in this chapter). The precipitating cause, however, lies within the person rather than without.

In another type of full-blown neurosis the person has a compulsion to perform certain ritualistic acts, for example, frequently repeated washing of the hands. He is afraid that erotic and aggressive instinctual impulses within himself will make him commit a sin or harm himself or others unless he erects some kind of ritualistic defense against them.

In mild forms of neurosis most sufferers under ordinary circumstances can attend to their personal affairs and carry on their work. Often they do not even know that they are neurotic. Although they feel more or less constantly tired, unhappy, worried, nervous, confused, at odds with life, or ill without apparent physical cause, they do not realize that some underlying emotional conflict may be to blame. Often they go from doctor to doctor or from quack to quack, trying every brand of patent medicine guaranteed to alleviate their symptoms, change jobs frequently, or seek peace of mind in changes of scene.

If one of these unhappy people is fortunate enough to consult a doctor who understands him and can help him to understand himself, he is usually greatly relieved to find that his emotional or nervous disorders have causes as real as those of physical illnesses like pneumonia or appendicitis. Freed of his anxieties, tensions, and fears, his distressing symptoms often disappear because their causes have been eradicated.

Helping Children to Avoid the Neurotic Pattern. Teachers may seldom encounter full-blown neuroses in their students. However, neurotic trends are quite common in childhood. It is usually possible to arrest the development of such trends if the child's teachers and other adults intimately associated with him understand their significance and give him reassurement. All children should be helped to realize that it is natural to feel cross or resentful or fearful when confronted with disappointments or failures or strange or violent emotions. They should be encouraged to get rid of such feelings by talking them out to someone who understands. If a child who exhibits antagonistic tendencies is given opportunities through socially acceptable activities for gaining the attention and approbation or the sense of security that he needs, his teachers may help to keep him from growing up to be an "antisocial, egocentric, contentious, maladjusted adult." And if the shy, timid, dreamy, easily discouraged child is unobtrusively drawn out and given self-confidence through a series of small successes, his teachers may help to keep him from growing up into a neurotic, complaining, economically dependent adult.

Psychotherapy. Some children who have failed to get sympathetic help at home or in school may develop such pronounced neurotic trends that psychiatric study and treatment are advisable. The psychiatrist is a physician who has specialized in the study, prevention, and treatment of mental illness. The kind of treatment he gives is called psychotherapy, or treatment of the mind. The primary object of psychotherapy in the treatment of the neuroses is to make the conscious self aware of the unconscious conflict and permit the Ego to solve in a healthy way the problems it was too weak to solve when the neurotic pattern developed.

Unfortunately, on a country-wide basis, there are not nearly enough mental-hygiene clinics or child-guidance clinics available for all the children who would benefit by psychiatric guidance. The great majority of these youngsters must look to their teachers, their pastors, or their family physicians for the friendly teamwork with themselves and their parents which will help them to escape mental illness.

In many cases of emotional distress in young people, healing has come through talking over and sharing problems with an understanding teacher. We all know the relief obtained merely by getting our troubles off our chests. If hand in hand with this catharsis, or emotional release, go reassurance and the wise use of suggestion, the way is open for education or reeducation directed toward giving the disturbed youngster an understanding of how his emotions and poor mental habits are interfering with his health and behavior.

Psychotic Patterns

The psychoses are far more serious forms of mental illness than the neuroses. They account for the great majority of the mentally ill who require institutional care.

We are all familiar with the age-old conception of serious mental illness as demonic possession. The neglect and even physical abuse of its victims, cruel as they were, seemed to be justified on the principle that demons would leave a body, as tenants would leave a house, which had been made untenable. Philippe Pinel's act in striking the chains from the limbs of the insane in the Salpêtrière in 1793 has become symbolic of the setting free of the minds of the sane from the prejudice and superstition that so long delayed advances in an understanding of mental illness.

We now know that mental illness in all its forms is real, treatable, and in many cases preventable. Removing through education the age-old stigma attached to it is one of the principal aims of the mental-hygiene movement. Early diagnosis and treatment offer the best chance of avoiding much of the human suffering and economic cost of mental illness. The outlook for recovery has become more hopeful with the advent of various physical forms of treatment for use as adjuncts of psychotherapy, for example, electroshock therapy and drug therapy.

There are many different forms of functional psychosis, as serious mental illness without apparent organic cause is called. The two most common patterns of psychotic behavior are the manic-depressive and the schizophrenic.

Manic-depressive Illness. Happiness and unhappiness in the lives of most individuals are as fleeting as the play of sunshine and shadows when clouds form and disappear in the sky on a fair day. The terms in which we try to define these qualities are as elusive as the qualities themselves. All we know is that sometimes we're happy and sometimes we're blue. In some people, however, a peculiar combination of unpleasant events or a loss or reversal in fortune may bring about a prolonged state of deep blueness. In mentally healthy people this period of profound unhappiness is usually comparatively short. In others less stable mentally it may last much longer. Psychiatrists call such a state a "depression." If there is a swing from depressed periods of greatly reduced activity to excited "manic" periods of greatly increased activity, the condition is called a manic-depressive psychosis.

Depressions in young people are uncommon and when they do occur are normally short-lived. However, they should always receive professional attention, as they may be the harbingers of manic-depressive disease.

Schizoid States. There is no more puzzling problem in psychiatry than that of determining what factors in queer, ingrown people make the world as seen by most people so different to them. There are a very great many different varieties of "schizoid" states. It is only when an individual shows by his actions and words that he has left the practical world about him to live in a world of phantasy that he is considered to be psychotic. Psychoses that occur in dreamy people far outnumber any other one type of psychosis.

The best known mental illness of the withdrawing type of personality is dementia praecox, or schizophrenia. The term "dementia praecox" was first used to designate this psychosis because its onset so often occurs in adolescence (*praecox,* in Latin, means "early ripe," and *dementia* means "madness"). However, this name later was considered to be something of a misnomer. Dementia praecox does not always begin in youth and early maturity, and its victims do not always develop madness. Both to meet these objections and to describe the splitting of the personality that is characteristic of this psychosis, the term schizophrenia was introduced in 1924. This term is derived from two Greek words: "schizo-" from a word meaning "to divide or split," and "-phrenia" from a word meaning "the mind." At present, the terms dementia praecox and schizophrenia are used interchangeably.

It should be emphasized again that all people indulge to some extent in daydreams and in other forms of escape from reality, but of these comparatively few retreat wholly or even in part into a dream world of their own. Some individuals with definite schizoid tendencies are able to make good adjustments and even to do highly useful work. It is not safe to assume, however, that children who show pronounced forms of withdrawing behavior will outgrow them or that they are of no significance.

Anyone who has indulged in daydreams—and who has not!—knows how rough the coming back to reality can be. Young inexperienced lotus-eaters who hug the cloak of phantasy that gives them some protection from the rigors of actuality feel more keenly than their weathered companions the discrepancy between the ideal and the real. Even if their tendency to dream never makes them lose touch with reality, they are bound to be unhappier than those whose ideals are not so far out of reach that they can be attained only in made-to-order phantasies.

IDENTIFYING CHILDREN WITH EMOTIONAL AND SOCIAL PROBLEMS

The attitude of teachers toward their children's behavior is important because attitudes determine reactions, and reactions in turn determine how behavior problems are handled. Although a teacher may realize that a child is emotionally disturbed, her own feelings may stand in the

Table 5. SOME COMMON INDICATIONS OF MALADJUSTMENT IN SCHOOL CHILDREN

Attacking behavior . . . .   Temper outbursts

Aggressiveness, defiant attitude, resistance to authority, disobedience

Quarrelsomeness, fighting, boasting

Rejection of school routine; wanting always to be the leader in school activities or to pursue own methods of work

Contentiousness, poor sportsmanship

Overactivity

Delinquency, truancy

Withdrawing behavior . . . .   Shyness, timidity, cowardliness

Unsocialness, solitariness, inability to make friends

Dreaminess

Extreme docility, overdependence on adults or on routine

Sensitiveness to criticism, feelings easily hurt

Fearfulness, suspiciousness

Pedantry, overdiligence in schoolwork

Inability to carry responsibility

Somatic manifestations . . . .   Nail biting

Finger sucking

Pencil chewing

Blinking

Facial twitching

Infantile speech

Unestablished toilet habits

Educational problems . . . . .   Difficulty with reading despite normal intelligence and vision

Difficulties with arithmetic

Lack of application

Speech difficulties

---

way of giving the right sort of help. It is extremely difficult to be objective about the behavior of others. That has always been the principal drawback in getting symptoms of maladjustment recognized for what they are. It is easy to feel personally affronted or disgusted by behavior we dislike—hard to realize that our feelings may lead us to make serious mistakes in interpreting and dealing with such behavior— still harder to admit that we may dislike a person because he possesses attributes that we dislike in ourselves.

Teachers who understand children know that all forms of behavior have underlying causes. If there is one sure thing that has been learned in the study of the mind, it is that no one lives in a vacuum. Every pattern of behavior in a child is the result of the reactions of that particular child to a series of particular environmental situations. Knowing this, the understanding teacher will not reject any child whose behavior differs markedly from that of the average healthy well-adjusted child. This does not mean that she will condone his undesirable behavior. Rather she will seek to understand its significance so that her methods of dealing with him will serve to counteract rather than to entrench unsatisfactory ways of meeting life.

It is agreed that teachers have a unique opportunity to observe deviations from normal behavior in children which indicate that professional advice is needed. The most helpful observations are those in which specific descriptions are given of how the child acts in concrete situations. Instead of giving snap judgments, colored by what the teacher personally thinks about the child's behavior, it is better to record incidents that will give a clear picture of how the child is failing to react adequately to the requirements of social living. It takes practice to do this, because most of us are in the habit of interpreting and judging behavior, often without sufficient evidence, instead of recording simply what we hear and see.

In deciding what children need to be studied, it is important to keep in mind the stage of personality development* through which all the children under observation are passing. As we have learned, children normally and characteristically have different emotional reactions at different periods in their lives. Although understanding teachers and parents know this, they are sometimes hard put to it not to show their embarrassment or anxiety when children fail to make a good impression on less understanding outsiders. Because of fear of criticism from "visiting firemen" or from relatives with antiquated notions of child upbringing, they may try to force the children into patterns of behavior for which they are not yet ready. At least part of the feelings of frustration or even of guilt which children suffer come from such attempts on the part of those who love and understand them.

Knowing that children go through various stages of personality development helps us to determine whether behavior at a certain age should be tolerated as "natural" or tackled as a problem. For example, lying, stealing, and temper tantrums are natural in young children, but undesirable in older children. We may adopt as our definition of children who should be reported for study, then, those whose pattern of acting at a certain age is markedly different from that of the average child in that age period.

It is possible to give here only general descriptions of some of the characteristic ways of behaving which indicate that a child may need help in adjusting to his life situation.

The Different Child

In her initial contact with the children in a class, the teacher will notice whether there are any children who "stand out like sore thumbs" in appearance or behavior. Children of school age normally are conformists. They want to look and act as much as possible like the other children of their age and social status.

Of course, the teacher knows from her training and experience that there is a wide variation within normal limits in social behavior, intelligence, and appearance, just as there is in physical body measurements. Children intuitively know this, too. They will not reject another child simply because he is a little cleaner or neater, or a little dirtier or more slovenly, or a little more withdrawn or aggressive, or somewhat brighter or duller than the average. It is the Little Lord Fauntleroys and the Ugly Ducklings, the sissies and the bullies, the highly gifted or the extremely backward who frequently find themselves misfits in the school community. A child who is radically different from the others in his group may need special attention in order to keep him from becoming permanently stigmatized as an outsider during his school life.

The Suddenly Changed Child

As the teacher becomes acquainted with her students, she knows what to expect of them in appearance and behavior. She also knows the child's record of previous scholastic attainments and, in most schools, his health record. When a child who has always been clean and neat *suddenly* becomes slovenly and unkempt for several days; or a normally cooperative child suddenly becomes hostile or negativistic for any length of time; or a child who has done adequate schoolwork begins consistently to fail; or a child who has hitherto shared the enthusiasms, fads, and prejudices of his classmates suddenly shows little interest in school activities, there may be something wrong physically or some alteration in personality or in the home situation or in relationships in the child's life which ought to receive attention.

Sudden changes in the other direction—from bad behavior to good— also may have psychiatric significance unless the change is the result of the correction of some physical disability like poor eyesight or malnutrition. Although such a change may come as a relief to the teacher, it sometimes is a sign of an alteration in attitude or in relationships which presages a more profound alteration in personality.

The Unhappy Child

Young people, like their elders, have fits of the "blues," but it is not natural for them to act "broody" for any length of time.

Sometimes, however, particularly during adolescence, a boy or girl may go through a prolonged period of depression. Any one or more of a great variety of factors in the environment or some inner duel between warring impulses may be responsible. Being like everyone else in appearance, in attitudes toward the other sex, in enthusiasms and "pet hates" is extremely important to adolescents. It may be that a despondent girl is not able, for some reason, to meet the standards of her school group. Perhaps she cannot dress like the other girls for economic reasons or parental foibles and feels sensitive about her appearance. Or special skills or talents may not give her the prestige they did earlier and will later. A boy may be hiding rebellious impulses under his cloak of gloom. Perhaps he resents the fact that he is not allowed as much freedom as his companions. Or some physical disturbance of metabolic origin may be the trouble. Or he may be developing physically at a much slower or faster rate than the other boys of his group. Whatever may be the cause, these unhappy youngsters may develop a stubborn or sulky or morose manner, or consistently fall below their demonstrated ability in their schoolwork, or take no interest in school activities, with the result that their relations with their group deteriorate.

The chances are that they will recover spontaneously, but even so they need understanding, special guidance, and perhaps psychiatric attention. The teacher and the parents cannot know whether the depression is transitory in nature—"just one of those things"—or whether repeated episodes may be expected to occur.

Nothing will be gained by trying to kid a youngster out of a prolonged fit of blueness. An older wiser person may talk herself hoarse about the advantages of distinction, of being different, or of making the best of things for the time being, without giving the slightest help to the unhappy girl or boy who is depressed because of repressed feelings of inferiority or guilt or insecurity. Making light of things, because they really do seem of little importance from the adult point of view, only aggravates the young person to whom they are of great importance.

The Solitary Friendless Child

During elementary school age, particularly, children normally are friendly and gregarious. They want intensely to "belong," to be chosen when sides are being chosen in a game, to have chums or good pals. Hence, manifestations of pronounced withdrawal behavior should be viewed with suspicion. At best, they may clear up spontaneously; at worst, they may indicate emotional trends that may sweep the child from the safe harbor of actuality.

The withdrawn child is usually very timid. He may shun his class-mates—refuse to take part in group games—have no close friends—sit dreamily staring into space when the others are playing or studying. He is likely to be docile and give the teacher no trouble except for his extreme sensitiveness. He may be easily embarrassed while reciting and stutter when asked to "speak up" or when his recitation is criticized. However, he may do well in his written work and test above average in intelligence.

It is a great mistake to allow the solitary, friendless, dependent child to drift further and further out of touch with the real world of social and economic competition in which he must eventually make a place for himself. He is already failing to meet the social requirements of his companions. He may long to "get in," to be acceptable to his group, but he gives the impression that he prefers to be "out." Left to himself he is often helpless to overcome this impression. He literally doesn't know how to break in, and so he doesn't try. But since he has to be "in" somewhere, he retreats more and more frequently into his own private world, and makes his bids for approval from the outside world to adults. The adults, however, cannot or will not go on indefinitely giving him sympathy and protection when he has reached the age at which society expects an individual to stand on his own feet. Also he is acquiring a taste for the delights to be found in getting what he wants in dreams without having to go to all the bother of working for it in a hard, cold world which in his experience is as likely as not to reward his best efforts with failure.

The Social Rebel

As we have seen, aggressiveness is normal in school children in the latent period. This is largely because they want to feel important, to boss others or at least to feel that they can do so. This is a period of intense likes and dislikes, and it is natural for children to pick on or gang up against those they dislike when they feel they can get away with it. This is especially true of children who have seen parents or teachers use bullying or tyrannical methods successfully to gain power over others, or who have never learned by experience the value of kindness and consideration in human relations.

Consistently defiant attitudes and extreme egocentricity may lead later on to definite antisocial tendencies. The destructive effects of chronic aggressive reaction states are shown in delinquents, criminals, and psychopathic personalities.

Children whose social maladjustment is manifested in various forms of overaggressiveness usually need psychiatric help. Very often the parents as well as the children will require treatment.

Overdependence upon one or both parents or repressed feelings of guilt or inadequacy or unfortunate experiences with authority in the home usually lie back of personality disorders characterized by overaggressiveness. Perhaps a boy may be boastful and quarrelsome—always wanting to be the leader in every activity, constantly looking for ways of securing attention—because he is not so good as the other children in his schoolwork and in playing games and hence has failed to gain the approval of his schoolmates or his teacher. Making a nuisance of himself is his way of gaining prestige—of excelling in *something*. Asked why he acts as he does, he cannot possibly give the real reason because he doesn't know it himself.

Another child may be a trouble maker—a bully and poor sport with his classmates—a "tattletale" and "apple polisher" with his teachers— because he has learned that the easiest way to deal with authority is to placate it. But he must have some outlet for his outraged feelings, and so he takes out on his smaller or weaker classmates the impulses he is obliged to repress in the more complicated home situation, where the love of family he thinks he ought to have conflicts with the hate he would be ashamed to admit even if he knew it existed.

Still another child may be a chronic truant, showing that he hates school by staying away whenever he gets the chance and by defying the teacher when he is present. Investigation may show that he has a stern, unbending father, or a domineering, selfish, exacting mother, or a bossy older brother or sister. The deep-seated resentment he feels is unconsciously transferred to his teacher, toward whom he can show his hostility without feeling guilty because he does not have to love as well as to obey her. In many cases of truancy or delinquency it has been shown that the children involved are letting off emotional steam in their relationship with persons or institutions which may be entirely blameless in their dealings with the children, but which have the misfortune to stand for authority.

The Accident-repeater Child

A history of repeated accidents indicates a need for studying a child and his environment (see Accident-proneness under Psychogenic Reactions in this chapter). Perhaps he *is* simply having a run of bad luck. Or he may have some physical defect like poor eyesight or poor hearing. Or his history of repeated accidents may be explained by a tendency to be over-active and impulsive combined with a poor reaction to stress or by in-different parental supervision or possibly by pent-up feelings of hostility and aggression.

Whatever may be at the bottom of repeated accidents, the child's teacher can be of real help in preventing the establishment of the acci-dent habit by recognizing it as a symptom that should be brought to the attention of those responsible for the child's well-being.

Meeting the Need for Guidance in School-age Children

In recent years rapid progress has been made in the science of psychology, upon which the recognition and treatment of unhealthy emotional pat-terns are based. Unfortunately, however, the facilities for applying this science in the guidance of school children with behavior problems are at present very inadequate. A few school systems do have a bureau or department of child guidance, together with a mental-hygiene clinic or child-guidance center to which children requiring psychiatric study and treatment may be referred by the teacher, school nurse, or school phy-sician. Lacking such an arrangement, it is possible in some of the larger cities to obtain psychiatric services for school children with behavior problems from child-guidance or mental-hygiene clinics in the com-munity. Even where professional services are available, it is agreed that administrators, teachers, and parents must cooperate closely with the specialists in dealing with a particular child so as to avoid conflicts in methods of handling which would confuse the child still further.

Important as it is to have specialists to treat the serious problems of emotional disturbance among school children, it is more important to use the time and skill of these specialists to help teachers and principals to understand the emotional health of all children so that, in the day-to-day contacts that the educational staff has with children, they may pre-vent serious disorders from developing.

One of the great advantages of clinic guidance is the opportunity it affords for getting at the source of the trouble in problems arising out of the home situation. Even if the teacher knows that parent-child rela-tionships or family conflicts of one kind or another or economic difficul-ties are the cause of a child's behavior problem, the home environment is seldom within the sphere of her influence. In the mental-hygiene clinic, parents are encouraged to talk over with trained persons their own problems and those of their children. Conferences also may be arranged to give teachers, school nurses, parents, social case workers, child psychologists, and child psychiatrists opportunities to work together on plans for changing misunderstood unhappy children to well-adjusted happy children.

Above all is the need for a climate in the school which permits healthy mental and emotional development of all children. The teacher, herself, is the key to this situation. Serenity, stability, understanding, patience, and tolerance are essential attributes in all teachers if the need for psychiatric study and treatment in childhood is to be reduced to a minimum.

DO YOU KNOW?

1. Tell the difference between the words or terms in each of the following pairs:
    a. Cerebral cortex and autonomic nervous system
    b. Vasodilators and vasoconstrictors
    c. Parasympathetic division (of the autonomic nervous system) and sympathetic division
    d. Psyche and soma
    e. Organic illness and functional illness
    f. Stimulus and impulse
    g. Signs and symptoms
    h. Adrenaline and insulin
    i. Antigen and antibody
    j. Phagocytes and hormones
    k. Immunity and susceptibility
    l. Vaccine and toxoid
    m. Infection and allergy
    n. Allergen and histamine
    o. Scratch test and patch test (for allergy)
    p. Diabetic coma and insulin reaction
    q. Chills and fever (give physiological distinction)
    r. Referred pain and psychogenic pain
    s. Neurosis and psychosis

2. In each of the following groupings of diseases or conditions, there is one that does not belong with the group. Select the one that does not belong and tell why it is out of place.

    a. Simple goiter, hay fever, diabetes, acromegaly
    b. Poliomyelitis, epidemic encephalitis, cerebral palsy, meningococcal meningitis

c. Epilepsy, schizophrenia, manic-depressive psychosis, conversion hysteria

d. Eczema, hives, allergic rhinitis, appendicitis

SUGGESTED ACTIVITIES

1. Have committees of the class report on the lives and work of the following men:

> Louis Pasteur (1822–1895)
> Elie Metchnikoff (1845–1916)
> Ivan Pavlov (1849–1936)
> Sigmund Freud (1856–1939)
> Walter B. Cannon (1871–1945)

After hearing the reports, have a class discussion on the contributions made by one or more of these men to

a. Our knowledge of the defense forces of the body

b. Our understanding of the mind

c. Our understanding of habit formation

2. To learn the effects of emotions from (a) experience and (b) observation—

a. The next time a situation arises in which you become angry or frightened, write down immediately afterward all the physical changes you experienced and what physiological processes were responsible for these changes.

b. Observe the actions, speech, and appearance of a child who is angry or scared. Write a description of what actually took place—why the child got angry or scared; what he did; what he said; how he looked.

Knowing from experience and observation that emotions have physical consequences, discuss these statements in class:

a. Physical health and mental health are interdependent.

b. Behavior patterns caused by consciously felt anger or fear and behavior patterns caused by repressed hostility or anxiety resemble each other because the same mechanisms operate to produce them.

3. Have a committee of the class find out and report on the treatment of mentally ill persons before and after present methods of treatment were put into practice. Some students may be interested in preparing reports on the life and work of Philippe Pinel and Dorothea Lynde Dix (founders of the movement for the humane treatment of the

insane) and Clifford Beers (founder of the modern mental-hygiene movement). Discuss in class the reasons for the emphasis now being placed on the teacher as a key person in the prevention of neurotic trends and in the detection of danger signals which indicate that professional help is needed.

4. To gain practice in reporting your observations in as helpful a manner as possible, keep a record over a period of time of the behavior and appearance of one or more children whom you have an opportunity to observe over that period. Make your notes explicit and concrete. For example, instead of noting that Philip looked (or acted) tired today, give the details which made you draw that conclusion— for example, "Philip went to sleep over his work," or "Philip's face looked drawn and pale," or "Philip didn't want to go out to play at recess." Instead of writing "Mary was naughty today," or "Tom was uncooperative," or "Jim was quarrelsome," or "Alice was inattentive," report what the child actually did and said that made you draw the conclusion you did. A book which you will find helpful in learning to make and record your observations objectively is "Helping Teachers Understand Children" (see References).

5. Make up a story about a child who presents a problem in school because of overaggressiveness, excessive shyness and timidity, or some other undesirable behavior pattern. Describe the child's family and home background, his career so far in school, and his health record; give examples of specific situations in which the child exhibited signs and symptoms indicating the form of maladjustment you have assigned to him. On the basis of the history you have invented, explain "how the child got that way." Then decide how you would help the child. Could you handle the problem yourself, or should you refer the child for professional help of some kind? If you think you could handle it yourself, make a plan showing how you would do so.

6. If there is a child-guidance center or mental-hygiene clinic in your school or community, arrange to have one student, or a committee, visit it and report to the class on its organization, personnel, methods of interviewing children and parents, and other points of interest.

7. Write to the Education Service of the National Foundation for Infantile Paralysis for publications of use in social studies classes and as background material in answering the questions of pupils about polio as these arise. After studying this material plan a unit for giving children information that will help to allay their fears during a polio epidemic and also motivate them to follow the precautions advised.

8. Suppose you had a crippled child in your class, or a child suffering from epilepsy. Plan what you would say to the other children to help

them to understand the handicapped child's problem and to cultivate the right attitude toward all handicapped children.

SELECTED REFERENCES

AMERICAN COUNCIL ON EDUCATION, COMMISSION ON TEACHER EDUCATION: *Helping Teachers Understand Children,* Washington, D.C., 1945. (Prepared by the staff of the Division on Child Development and Teacher Personnel as a study guide; helpful for teachers who wish to gain experience in making concrete and worth-while observations of child behavior.)

ASSOCIATION FOR SUPERVISION AND CURRICULUM DEVELOPMENT (a department of the National Education Association): *Fostering Mental Health in Our Schools; 1950 Yearbook,* Washington, D.C.

BEERS, CLIFFORD W.: *A Mind That Found Itself,* New York, Doubleday & Company, Inc., reprinted with additions, 1953. (The fascinating autobiography of the founder of the modern mental-hygiene movement.)

BURTON, MARY L. H.: *Your Child or Mine: The Story of the Cerebral-palsied Child,* New York, Coward-McCann, Inc., 1949.

CANNON, WALTER B.: *The Wisdom of the Body,* New York, W. W. Norton & Company, Inc., 1939. (A classic by a distinguished physiologist on the relation of the autonomic nervous system to the preservation of stability within the body.)

CANNON, WALTER B.: *Bodily Changes in Pain, Hunger, Fear and Rage,* an account of recent researches into the function of emotional excitement, 2d ed. Boston, Charles T. Branford Company, 1953.

CONKLIN, GROFF: *Good News about Diabetes,* Public Affairs Pamphlet No. 138, rev. ed. New York, Public Affairs Committee, 1954.

DUNBAR, FLANDERS: *Your Child's Mind and Body: A Practical Guide for Parents,* New York, Random House, Inc., 1949. (A detailed discussion of the emotional problems of infancy and childhood with suggestions on how to meet them effectively.)

ENGLISH, O. SPURGEON, and GERALD H. J. PEARSON: *Emotional Problems of Living; Avoiding the Neurotic Pattern,* New York, W. W. Norton & Company, Inc., 1945.

ENGLISH, O. SPURGEON: *Emotional Problems of Growing Up,* Chicago, Science Research Associates, 1951. (Better Living booklet.)

FEINBERG, SAMUEL M.: *Allergy: Facts and Fancies,* New York, Harper & Brothers, 1951.

GALLAGHER, J. ROSWELL: *Your Children's Health;* a handbook for parents and teachers, Chicago, Science Research Associates, 1952.

HYMES, JAMES L., JR.: *Behavior and Misbehavior;* a teacher's guide to action, New York, Prentice-Hall, Inc., 1955.

LANGDON, GRACE: *The Discipline of Well-adjusted Children,* New York, The John Day Company, Inc., 1952. (How hundreds of successful parents manage the big and little problems of rearing a family.)

OVERSTREET, HARRY A.: *The Mind Alive,* New York, W. W. Norton & Company, Inc., 1954.

SWARTZ, HARRY F.: *Allergic Child,* New York, Coward-McCann, Inc., 1954.

THORMANN, GEORGE: *Toward Mental Health,* Public Affairs Pamphlet No. 120, 8th ed. New York, Public Affairs Committee, 1950.

WALLEN, E. W.: *Children with Mental and Physical Handicaps,* New York, Prentice-Hall, Inc., 1949.

WICKMAN, E. K.: *Teachers and Behavior Problems,* New York, National Association for Mental Health, 1938. (A 40-page condensation of *Children's Behavior and Teachers' Attitudes* by the same author.)

WITTENBERG, RUDOLPH M.: *How to Help People;* the mental hygiene approach in your work with youth, New York, Association Press, 1953.

YAHRAES, HERBERT: *Epilepsy—The Ghost Is Out of the Closet,* Public Affairs Pamphlet No. 98, rev. ed. New York, Public Affairs Committee, 1954.

YAHRAES, HERBERT: *Gains for Handicapped Children,* Public Affairs Pamphlet No. 212, New York, Public Affairs Committee, 1954.

YOST, ORIA R.: *What You Should Know about Mental Illness,* New York, Exposition Press, 1953.

Organizations

American Diabetes Association
National Association for Mental Health
National Epilepsy League
National Foundation for Infantile Paralysis (Education Service)

Chapter 4 WHAT TO KNOW ABOUT THE HEART, BLOOD, AND LYMPH

Circulation Survey
Signs and Symptoms of Circulatory Disorders
Rheumatic Fever
Blood and Its Composition
Blood Disorders
Tissue Fluid
What to Do in Case of Circulatory Emergencies
Diseases Spread by Blood-sucking Insects

CIRCULATION SURVEY

The more or less solid tissues of the body may be compared to an expanse of wet sand on the seashore. The grains of sand are the cells, and the sea water that moistens them is tissue fluid, or lymph. The cells are fixed in their places. They cannot forage for the supplies they need or conduct the waste materials that result from their activities to the appropriate dumping grounds for removal from the body. Two moving streams within the body—one swiftly flowing, the blood; the other sluggish, the lymph—serve continuously as carriers between the fixed secluded cells and the places in the body where provisions are stocked and wastes are removed. Only by understanding the significance of these remarkable fluids and the manner in which they are kept in circulation can teachers appreciate the meaning of much of what they observe in healthy children as well as in those in need of medical attention.

The Heart

The blood moves swiftly in a completely enclosed system composed of miles upon miles of tubular vessels. The sole function of the heart is to act as a pump to keep the blood in motion. It is a powerful, highly specialized muscle containing two chambers, a right and a left. Each chamber is equipped with valves to keep blood flowing through the heart in the right direction. These valves are located at the inlet and outlet of each of the heart chambers, and at the opening in the partition

that separates each heart chamber into two compartments, an upper
(auricle) and a lower (ventricle).

When the Heart Beats. . . . At each beat or contraction of the heart
(the systole) the inlet valves close and blood is driven through the outlet
valve of the left ventricle into the great main arterial trunk of the body,

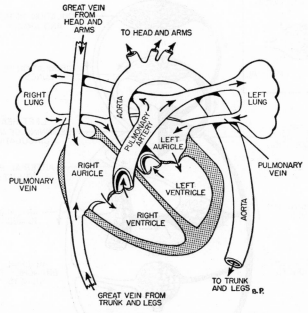

Fig. 24. The circulation through the heart and lungs. Blood flows into the right
side of the heart from the two grand trunks of the tree of veins. From there it is
pumped to the lungs, through the pulmonary artery and its branches. It returns
to the left side of the heart through the pulmonary veins and is pumped into
the aorta (the grand trunk of the arterial tree) for distribution to all parts of
the body.

and through the outlet valve of the right ventricle into the vessels that
carry it to the lungs. The heart must then rest before it can contract
again. The split second of rest between beats makes it possible for the
healthy heart to keep up its work of driving out a heavy load of blood
seventy times a minute or faster for 70 years or more without noticeable
fatigue. During this period of relaxation (the diastole), the outlet valves
of the heart chambers close and the inlet valves open, permitting blood
to flow from the great veins into the right auricle from all the remote
regions of the body and into the left auricle from the lungs.

The Circulatory Trees

The blood vessels are arranged in two distinct but continuous systems. Because of their elaborate branchings they are often compared to luxuriantly growing trees. The arterial tree carries blood *away* from the heart.

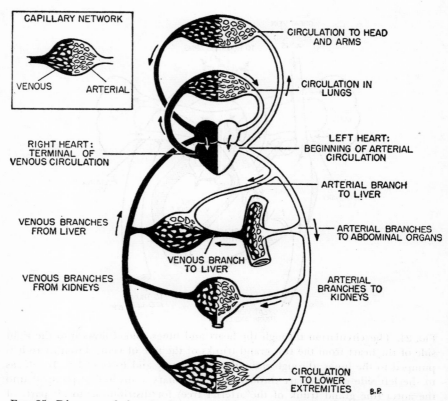

FIG. 25. Diagram of the circulatory system. Arterial blood is pumped from the left side of the heart into arteries, which lead into capillary networks. Venous blood is collected from the capillary networks and returned to the right side of the heart through veins. Then it is pumped to the lungs for oxygenation and returned to the left side of the heart.

The venous tree carries blood *toward* the heart. The blood finds its way into the tree of veins from the tree of arteries through delicate networks of minute blood vessels called capillaries.

The Greater, or Systemic, Circulation. The grand trunk of the arterial tree is the aorta, into which blood is forced directly from the left ventricle of the heart. Its big branches run to the arms and legs, the head, and the organs of the abdomen—the stomach, intestines, liver, kidneys, and spleen. In these regions the large arteries in their branchings get smaller and smaller until finally they dwindle to the size of minute twigs. These twigs of the arterial tree are the arterioles.

Blood flows from the arterioles into the exceedingly thin-walled capillaries which wind in and out among the cells in all tissues. The capillary meshworks may be compared to a vast irrigation system of closed canals through the walls of which water, food, oxygen, and other materials for the cells are exchanged for the wastes produced by the cells. After passing slowly through the capillaries, the blood with its load of waste products flows into the first tiny branches, or twigs, of the tree of veins. These little veins, or venules, merge to form veins which become increasingly larger until finally they join the two grand trunks of the venous tree, through which the blood is returned to the right auricle of the heart.

The Lesser, or Pulmonary, Circulation. The beat of the heart which forces arterial blood from the left ventricle into the aorta for its grand tour of the body also forces venous blood out of the right ventricle into another artery for a side trip through the lungs. The venous blood in the right chamber is blood that has been robbed in the tissues of the oxygen with which arterial blood is loaded. Also venous blood is heavily charged with carbon dioxide (CO_2). This gas is one of the end products of energy metabolism. The other end product is heat, the mechanical equivalent of which is energy. The carbon dioxide is a waste product and hence must be removed from the body. The heat is a vital product which keeps the fires of life burning and supplies the energy for all the work of the body.

Venous, or deoxygenated, blood is pumped from the lower right chamber of the heart through the capillary networks in the lungs. There the carbon dioxide is exchanged for oxygen, and the aerated, or oxygenated, blood flows on through veins into the upper left chamber of the heart.

It takes less than half a minute for blood to make its round trip through the greater and lesser circulations—from the right side of the heart through the lungs to the left side, and from the left side through the body and back to the right side.

The Pulse. Arteries have relatively thick elastic walls which are provided with a layer of circular muscle. Hence they can stretch and rebound to drive the blood along after the initial push given it by the heartbeat. Each time the heart forces a load of blood into the already full arterial tree, it starts a distending wave that can be felt as "a pulse" in any branch that lies comparatively close to the surface of the body. The principal places are in the wrist at the base of the thumb, at the temple in front of the ear, and at the back of the ankle on the inner side of the foot. The pulse rate is best taken by placing three fingers on the inner side of the wrist below the base of the thumb.

The pulse rate is regulated by the autonomic nervous system according to the needs of the body for oxygen and fuel food and for conserving or getting rid of heat. Vigorous physical activity, fever, and emotional excitement all make the heart beat faster than usual. The resting rate is normally more rapid in childhood than in adult life.

Blood Pressure. Any fluid that fills to capacity any closed system of tubes will exert pressure on the walls of the tubes. Blood actually over-fills the closed system of tubes consisting of the blood vessels through which it circulates. Arterial blood pressure—which is the pressure measured when a physician takes a person's blood pressure—varies rhythmically with the beating of the heart. It rises during contraction, when a fresh load of blood is driven into the arterial system (the systolic blood pressure), and falls during relaxation (the diastolic pressure), when the heart pauses to fill up between beats.

Except for the tempo and force of the heartbeat, the factor that has the greatest influence on arterial blood pressure is the resistance offered by the arterioles and capillaries (particularly the former) to the passage of blood from the tree of arteries to the tree of veins. The slightly elastic walls of the arterioles are composed mostly of rings of muscle. Nerves running from the autonomic nervous system to the muscles carry the impulses that make them contract or relax. Thus the bores of the arterioles may be made narrower or wider by nervous influences, as the occasion requires, to regulate the quantity of blood passing from the arteries to the veins by way of the capillaries.

The narrowing of the arterioles acts like a dam to back up the blood in the arteries. Naturally, the pressure in the arteries then goes up. The widening of the arterioles lowers the level of the "dam" and the pressure then goes down.

Temporary rises of blood pressure accompany muscular exertion and digestion (which increase the rate and force of the heartbeat) and periods of worry, joy, fear, anger, or other emotions (which give rise to nervous impulses that cause the arterioles to tighten up).

The Traffic Back and Forth between the Blood and the Tissues

The most important thing to remember about the circulation is the fact that the whole elaborate system of pump and tubes exists solely for the purpose of getting blood into the capillaries where the exchanges between the body cells and the blood take place. The walls of all the blood vessels, except those of the capillaries, are too thick to permit the passage of materials from the blood into the tissue fluid surrounding the cells or from the tissue fluid into the blood stream. The walls of the capillaries, on the other hand, are exceedingly thin. They are composed of a single layer of flat cells fitted together like paving stones. Digested food and oxygen and other dissolved substances can readily pass into the blood stream through the capillary walls in the loading stations of the digestive tract and lungs and out again into the tissues. And wastes from the tissues can readily pass into the blood stream and out again in the unloading stations of the lungs and kidneys.

SIGNS AND SYMPTOMS OF CIRCULATORY DISORDERS

Circulatory disorders in children are for the most part due to congenital defects of the heart or large blood vessels leading into or out of it, or to rheumatic fever (see Rheumatic Fever, further on) or other infections that damage the heart. The lay observer has no means of checking up on the condition of the heart and blood vessels. Only the physician can do this in the course of a thorough cardiac examination. However, information about various signs and symptoms commonly associated with heart trouble may be helpful to teachers in their observation and guidance of children.

Heart Murmurs

Heart murmurs are sounds produced as blood flows past the heart valves. By using his stethoscope, which amplifies chest sounds, the physician is able to detect heart murmurs or other sounds that indicate deviations from normal in the heart's action.

The presence of a murmur does not necessarily mean that the heart is diseased, damaged, or defective. A large percentage of healthy children have innocent murmurs. When the murmur is caused by some defect or deformity, it is called an organic murmur. Organic murmurs may be congenital or acquired. That is, a child may be born with a valvular deformity or may acquire one as a result of a disease that attacks the heart. Rheumatic fever is the commonest cause of acquired heart disease.

Hypertension

Hypertension (high blood pressure) means that through some nervous or toxic influence the arterioles throughout the body are kept in a more or less constantly constricted, or tightened-up, state. Hypertension increases the resistance that the heart must overcome in pumping blood into the arteries and thus greatly increases its work. This extra work tends to cause enlargement of the heart muscle. Hypertension is most often first encountered in middle age. It is rare in children. Only a physician can tell whether a person has high blood pressure. He uses an instrument called a sphygmomanometer to measure the pressure of the blood against the walls of the arteries.

Shortness of Breath

The medical name for difficult breathing is dyspnea (from two Greek words meaning "ill" and "breath"). It may be caused by anything that interferes with the oxygenation of the blood in the lungs or with the transport of the respiratory gases (oxygen and carbon dioxide). In children its most common cause is asthma.

Breathlessness during or after moderate exertion that has not previously caused breathlessness may be an early symptom of a weakened heart muscle. It most commonly occurs when the left side of the heart fails to pump on all the blood it receives from the right side by way of the lungs. As a result the lungs become congested with blood and their ability to distend during breathing is diminished.

Children who consistently "lose their breath" or get tired more quickly than their playmates do, or who consistently have trouble breathing during physical activities that give most children no respiratory distress, should be referred for a medical check-up.

Blueness

Cyanosis (from the Greek word *cyanos*, meaning "blue") is the medical name for the spreading dusky or bluish color given to the skin by the presence in the superficial blood vessels of blood that contains less than its normal quota of oxygen. This happens if the blood leaving the lungs contains less than the normal amount of oxygen, or if the blood circulating through the skin gives up more than the normal amount of oxygen, or if both events occur. Cyanosis is more clearly evident in regions where the skin is thin and unpigmented, such as the lips and under the fingernails, and also in regions where the skin blood vessels are normally well filled with blood, such as the face, ear lobes, and hands.

Conditions in which cyanosis might be expected to appear include (a) any defect or disease of the heart or blood vessels which might sidetrack or obstruct the flow of blood through the lungs or slow up the circulation in the tissues, and (b) any interference with the mechanics of breathing which might hold up the delivery of oxygen to the lungs or reduce the amount of lung tissue capable of receiving and passing on oxygen to the blood. Most people are familiar with the term "blue babies," applied to infants who are born with a heart or blood-vessel defect that interferes with the oxygenation of the blood. The cyanosis of pneumonia is an example of a condition in which the functioning area

Joseph G. Dzenowagis

of the lungs is reduced. Blueness also may be associated with a chill, a convulsion, or an epileptic seizure (see Epilepsy, in Chap. 3).

Hysteria accompanied by breath holding is a familiar example of cyanosis caused by sudden interference with breathing. A young child in a fit of temper may hold his breath until he is "blue in the face." Usually there is nothing to worry about in this, because the child will be forced to take a breath before his oxygen supply becomes dangerously low.

Cardiac Misbehavior

The heart may act queerly without having anything organically wrong with it. Sometimes children, like their elders, experience common but annoying sensations such as skipped beats, palpitation, and very rapid beating of the heart. A child who complains of noticeable misbehavior of the heartbeat, pain or discomfort in the chest region, or any other annoying symptoms should always be referred for medical attention. If the physician after a careful examination can find nothing wrong with the heart, every effort should be made to reassure the child. Young people with sound hearts can be made very miserable and even develop emotional disturbances if they are allowed to grow up with the mistaken notion that something is wrong with their hearts.

RHEUMATIC FEVER

Rheumatic fever, combined with the organic heart disease it so often causes, is a leading cause of death by disease in the primary and elementary school ages (Fig. 2). In fact, it is responsible for most of the organic heart disease before age forty. Rheumatic fever is an acute disease marked by fever and the migration of heat, pain, and swelling from joint to joint (usually the knee, ankle, hip, and wrist).

Streptococcal infections (see Respiratory Infections, in Chap. 5), for example, tonsillitis, scarlet fever, or a streptococcal cold, are responsible for lighting up rheumatic fever in children or young adults who are susceptible to it. There is more in the picture than infection, however. Rheumatic fever occurs particularly in certain families, and it appears certain that a hereditary factor is involved. However, it has been impossible so far to find any mechanism by which the streptococcus exerts its effects. Lacking this knowledge, it is impossible to determine whether the hereditary factor is a familial allergy to one or more products of the streptococcus or some other kind of inherited sensitivity. All that can be said with certainty is that children of some families are more susceptible to rheumatic fever than are children of other families.

Also, it has been impossible to find thus far any constituent or product of the streptococcus which acts as the immediate cause of rheumatic fever. Until this hypothetical agent and its mode of operating have been discovered, no method of active immunization can be devised. Fundamental research on this problem is being carried on in several universities and hospitals.

In the meantime the well-known antagonism between *Streptococcus hemolyticus* and the sulfonamides and penicillin furnishes us with a makeshift method of preventing recurrences of rheumatic fever in susceptible children. These recurrences are one of the worst features of the disease. A child doesn't "catch" rheumatic fever and set up an immunity as he does when attacked by measles, chickenpox, and other childhood diseases. Rather, a first attack makes him more vulnerable to a second; a second, to a third; and so on. Each attack provides a fresh opportunity for damaging the heart. To prevent these recurrent attacks, the Committee on the Prevention of Rheumatic Fever of the American Heart Association recommends that prophylactic treatment with penicillin or sulfadiazine be started as soon as the diagnosis is made and continued until new knowledge makes such a course unnecessary.

Cortisone, an adrenal cortex hormone recently made available for use in medical practice, and ACTH, an anterior pituitary hormone which stimulates the adrenal cortex to produce cortisone, have given favorable results in relieving the symptoms of acute rheumatic fever. Longer experience with these hormonal substances is necessary before we shall know definitely whether or not they prevent or decrease the development of chronic heart injury.

Sydenham's Chorea

Sydenham's chorea is in many cases either a forerunner or a follower of acute rheumatic infection. Apparently, it has the same cause as rheumatic fever, tends to run in families, and most frequently occurs in the winter and spring.

The popular name for Sydenham's chorea is St. Vitus's dance. It is a convulsive nervous disease, especially common in girls, which is marked by involuntary jerky movements involving the muscles of the limbs and face. In a large percentage of the cases rheumatic joint symptoms develop later. When this happens the heart is often but not always affected.

Signs and Symptoms of Acute Rheumatic Fever

The school occupies a unique position in relation to rheumatic-fever control. This was pointed out in a special report [1] from the Committee on School Health and the Committee on Rheumatic Fever of the Ameri-

[1] *Pediatrics,* Vol. 2, No. 3 (September), 1948.

can Academy of Pediatrics. A first attack of rheumatic fever usually occurs in children at the age when they enter the first or second grade, and recurrences are most common up to the age when children are leaving high school. The insidious onset of so many cases of rheumatic fever during the school years suggests that teachers should be familiar with the signs and symptoms that may mean acute rheumatic fever. Those to which teachers should pay special attention were listed as follows in the special report referred to above:

1. Failure to gain weight
2. Pallor
3. Poor appetite
4. Fatigue
5. Frequent colds and sore throats
6. Tonsil and adenoid operations (because they may indicate previous sore throats)
7. Scarlet fever or any known streptococcal infection
8. Unexplained nosebleeds
9. Unexplained fever
10. Pains in arms, legs, and joints
11. Unusual restlessness, irritability, twitching or jerky motions
12. History of previous rheumatic fever
13. Behavior and personality changes
14. Decreasing accomplishment in school by a child who has previously done well

Of course, rheumatic fever does not have a monopoly on the signs with which its early development is associated. Some of the signs—for example, pallor, loss of appetite, failure to gain weight, and nervousness or irritability—are similar to those of other slowly developing childhood illnesses. None the less, vague conditions of this kind may, if properly investigated by a physician, disclose early cases of acute rheumatic fever. Even if rheumatic fever is not found, it is all to the good to have secured medical attention for school children with signs and symptoms of substandard health.

More definite signs of rheumatic fever are pain in joints and muscles; twitching or jerking of the face, arms, or legs (St. Vitus's dance); unexplained nosebleeds; and sometimes a patchy reddening or mottling of the skin. A period of medical observation and special tests may be necessary to determine whether rheumatic fever is or is not the cause of these manifestations.

If the diagnosis is rheumatic fever, the child will be kept in bed to protect his heart until the doctor says it is safe for him to get up. After that he may lead a normal or near-normal life unless his heart has been severely damaged.

The Rheumatic Child in School

In the special report of the committees on school health and rheumatic fever of the American Academy of Pediatrics, it is pointed out that schools in the past have tended to place too much emphasis on restricting the activities of rheumatic children. Yet relatively few rheumatic children attending regular school in the intervals between attacks need to have their physical activity restricted except, perhaps, in competitive sports. The overanxious supervision of parents and teachers can quite easily make chronic invalids out of these children or engender fears that may lead to serious emotional disturbances. On the other hand, rheumatic children need regular medical supervision and also the common-sense health guidance that teachers are in an excellent position to give.

It goes without saying that the teacher should know whether any child (or children) in her group has had an attack of rheumatic fever with or without heart damage. She can then cooperate with the parents, physician, and nurse in efforts to prevent recurrences. She ought also to know if the child is taking a rheumatic-fever preventive such as a sulfa drug or penicillin. It is especially important for the rheumatic child to learn and practice good health habits so that he can help to protect himself from respiratory infections. By her unobtrusive supervision the teacher can make sure that he practices what he has learned from his doctor, his parent, and herself. And she can be on the alert for signs suggestive of a recurrence and see that he gets prompt medical attention.

BLOOD AND ITS COMPOSITION

Until William Harvey announced his discovery of the circulation in 1628, nothing actually was known about blood except that it is essential to life. Now a great deal is known about this extraordinary fluid.

Blood Plasma

If you will look at the diagram in Figure 26, you will see that more than half the total volume of whole blood is made up of a thickish liquid called plasma. Plasma is mostly water. The solid substances dissolved in it are proteins (which make up about 7 per cent of plasma) and a smattering of fats, sugar, and mineral salts. In recent years the proteins of plasma have been broken down into many different fractions, which are proving to be of the highest value in medical and surgical practice. One of these fractions is gamma globulin which carries the antibodies developed by the body to fight germ-invaders.

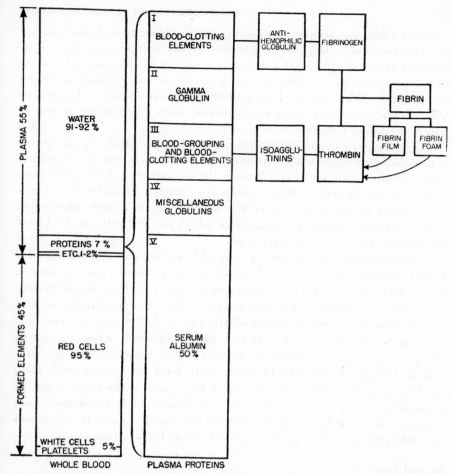

FIG. 26. Principal medical uses of blood and its derivatives. The size of the blocks indicating Fractions I, II, III, IV, and their subgroups is arbitrary. (*From "Health Bulletin for Teachers," February, 1949, Metropolitan Life Insurance Company.*)

Whole blood. To replace blood lost through hemorrhage.

Red cells. To treat anemias except those due to blood loss or infection.

Plasma. To prevent or treat (*a*) shock and (*b*) hypoproteinemia (a decrease in the normal amount of protein in the blood).

Fibrinogen and thrombin (blood-clotting elements). To make *fibrin foam* and *fibrin film* for the control of bleeding and for tissue repair in surgery.

Antihemophilic globulin. To shorten temporarily the blood-clotting time in hemophilia (a hereditary disease in which the blood fails to clot normally).

Gamma globulin (immune serum globulin). To prevent temporarily, or modify, measles infectious hepatitis, and polio.

Isoagglutinins. To obtain anti-A, anti-B, and anti-Rh typing serums.

Serum albumin. To prevent or treat shock and hypoproteinemia.

Blood Clotting. Another group of protein elements in blood plasma are the substances responsible for the highly complicated process of blood clotting. If blood did not have the ability to clot over a break in the skin or mucous membrane and plug it, we might bleed to death from a very slight wound. This actually has been known to happen in hemophiliacs, that is, boys or men suffering from a hereditary disease in which the blood fails to clot normally.

The changes in blood which make it clot begin with the formation of a protein substance, called thrombin, from another protein substance, called prothrombin. Quickly following the formation of thrombin, fibrinogen, another protein in blood plasma, is changed to fibrin. The fibrin is deposited in the form of very fine needles, which rapidly increase to make a network in the membranes of which the red cells of the blood are caught, thus forming a red clot.

Serum Albumin. About 50 per cent of blood plasma is made up of a watery solution of albumin (white of egg is practically pure albumin). Serum albumin was the last protein to be separated from blood plasma in the famous blood fractionation program that was started in the Second World War under the direction of Dr. Edwin J. Cohn of the Harvard Medical School. It is often used now instead of whole blood plasma in the prevention or treatment of the shock that frequently occurs after serious injury. In this type of shock more fluid than usual seeps from the blood capillaries into the tissues. A large part of the effectiveness of plasma in transfusions given to prevent or treat shock is due to the serum albumin, which helps to hold water in the blood stream. Hence serum albumin can be used as a substitute for whole blood plasma.

Formed Elements

The Red Cells. A little less than half the total volume of whole blood is made up of formed elements. Of these, by far the most numerous are the red cells. There are about 5,000,000 red cells in 1 cubic millimeter of blood (a small drop). Yet small as they are, one now and then has to squeeze to get through a capillary which is fifty times smaller than one of the hairs of your head.

The red cells are the oxygen carriers of the blood. Technically they are called erythrocytes ("erythro-," meaning "red," plus "-cyte," meaning "cell"). Erythrocytes are born in red bone marrow, where they go through several stages of development from infancy to maturity. When they are mature, capillaries in the red bone marrow open up and release them in batches into the blood stream.

The mature red cell is an extremely small disk without a nucleus. Its groundwork is a spongelike jelly in which hemoglobin is enmeshed. Hemoglobin consists of an iron-containing red pigment (heme) combined with a protein substance (globin). The iron in hemoglobin gives it its red color and its property of combining with oxygen in the lungs and releasing it in the tissues.

The Red-cell Population. In health the population of the red cells is kept within normal range by a nice balance between their birth rate and their death rate. The total number of red blood cells in the blood of the average man is about thirty trillion (30,000,000,000,000). This is about 200,000 times the population of the United States. The average length of life of each red cell is about 80 days, but some old-timers sur-

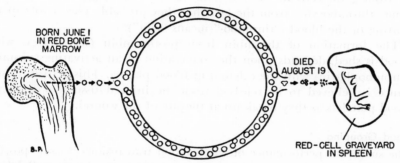

FIG. 27. Red cells born in red bone marrow circulate on the average for 80 days and then break up and are removed from the blood by the spleen.

vive for 120 days or more. The average length of life of United States citizens at present is about 70 years. In health about 10,000,000 red cells are destroyed every second, or an average of 864,000,000,000 every 24 hours. This is a daily death rate per 1,000 of about 28. The annual death rate per 1,000 of the United States population at the present time is less than 7.

The White Cells. The white cells of the blood are called leukocytes ("leuko-," meaning "white," plus "-cyte"). They belong to a class of cells widely distributed throughout the body which act as phagocytes (literally "cell eaters"). To the army of phagocytes all substances foreign to the body, including bacteria, are legitimate prey. Hence, phagocytosis (the eating up of bacteria by phagocytes) is one of the most powerful of all bodily defenses against infection.

Most white blood cells, as well as all red blood cells, are normally produced in red bone marrow. In one small drop of blood (1 cubic millimeter) the number of white cells normally ranges from 5,000 to 10,000. Hence, for each white cell there are from 500 to 1,000 red cells. Unlike the red cells, to which the blood stream is home, the white cells are transients in this stream. They use it as a highway in getting to places where they are needed to fight infection.

The White-cell Population. Normally the proportion of white cells to red cells is fairly constant. However, the white blood cells usually increase in number under the stimulus of an infection. This is an orderly mobilization set in motion by the body's need for new recruits to fight invading bacteria. When there is a wild disorderly overgrowth of white cells, leukemia (see Blood Disorders, further on) is the result.

The Blood Platelets. The blood platelets are infinitesimally small bodies which are generally believed to be fragments of protoplasm broken off from giant cells in the red bone marrow. They get their technical name, thrombocytes, from the fact that they probably play a role in the clotting of the blood ("thrombo-" means "clot").

The formation of thrombin from prothrombin (see above), when blood is shed, depends upon the cooperation of an activating substance (thromboplastin) with the calcium in blood plasma. This activating substance is believed to be released from the injured tissues or from the blood platelets as they break up at the site of the wound.

Blood Grouping

The successful performance of whole-blood transfusions became possible when the discovery that every person belongs to one of four well-defined blood groups was announced by Dr. Karl Landsteiner in 1901. Each individual inherits the blood group to which he belongs. The four major blood groups (see Fig. 28) are characterized by different combinations of two factors capable of being agglutinated (agglutinogens A and B) in the red blood cells and two agglutinins (anti-A and anti-B) in the serum.

Compatibles and Incompatibles. In a whole-blood transfusion, the bloods of donor and recipient must be compatible (match) to avoid the agglutination, or clumping together, of the red cells in the donated blood with serious and often fatal results. By referring to Figure 28 it is easy to see that blood groups A and B are incompatible. If group-A blood is transfused into a group-B recipient, its red cells, which contain agglutinogen A, will be agglutinated by the anti-A agglutinin in the recipient's blood serum. A similar reaction will take place if the donated blood belongs to group B and the recipient to group A. The blood of a donor belonging to group O, however, can *as a rule* be given safely to a recipient in any of the other three groups because its red cells contain no agglutinogen to react with an anti-A or anti-B agglutinin. On this account, persons belonging to group O have been called "universal donors." As a person belonging to group AB has no agglutinin in his blood serum, he can *as a rule* receive blood safely from persons belonging to any of the other three groups. Persons belonging to this group, therefore, have been called "universal recipients."

It has been pointed out, however, that the terms "universal donor" and "universal recipient" may be dangerously misleading. To be on the safe side, blood of the same group to which the recipient belongs is employed in whole-blood transfusions unless it is unobtainable and the emergency does not brook delay.

GROUP	AGGLUTINOGEN IN RED CELLS	AGGLUTININ IN SERUM
A B	A AND B	NONE
A	A	ANTI - B
B	B	ANTI - A
O	NONE	ANTI - A AND ANTI - B

FIG. 28. The four major blood groups.

The Rh Factor. In 1940, shortly before his death, Dr. Landsteiner and his coworker, Dr. Alexander S. Wiener, reported the discovery of another blood factor which they named the Rh factor because they first identified it in the blood of rhesus monkeys. This hereditary factor is attached to the red cells of approximately 85 per cent of white persons regardless of blood group. These persons are called Rh-positive. The 15 per cent who do not possess it are said to be Rh-negative. The Rh factor is important clinically because of its antigenic activity. That is, it has the power to stimulate the development of anti-Rh antibodies (agglutinins) in the serum of Rh-negative blood.

At least 11 separate antigenic members of the Rh family have been identified since its discovery, and a great deal of detailed information regarding the inheritance of the Rh antigens has become available. The commonly used terms "Rh-positive" and "Rh-negative," however, refer to the presence or absence of one antigen only (the D antigen) because it is clinically the most important factor.

Rh-negative individuals may become sensitized to Rh-positive blood in two different ways. The first way is by whole-blood transfusion. If the blood of an Rh-positive donor is transfused into an Rh-negative recipient, the development of Rh antibodies may be stimulated in the blood serum of the recipient. If an Rh-negative individual who has been sensitized in this way should be transfused later on with Rh-positive blood, the Rh antibodies in his serum will agglutinate and dissolve the red cells in the donated blood. It has been made an invariable rule, therefore, never to give Rh-negative persons Rh-positive blood by transfusion.

The second method of sensitization may take place during pregnancy, when the unborn child of an Rh-negative mother has inherited the Rh-positive factor from his father. In that case, the Rh factor in the child's blood may stimulate the development of Rh antibodies in the mother's blood. If that happens, the Rh antibodies in the mother's blood may clump the Rh-positive red cells in the child's blood. As a result the child may be born dead (stillborn) or born with erythroblastosis, a blood disease of the newborn in which the red cells are damaged. This "accident" seldom happens, as only about 1 in 50 Rh-negative mothers will become sensitized even if the unborn baby is Rh-positive.

It is now possible to be prepared for approaching trouble by testing pregnant women and their husbands for the Rh factor. If it is found that the husband is Rh-positive and the wife Rh-negative, and the wife shows evidence of sensitization during pregnancy, the physician will be ready to exchange part of the newborn baby's blood for blood from an Rh-negative donor. As exchange transfusions will temporarily make the child Rh-negative, the Rh antibodies in his blood serum can no longer hurt him. Later the baby makes his own fresh Rh-positive blood and becomes an Rh-positive individual.

BLOOD DISORDERS

Blood does so many things for us, as it courses through the body on its rapid rounds from the heart and back to it, that any change in its own composition or in the freight or passengers it normally transports has significance from a health point of view. Information regarding such changes can be gained only by submitting a blood specimen to various types of laboratory examination, depending upon what the physician wishes to find out.

Teachers, parents, and other lay observers have no means of checking up on the condition of the blood, but they may be of service in getting medical attention for children who show persistent changes in skin color (see Observing Cutaneous Deviations from Normal, in Chap. 7) or easy fatigability or some other possible indication of a deviation from normal in the composition of the blood. The more common disorders in which such changes occur are described here.

The Anemias

It sometimes happens that the balance between the death rate and the birth rate in the red-cell population is tipped one way or another. The number of red cells turned out by the red-cell factories in red bone marrow may be below normal; or the number of red cells destroyed or lost from the circulation (as in hemorrhage) may be above normal; or the quality of the red cells may be below standard—for example, too large or too small or deficient in hemoglobin. When any of these things happens the capacity for transporting oxygen to the tissues is inadequate.

Anemia means literally "bloodless" (Greek *an,* meaning "not," plus *haima,* "blood"). Any disease in which the red-cell population, or the quality of its individual members, is adversely affected may be characterized by anemia.

The many different types of anemia fall roughly into two broad classifications: (*a*) anemias in which the red cells are abnormally large and contain an abnormally large amount of hemoglobin; and (*b*) anemias in which the red cells are abnormally small or normal in size but deficient in hemoglobin. Anemias in the first class include pernicious anemia and other anemias which are caused by anything that interferes with the normal manufacture of red cells in the red-cell factories. These anemias are very rarely found in school children. Anemias in the second class include those caused by a deficiency of iron and other blood-building substances (the so-called "nutritional anemias"). Iron-deficiency anemia is fairly common in infancy, early childhood, and about the age of puberty.

Examination of a blood specimen is the only sure way of telling whether a child is anemic and, if so, which one of the manifold forms of anemia is present.

The Leukemias

The name leukemia means literally "white blood." It was invented about a century ago by Rudolph Virchow, a famous German pathologist, who found some cases in which the blood had turned white as a result of the replacement of red cells by white ones.

Actually, cases of leukemia in which this phenomenon occurs are extremely rare. In many, however, the blood is paler than normal, because the wild uncontrolled overgrowth of the white blood cells crowds out the red cells and eventually destroys their manufacturing centers and those of the blood platelets as well.

There are several different types of leukemia, but they are all characterized by runaway growth of the white cells. For this reason leukemia is sometimes referred to as cancer of the blood. Largely because of the decrease in deaths from the communicable diseases of childhood, leukemia (classified under cancer) has advanced to second place in the ranks of the leading causes of death in the school ages (ages five to nineteen). It is one of the diseases for which there is as yet no cure. However, it is being studied intensively with good hope that some day some group of workers will "hit the jackpot."

Changes in Skin Color Associated with Blood Disorders

Pallor. In the popular mind pallor [2] is so often associated with anemia that it is tempting to think or say of any persistently pale child that he is "anemic." As a matter of fact, the color of the blood may be normal, greatly reduced, or raised, according to the type of anemia from which an individual is suffering.

It is chiefly in the nutritional anemias, especially those caused by iron deficiency, that the blood is paler than usual. The low color index of the blood is due partly to the smaller size of the red cells and partly to the fact that each red cell has received less than its normal quota of pigment. The iron deficiency responsible may result from not getting enough iron in the diet or from defective absorption of iron from the food.

One form of nutritional anemia, once very common in girls and young women, is called chlorosis ("green sickness") because of the peculiar greenish pallor of the skin which characterizes it. A favorite explanation of green sickness, before its true nature was discovered a few decades ago, was "love-sickness" (*mal d'amour* or febris amatoria). No less than 15 paintings by seventeenth-century Dutch painters were on this theme. Garrison points out that in these canvases "the representation of the pallor and feverish discomfort of the greensick lovelorn maidens is very life-like." [3] Chlorosis is now very rare, not, one surmises, because the course of young love runs smoother, but rather because the diets of young maidens are now much better than they were one or two generations ago.

While pallor is frequently misleading as an indication that anemia is present or, if so, in what degree it exists, its presence is a valuable diagnostic aid to the physician. The history of its onset as obtained from parents is occasionally vague and unsatisfactory, especially in the chronic forms of anemia. Physiological adjustments in chronic anemia may be

[2] Pallor is also associated with constriction of the surface blood vessels. Withdrawal of blood from the surface blood vessels takes place under all circumstances in which the body must conserve blood to carry on the vital activities of its internal organs. This explains the pallor in extensive hemorrhage, in shock, and in fainting. See also Normal Temporary Changes in Skin Color, in Chap. 7.

[3] GARRISON, FIELDING H., "An Introduction to the History of Medicine," 3d ed., pp. 304–305, Saunders, Philadelphia, 1924.

so efficient that physical activity can be carried out for long periods of time with a decidedly lowered hemoglobin level. Hence, a teacher who observes that a child is beginning to look paler than usual and seems tired or generally not up to par will be doing that child a great service by referring him for a medical examination.

Purpura. Purpura is the term applied to the formation of purple patches on the skin and mucous membrane. These patches are caused by spontaneous bleeding beneath the skin (subcutaneous hemorrhage) or mucous membrane (submucous hemorrhage). The purplish spots may be small (petechiae) or large. They gradually pass through the color changes characteristic of a bruise (see Skin Injuries, in Chap. 7). Purpura occurs in many widely different diseases and conditions. Hence it is considered as a symptom rather than a disease in itself.

Subcutaneous hemorrhages are features of scurvy, leukemia, and certain anemias. Also, they may follow infections or poisoning with various toxic agents (snake venoms, for example). One type of purpura (purpura hemorrhagica) is associated with a great reduction in the number of blood platelets (see The Blood Platelets, above) in circulation.

Needless to say, the appearance of purplish spots in the skin or mucous membrane should be immediately reported to the nurse or physician.

TISSUE FLUID

The cells that form the tissues of the body are water dwellers. They must be surrounded by fluid or they would surely dry up and die. Even the living tissues that must of necessity be in contact with the air are all kept moist. You see the lines you are now reading, for example, through a film of salty water covering the living "windows" of your eyes. The fluid that occupies all the cracks and crannies between the closely packed cells is lymph. It drifts slowly in thin streams like sea water in wet sand until it enters the lymph vessels, which empty it into the blood stream.

Fluid Interchanges between the Blood and the Tissues

Tissue fluid, or lymph, and all other special body fluids come from blood plasma. The hydraulic (water) pressure of the blood within the capillaries tends to squeeze fluid out of the capillaries. Too steady a seepage, however, not only would deplete the water content of the blood but also would swell and waterlog the tissues. The counterforce that keeps this from happening ordinarily is osmotic pressure.

Osmotic pressure may be simply defined as the drawing force that salt, sugar, and many other substances dissolved in water exert upon the water molecules when water and a solution of any of these substances are separated by a semipermeable membrane. Here you see water separated from a solution of sugar by such a membrane:

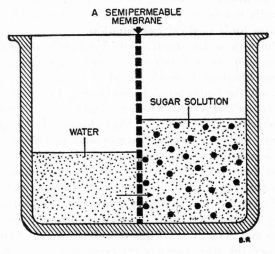

The water molecules (represented by small dots) can pass through this membrane into the sugar solution, but the sugar molecules (represented by large dots) cannot pass into the water. However, the sugar molecules exert a force which attracts, or draws, the water molecules across the semipermeable membrane into the sugar solution. As a result, the volume of the sugar solution increases and its pressure rises. This pressure is called osmotic pressure.

The blood plasma inside the capillaries contains in solution more protein particles than are contained in the tissue fluid outside the capillaries. As a result, the protein particles exert a drawing force which tends to draw water into the blood stream through the semipermeable capillary walls. Thus a nice balance is achieved between the hydraulic pressure tending to force water out of the capillaries and the osmotic pressure tending to draw it in.

Edema. Edema, which literally means "swelling," is the term applied to an excessive accumulation of fluid in the tissue spaces. The old-fashioned name for it is dropsy, which literally means "water." Edema occurs when the balance between the inward and outward flow of fluid through the capillary walls is upset. Among the possible causes of edema are (*a*) an abnormally low concentration of protein particles in the plasma as a result of kidney disease (see The Kidneys, in Chap. 6); (*b*) a rise in the pressure of blood in the capillaries which takes place when the blood flow is abnormally slow because of a weakened heart muscle; (*c*) increased permeability of the capillary walls as a result of bacterial toxins or other injurious agents; and (d) obstruction of the lymph channels.

It is important to remember that shifts in tissue fluid take place constantly in health. Just standing up for a long time, for example, may make the legs or ankles swell, because of an increase in the amount of fluid outside the blood vessels. However, any persistent swelling of the legs and ankles or of any other part of the body open to observation indicates the need for medical attention.

The Lymphatics

Fluid does not normally collect in stagnant lakes in the tissues. It is kept moving slowly in thin streams by the rhythmical pressure of working muscles and also by the currents set up by the constant shifting of tissue

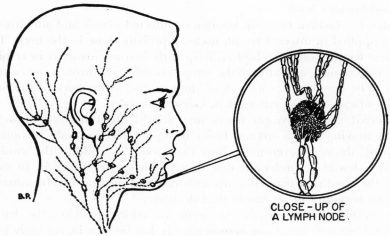

CLOSE-UP OF
A LYMPH NODE

FIG. 29. Lymph vessels and nodes in the face and neck.

fluid out of and into the blood stream through the capillary walls. These sluggish streams eventually enter channels of their own which drain directly into the blood stream. The lymph channels are called the lymphatics, or lymph-vessel system. The lymph capillaries originate as tiny blind tubes in the tissues in the close neighborhood of the blood capillaries. They converge to ever-larger vessels with ever-thicker walls. Through these vessels the tissue fluid drifts eventually into two large lymph vessels draining into veins of the blood-vessel system.

The Lymph Nodes. The lymph-vessel route is also the one chosen for removing from the tissues all sorts of foreign particles, including bacteria. Tiny ductless glands, called lymph nodes, are placed at intervals along the course of the lymph vessels to filter out these foreign particles. One of the most amazing features of the lymphatic system is the rapidity with which even large-sized particles can travel from the blood stream or the tissues into the lymph vessels. The mechanism of such a transit is wholly mysterious. However it is managed, little or no foreign material that reaches the tissues either through the blood capillaries or by accidental entrance from without fails to pass into the lymph vessels and on into the lymph nodes.

The lymph nodes act as very effective filters. On passing into a lymph node from an incoming lymph vessel, lymph spreads out in a relatively large umbrella-shaped lake where the rate of flow at once becomes exceedingly slow. Thus there is every opportunity for the settling of bacteria or other small particles. In this water trap, so to speak, bacteria become an easy prey for the phagocytes in the lymph nodes.

Infected Lymph Glands

Adenitis (Swollen Glands). Swollen or infected glands and adenitis are terms applied to infected lymph nodes, especially those in the neck. The cervical lymph nodes in children frequently become involved in respiratory infections, especially colds, streptococcal sore throat, and scarlet fever. The lymph nodes in back of the ears and at the back of the neck nearly always become enlarged in German measles.

Infected cervical lymph nodes may steadily feed bacteria into the slowly moving lymph stream. From being a filter the node becomes a cesspool, draining eventually into the blood. A child with "swollen glands" should be under the care of a physician (see Plate 5). In some cases the condition may clear up with rest and medication. In others it may be necessary to set up surgical drainage.

Infectious Mononucleosis. An acute infection involving the lymph glands, known as infectious mononucleosis, has become increasingly common in recent years. Its incidence is greatest among children and young adults. Epidemics are most frequently recognized in schools and institutions for children.

The cause of infectious mononucleosis is unknown, but a virus is suspected. One form, commonly called "glandular fever," is characterized by fever and enlargement of the lymph glands (especially those at the back of the neck) and the spleen. Glandular fever is common in children. Another form in which the physical signs are fever and sore throat with or without lymphatic gland involvement is common in older children and adults.

A great variety of unusual manifestations occur often enough in infectious mononucleosis to make doctors keep it in mind when confronted with any fever of unknown origin. A diagnosis can be made only by the laboratory examination of blood samples.

Although there is no specific remedy for the disease, most cases end with complete recovery. Serious complications may arise, however, particularly if the central nervous system becomes involved in the infection.

Tuberculosis of the Cervical Lymph Glands. Early in the twentieth century, tuberculosis of the cervical lymph glands was a fairly common form of tuberculosis among young children. The tubercle bacillus responsible for most of the tuberculosis of these glands (and of bones and joints as well) is the bovine type. By far the most important source of bovine-type infections in human beings is raw milk from tuberculous cattle. With the adoption and enforcement of laws requiring the pasteurization of milk sold in large cities and the progress made in detecting tuberculous cattle and eliminating them from dairy herds, tuberculosis of the cervical lymph glands in children has become exceedingly rare in our country.

Tonsils and Adenoids

Tonsils are olive-shaped masses composed mainly of lymphoid tissue and covered with mucous membrane. They contain various crypts and many lymph follicles. It is believed that they act as sources for the supply of phagocytes to the mouth and throat which destroy bacteria entering the mouth. However, this function is not a vital one, as we can get along quite well without tonsils.

One tonsil stands guard between the pillars (folds of mucous membrane) on each side of the passage leading from the mouth to the pharynx (Fig. 38). Another mass of lymphoid tissue known as the pharyngeal tonsil is normally present in the nasopharynx between the openings of the eustachian tubes. Overgrowth of the pharyngeal tonsil is popularly called "adenoids" (adenoid means "resembling a gland"). The tonsils, located as they are at the portal of entry from the mouth to the throat, are exposed to frequent mass attack by bacteria. As a result they often become infected, especially in childhood, when they are larger than in maturity. Adenoids also are practically a childhood monopoly. The pharyngeal tonsil normally is much larger in children than in adults, and frequently becomes abnormally enlarged or infected, with consequent blocking of the throat openings of the nose and eustachian tubes.

Selection of Children in Need of Operations. The recorded observations of teachers and nurses are of the greatest help to physicians in making decisions when there is doubt as to the advisability of removing tonsils and adenoids. A history of recurrent colds, earache or discharge from the ears, frequent sore throats, or swollen glands have direct bearing on the problem. The child's manner and appearance also are significant. Persistent mouth breathing (almost the sign manual of the adenoidal child), mannerisms suggesting hearing loss (see Hearing Right and Hearing Wrong, in Chap. 8), easy fatigability, slowness in gaining weight, and listlessness are among the signs that the examining physician will wish to consider in interpreting his physical findings.

Prevention and Treatment. In the past few years significant advances have been made in both the prevention and the treatment of chronically infected tonsils and adenoids. The use of chemotherapeutic and antibiotic drugs in clearing up acute bacterial infections of the ear, nose, and throat has been of great help in prevention. As for treatment, there is no question but that the surgical removal of chronically infected tonsils and adenoids results in great physical improvement in most children. Infection of this lymphoid tissue plays a major role in the causation of some loss of hearing and many acute and chronic infections throughout the respiratory tract. Adenoid tissue can be satisfactorily and permanently removed by the use of radium. Irradiation in very small doses shrinks the adenoid tissue so that it finally disappears, leaving a smooth mucous-membrane covering over the nasopharynx, not unlike that which lines the nose.

WHAT TO DO IN CASE OF CIRCULATORY EMERGENCIES

Shock, external bleeding, and fainting are the principal circulatory emergencies with which the teacher may have to deal while the doctor, nurse, or someone trained in first aid is being summoned.

Shock

Shock is a condition associated with stagnation of the blood in the capillaries, principally in those in the organs of the abdomen, and the automatic reduction of the amount of blood in circulation. It may occur as a result of loss of blood, of damage to the tissues as in a severe burn or other injury, or of the effects of pain or strong emotion on the nervous system.

Practically all the signs of shock are produced by the reduction in the amount of blood circulating in the tissues and the resulting radical cut in their oxygen supply. These signs vary with the cause and degree of shock. Usually the face is pale and the skin cold and clammy. Breathing is rapid and shallow and the pulse rate rapid. The injured person acts dull and listless.

To prevent shock or lessen its severity, the following measures should be taken when any child (or older person) is severely injured:

1. Keep the child lying down, quiet, and comfortably warm with coats, blankets, or newspapers over and under him.
2. Control bleeding if it is present (see Bleeding from an External Wound, below) and support, splint, or otherwise protect injured limbs (see Broken Limbs, in Chap. 9).

3. Give warm sweetened drinks if the child is fully conscious and has no abdominal injury.
4. Relieve pain and allay fear as much as possible. If the child must be moved, see that this is done gently and skillfully.

Bleeding from an External Wound

It is customary to classify bleeding from a wound as arterial, venous, or capillary. In bleeding from an artery the blood is scarlet and flows in quick spurts, which keep time with the beats of the heart. In bleeding from a vein the blood is dark red and flows in a sluggish stream or wells up in the wound. When capillaries are cut, the blood flows briskly from points all over the injured area. As a matter of fact, it is very seldom that bleeding occurs from one type of blood vessel alone. A severe wound usually bleeds from capillaries, veins, and arteries at the same time.

Pressure Bandage. All bleeding should be stopped as soon as possible. The simplest method is to place a compress (a pad of sterile gauze, a clean handkerchief, or other clean cloth) over the wound and fasten it tightly in place by means of a bandage or adhesive tape. If this pressure bandage, as it is called, does not stop the bleeding, hand pressure applied directly over the compress may stop it. If the bleeding is from an arm or leg, elevating the limb may help to control the bleeding.

Pressure Points. If bleeding is severe, indicating that a major artery has been cut, or if it does not stop in 5 minutes after applying pressure over the wound, it may be controlled by pressing upon the appropriate pressure point. Pressure points are points on the body at or near the point where an artery crosses a bone. Pressure must be made at the pressure point nearest the wound between the wound and the heart (Figs. 30–35).

Tourniquet. A tourniquet (Fig. 36) should be applied only for severe life-threatening hemorrhage which cannot be stopped by other means. It is placed close to, but not at the edge of, the wound between the wound and the heart. After the tourniquet has been applied tightly enough to control bleeding it should not be released, except by a physician, no matter how long it has been in place.

Nosebleed

Bleeding from the nose is a common occurrence among school children. It may happen spontaneously without apparent cause, or it may result from a blow on the nose. "Bloody noses" and "black eyes" are popularly interpreted as almost sure indications that a child has been in a fight. Recurrent nosebleeds without apparent cause should always be reported

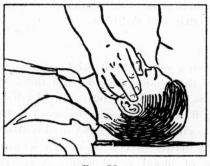

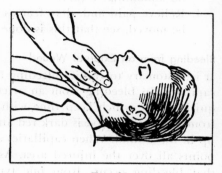

FIG. 30.   FIG. 31.

FIG. 30. Bleeding of the head above the eyes. Press with the index and middle fingers just in front of the ear. (*Figs. 30–36 from "First Aid," Metropolitan Life Insurance Company.*)

FIG. 31. Bleeding of the cheek below the eyes. Press in the notch on the side of the jawbone which is 1 to 1½ inches in front of the angle of the jaw.

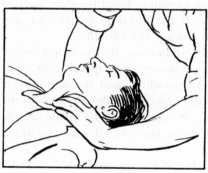

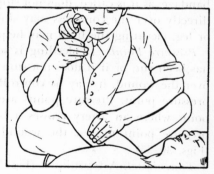

FIG. 32.   FIG. 33.

FIG. 32. Bleeding from the neck or throat. Place your thumb against the back of the victim's neck and your fingers in the depression at the side of the windpipe (not over it), with one finger above the wound and one finger below it. Press the fingers and thumb toward each other.

FIG. 33. Bleeding from the lower two-thirds of the arm and from the hand. Place your fingers halfway between armpit and elbow, on the inside of the arm, and press fingers and thumb toward each other with the arm bone between. (If the arm is fat, place your hand underneath it.)

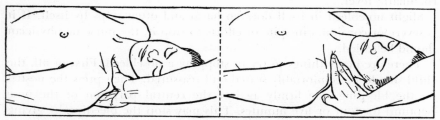

FIG. 34. Bleeding from the shoulder, armpit, and upper part of arm. Place your thumb or fingers in the hollow behind the victim's collarbone, and press against the upper surface of the first rib.

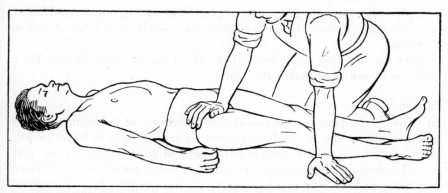

FIG. 35. Bleeding from the thigh, leg, or foot. Place the heel of your hand just below the victim's groin at the point indicated, and press downward.

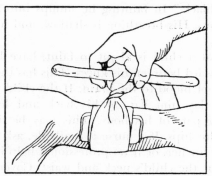

FIG. 36. How to apply a tourniquet to the arm.

to the physician serving the school, as they are one of the indications of rheumatic fever.

Slight nosebleed in itself does no harm and often stops by itself. If it is severe or continues in spite of efforts to stop it, the nurse or physician should be called.

There are many things to try in stopping a nosebleed. First of all, the child should be comfortably seated and reassured. Then press the nostril on the bleeding side firmly against the central partition of the nose (septum) for four or five minutes. This may stop the bleeding by giving an opportunity for a clot to form. Also placing a little pad of soft paper or cloth under the upper lip and pressing with the fingers laid across the lip may stop the bleeding by compressing the anterior (front) blood vessels of the nose.

If these measures do not work, apply cloths wrung out of cold water over the nose. It may also help to plug the nostril with a bit of cotton or gauze.

After the bleeding stops, instruct the child not to blow his nose for a while so as not to dislodge the clot.

Fainting

In fainting the person loses consciousness because of a lessening of the blood supply to the brain. Besides strong emotion such as fright or joy, other common causes of fainting are want of food, fatigue, pain, prolonged standing, and exposure to an overheated room. Some children may faint at the sight of blood or as a consequence of even a trivial injury. The face of a person about to faint gets very pale because of the constriction of the surface blood vessels, and perspiration usually breaks out on his forehead. He may say that he feels dizzy and weak, or that "everything looks black." In fainting he slumps into a chair or falls to the floor unconscious. His breathing is shallow, and his pulse weak and slow.

If you notice that a child is about to faint, have him sit down and thrust his head forward between his knees. This has the effect of improving the circulation of blood to the brain. If the child does not improve, or actually faints, lay him flat on his back and lower his head by elevating the lower part of his body. This may be done by placing a folded coat under his hips. If a nurse is available, ask someone to notify her. While waiting for her, or if no professional help is available, loosen tight clothing about the child's neck and waist. Cover him warmly and see that he gets plenty of fresh, moving air. Open a window or fan him. Also it may help to sprinkle cold water on his face.

Usually a victim of fainting revives in a very short time. After he regains consciousness he should lie still for a while in a quiet place. If aromatic spirits of ammonia is on hand, he may be given half a tea-spoonful in water.

If a fainting attack lasts for more than a few minutes, keep the child covered warmly and summon a physician at once. Any child who is subject to fainting spells should be referred for medical attention.

DISEASES SPREAD BY BLOOD-SUCKING INSECTS

The parasites responsible for several infectious diseases depend upon blood-sucking insects for their passage from host to host, and in some species for the completion of their life cycles. The most important insect-borne disease problems in our country are malaria, endemic typhus, and spotted fever.

The information given below and in Table 6 regarding these three diseases is for the use of teachers who live in areas where one or more of them are prevalent. These teachers and their students are often called upon to assist in the public health measures required for the control of insect-borne diseases. Also teachers may be of service in helping students and their families to learn about the things they can do for their own protection. Children who live in regions where the bites of possibly infected insects are a known hazard should have the benefit of the careful supervision required both for the prevention of infection and for the early recognition of indications of infection.

Malaria

Malaria is caused by any one of four different species of *Sporozoa* of the genus *Plasmodium*. *Sporozoa* belong to a class of parasites which repro-duce by forming spores. The *Sporozoa* of malaria spend part of their life cycle in mosquitoes of the genus *Anopheles* and part in the blood stream of human hosts.

About a week after entering the human blood stream, the parasites invade the red blood cells. The destruction of the invaded red cells as a result of the growth and development within them of the parasites is responsible for the periodic attacks of "chills and fever" characteristic of malaria. As large numbers of red cells cannot be destroyed time and again without causing anemia (see Blood Disorders, above), repeated attacks of malaria leave a person pale, tired, and often too weak to work. Children particularly suffer badly from malaria. They often become thin and pale, do not grow as they should, and have to miss a good deal of time from school.

Methods of Control. Malaria can be controlled—even wiped out—by getting rid of anopheles mosquitoes. This has been proved in the south-ern United States, where malaria has been reduced to a minimal public health problem. The methods chosen for destroying anopheles mos-

Table 6. THREE COMMUNICABLE DISEASES SPREAD BY BLOOD-SUCKING INSECTS

	Malaria	Endemic typhus	Spotted fever
Cause.	Any one of four species of malarial parasites (Sporozoa) of the genus Plasmodium.	Rickettsia prowazekii.	Rickettsia rickettsii.
How spread.	By the bite of infected anopheline mosquitoes. The mosquito is infected by biting someone who has malaria when the sexual forms of the malarial parasites are present in the blood. After going through certain changes in the mosquito's body for 10 to 14 days (21 days for the quartan type) the parasites appear in the mosquito's salivary glands ready to be injected into the blood stream of every person bitten thereafter.	By the bite of infected rat fleas commonly of the species Xenopsylla cheopis. The fleas are infected by biting rats suffering from the disease. Infected black rats (Rattus rattus) and infected brown rats (Rattus norvegicus) are the chief reservoirs of infection.	By the bite of infected ticks or contact of the unbroken skin with crushed infected ticks. In the East and South, the tick carrier of spotted fever is the dog tick (Dermacentor variabilis); in the Northwest, the wood tick (Dermacentor andersoni); in the Southwest, occasionally the lone-star tick (Amblyomma americanum). Even in highly endemic areas only about one out of every 200 to 300 ticks is infected.
Incubation period.	Varies with the species of infecting plasmodium; 14 days for the most common variety.	From 6 to 14 days; usually 12 days.	From 3 to about 10 days.
Character of the attack	Abrupt onset, with a shaking chill followed by a burning fever accompanied by severe aching, thirst, and nausea. A few hours later a drenching sweat sets in and the	Abrupt onset, with fever, chills, headache, and prostration. The fever rises rather rapidly for three or four days and then continues for 14 days, rarely for more	Abrupt onset, with chills, fever, severe headache, muscle and joint pains, and sleeplessness. About three or four days after the fever begins a pinkish skin rash

	fever goes down. Then there is a fever-free interval before the next episode. The variety of malarial parasite present in the blood determines whether the chills and fever recur every day, every other day, every third day, or at irregular intervals. Treatment with the appropriate antimalarial drug usually reduces the number of episodes of chills and fever. Without treatment the episodes may continue for some time before the attack runs its course.	than 16 days. On about the fifth day a skin eruption of small, pink or bright red spots develops. It usually begins with a few spots on the abdomen or on the inner surfaces of the forearms and within 24 hours becomes scattered. It seldom involves the face. Early treatment with the appropriate antibiotic usually shortens the course of the disease.	appears. The individual spots, which give the disease its name, are small and distinct and usually break out first on the ankles, wrists, forehead, palms of the hands, and soles of the feet, whence they spread rapidly over the entire body. Early treatment with the proper antibiotic usually shortens the course of the disease.
Prevalence..........	All over the world in tropical and semitropical regions.	World-wide in areas where man and rats occupy the same buildings. Most prevalent during summer months.	Occurs widely throughout the United States in the spring and early summer when the adult ticks become active.
Resistance..........	Individuals vary in their ability to resist malaria. Some may have light attacks with no chills and fever—just a dull, tired feeling. Others may have malaria parasites in their blood without feeling ill at all. Such persons act as malaria carriers. Relative immunity to the infecting species of Plasmodium (but not to other species) is usually acquired after repeated attacks.	No one is naturally resistant. Immunity (which is not always lasting) follows an attack.	No one is naturally resistant. Immunity (which may or may not be lasting) follows an attack.

quitoes and reducing their opportunities to breed depend on the particular species found in the locality. All anopheles mosquitoes do not have the same habits. Local public health officials know what methods are best for their areas.

Where it is difficult or impossible to wipe out anopheles mosquitoes in a locality, good results in controlling malaria can be obtained by screening homes and spraying both living quarters and outbuildings on farms with the appropriate insecticide (for example, DDT).

Education of the people regarding malaria and its anopheline carriers helps to gain their cooperation in taking the appropriate protective measures. Anopheles mosquitoes usually bite only after dark and prefer to have their victims sleeping or sitting quietly. People who live in malarious areas can usually avoid the disease by mosquitoproofing their homes and staying in them after dark as much as possible, and by using an insect repellent when it is necessary to remain out of doors after sundown. Suppressive drugs are available for preventing attacks in persons in malarious areas who are unable to protect themselves from the bites of anopheline mosquitoes.

Keeping persons who have malaria from passing on the parasites is another important part of malaria control. A child in school should be referred to the nurse or physician whenever malaria is even suspected. A simple blood test indicates whether there are malaria parasites in the blood, and if so, what type they are. The physician can then prescribe the treatment that will be most effective. Several newly developed antimalarial drugs are giving high rates of cure.

Typhus Fever

There are two kinds of typhus, one endemic, the other epidemic. A disease dubbed "endemic" is a disease that has a low incidence but is constantly present in a given locality. An epidemic disease, on the other hand, attacks many people at the same time but is only occasionally present in a given locality.

Both epidemic typhus and endemic typhus are caused by a species of bacterialike microorganisms called rickettsiae. They get their name from Howard Taylor Ricketts, the young American doctor who first described them in 1909 in his studies of Rocky Mountain spotted fever, another rickettsial infection (see Spotted Fever, below).

The rickettsiae that cause epidemic typhus are spread by lice, mainly body lice, which have fed upon infected persons. Prior to modern methods of control, epidemics were frequent among military and refugee populations and in areas suffering famine or war.

Endemic typhus is a much milder disease than its close relative, epidemic typhus. The great majority of persons who contract it recover completely. Primarily it is a disease of rats. For that reason it is sometimes called murine typhus, from *mus*, the Latin word for "rat." The rickettsiae causing it are carried from rat to rat and from rat to man by rat fleas that have become infected by biting a rat suffering from the disease. It cannot be transferred directly from person to person.

Endemic typhus originally occurred in the United States only in seaport cities along the southern and southeastern coasts. However, there has been a gradual spread to rural areas. The highest attack rates are in the Gulf and South Atlantic seaboard states.

Methods of Control. Active immunization with rickettsial vaccine is used to protect laboratory and field workers engaged in typhus work. However, it is not practical to protect persons generally from endemic typhus. Its prevention depends upon getting rid of rats or, if that is not possible, upon spraying rat runs, burrows, and harborages with insecticides or other agents for killing rat fleas.

In a community where typhus has become a serious problem, the public health authorities may launch a rat-control program, including the extermination of living rats, a cleanup of rat-infested premises, and the ratproofing of buildings. Such a program may involve an entire town or large sections of a town or city. Teachers and their students have often helped in this important work.

Spotted Fever

This serious rickettsial disease is transmitted by ticks. Although it is now known to occur widely throughout the United States, it was first recognized in the mountain states, particularly in Montana and Idaho. For that reason it is usually called Rocky Mountain spotted fever.

The infection is passed from generation to generation in ticks. The ticks probably become infected in the larval stage by feeding upon infected wild rodents. Adult female ticks hibernate during the winter months and do not become active until the first warm days of spring. They lay their eggs in the late spring and early summer after a meal of blood, and then die. That accounts for the fact that spotted fever is limited to the spring and summer months.

Once attached to an animal or human host, a tick may feed for several days. A blood meal seems to make the spotted-fever organisms increasingly active and virulent.

Methods of Control. In areas highly infested with ticks, a vaccine is available for immunizing persons most likely to be infected. For the general population the avoidance of tick bites is the only practicable means of prevention. The simplest means of avoiding tick bites is to stay out of underbrush and tall grass in tick-infested localities during the tick season. Some insect repellents are of value against ticks.

The dog tick is by far the most common carrier of spotted fever in the East. Families that keep dogs in Eastern tick-infested areas should take special precautions to avoid infection. The dogs should be examined periodically for ticks and the ticks carefully removed as described below.

Since spotted fever is usually not transmitted until an infected tick has been feeding for several hours, careful search for attached ticks and their prompt removal reduces the risk of infection.

Children in tick-infested localities who travel through wooded areas, underbrush, or tall grass on the way to school, or who belong to families that own dogs, or who have access to dogs, should be looked over carefully for ticks upon arrival in school. Their parents should be urged to do this at the end of the day. It is especially important to examine the nape of the neck and the scalp. The tick has a small-toothed probe on its head. In attaching itself to the skin of its victim it sinks in its probe and hangs on. The trick in removing ticks is to avoid crushing them with the bare hands and to make sure that the probe does not break off and remain embedded in the flesh.

Ticks should be removed with tweezers or with a bit of cotton or paper held between the fingers. The insect may be induced to withdraw its probe by holding the hot tip of a needle or knife near its rear end. After the tick has been removed, the tick bite should be painted with an antiseptic, such as iodine, and the tick itself should be burned or flushed down the drain.

If an engorged tick is crushed accidentally between the fingers, its contents should be washed thoroughly from the skin with alcohol or soap and water. This is important because it is possible to contract spotted fever by getting the blood or excreta of an infected tick on the skin.

DO YOU KNOW?

1. If you were given the task of labeling a "road map" of the circulation, where would you find and how would you label

    a. The points of arrival and departure for the round trip of blood through the body?

    b. The points of arrival and departure for the round trip of blood through the lungs?

    c. The highroads leading away from the heart?

    d. The highroads leading toward the heart?

    e. The loading stations where supplies for the tissues are delivered to the blood?

    f. The unloading stations where wastes from the tissues are removed from the blood?

g. The stations en route where supplies are delivered to, and wastes removed from, the tissues?

2. If you were on a hunting trip through the body, in which of the places named after each quarry should you expect to find it:

   a. Hemoglobin: phagocytes, erythrocytes, blood platelets
   b. Gamma globulin: blood plasma, spleen, red bone marrow
   c. Carbon dioxide: arterial blood, venous blood, serum albumin
   d. Trapped bacteria: lymph vessels, tissue fluid, lymph nodes
   e. Heart murmurs: auricles, heart valves, ventricles

3. Match each disease or condition listed in the box with the word or phrase below the box which you associate with it.

Nutritional anemia	Adenitis
Malaria	Cyanosis
Hypertension	Hemophilia
Rheumatic fever	Purpura
Shock	Endemic typhus
Spotted fever	Edema

Ticks
Swollen lymph glands
Streptococcal infections
Rat fleas
Tightened-up arterioles
Failure of blood to clot
   normally

Stagnation of blood in
   capillaries
Subcutaneous hemorrhage
Iron deficiency
Anopheline mosquitoes
Accumulation of fluid in
   tissue spaces
"Blue babies"

SUGGESTED ACTIVITIES

1. Arrange to have a physician demonstrate to the class the methods he uses to check up on the condition of a child's heart and how he measures blood pressure. Invite the child's parents to be present. In connection with the demonstration some students may be interested to look up and report to the class the histories of the stethoscope and sphygmomanometer.

2. If possible have a member, or committee, of the class visit:

    a. A cardiac clinic, to observe and report methods of examining the heart in children referred for possible heart trouble.

    b. A Red Cross blood center or mobile unit for collecting blood, to observe and report the methods used to collect blood and to obtain information on other phases of the American Red Cross National Blood Program. In connection with the report of this trip, it would be interesting to have reports from other students on the stories of blood transfusion, blood grouping, and blood fractionation.

3. Perform the following experiments to determine (*a*) the effect that size and age have on the rate of the heartbeat; and (*b*) the effect of activity on the rate of the heartbeat.

    a. Have each student in the class take the pulse of a baby, a child of three, a child of ten, a youth of fifteen, an adult of twenty-five, an adult of fifty, an adult of seventy. (Select subjects of approximately these ages, if necessary.) Have each subject sit quietly (reading, listening to soft music, or engaged in some other quiet occupation) for 15 or 20 minutes before you take the pulse. This is the resting pulse rate. Have a committee use the figures obtained by each member of the class to construct a table or graph showing the average resting pulse rate per minute in babyhood, early childhood, elementary school age, adolescence, early maturity, middle age, and old age.

    b. Have each student take the pulse of his or her ten-year-old subject when at rest, studying, standing up, after exercising hard, when excited, and after a meal. Construct tables or graphs to show the effect of activity and emotional state on the heartbeat. Explain these variations.

4. Have pairs of students demonstrate interviews between teacher and nurse in which sets of signs and symptoms suggestive of rheumatic fever, nutritional anemia, infectious mononucleosis, and chronically infected tonsils and adenoids are discussed with reference to particular children. Have the rest of the class guess which condition is indicated in each case.

5. Have demonstrations in class of the first-aid procedures to be followed to prevent shock following an injury; to stop bleeding by applying pressure at the appropriate pressure point; to stop a nosebleed; and to revive a child who has fainted.

SELECTED REFERENCES

AMERICAN MEDICAL ASSOCIATION: *Wonder Stories of the Human Machine: The Engine (Heart)*, Chicago, 1948. (Pamphlet 4 in a series explaining how the principal organs of the body work.)

AMERICAN NATIONAL RED CROSS: *The Story of Blood*, rev. ed. Washington, D.C., 1951. (A pamphlet describing the composition and functions of blood and the medical uses of blood and its derivatives.)

BLAKESLEE, HOWARD: *Know Your Heart*, Public Affairs Pamphlet No. 137, New York, Public Affairs Committee, reprinted 1955.

CABOT, B.: *Motion of the Heart;* the story of cardiovascular research, New York, Harper & Brothers, 1954.

GLYNN, JOHN H.: *Story of Blood*, New York, A. A. Wyn, Inc., 1948. (An interesting account of the nature and properties of human blood.)

MARVIN, H. M., T. DUCKETT JONES, IRVINE H. PAGE, DAVID D. RUTSTEIN, and IRVING S. WRIGHT: *You and Your Heart; A Clinic for Laymen on the Heart and Circulation*, New York, Random House, Inc., 1950.

YAHRAES, HERBERT: *Rheumatic Fever—Childhood's Greatest Enemy*, Public Affairs Pamphlet No. 126, rev. ed. New York, Public Affairs Committee, 1955.

ZINSSER, HANS: *Rats, Lice and History*, Boston, Little, Brown & Company, 1935. (A classic "biography" of typhus by a distinguished bacteriologist.)

Organizations

American Heart Association

American National Red Cross (National Blood Program)

Chapter 5   ON THE AIR ROUTE

The Respiratory Passages
Respiratory Infections in General
Respiratory Infections in Particular
Respiratory Allergies
The School and Respiratory-disease Control
What to Do in Respiratory Emergency
Speech Difficulties

THE RESPIRATORY PASSAGES

Of all the natural portals of entry into the body, the respiratory tract is the one most open to infection. Reference has already been made to the fact that colds and other infections of the breathing passages are the most common causes of illness among school children. A brief sketch of the plan and defensive arrangements of the air route into the body is given here to help teachers visualize the terrain, so to speak, of this most important beachhead.

The respiratory tract is the arrangement evolved for meeting the body's need for oxygen from the surrounding atmosphere and for removing from the body the waste gas (carbon dioxide) produced by the body's use of oxygen. Its plan is quite simple.

The Respiratory Tree

Air containing oxygen passes through an air-conditioning system (the nose) and enters what may be visualized as a hollow upside-down tree (the respiratory tree). The trunk of this tree is the windpipe. After passing through the windpipe, the air spreads out through its hollow branches (the bronchial tubes) and comes to a stop in the tiny blind air sacs (alveoli) at the ends of the hollow twigs (bronchioles).

A fine network of capillaries surrounds the alveoli, or air sacs. It is through the double partition represented by the exceedingly thin alveolar and capillary walls that the continuous, rhythmic exchange of oxygen and carbon dioxide between the air in the lungs and the blood in the capillaries takes place.

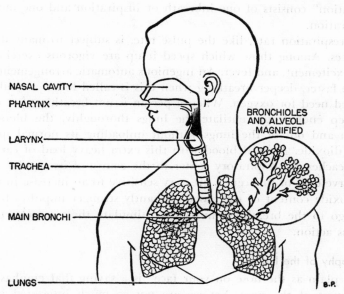

NASAL CAVITY
PHARYNX
LARYNX
TRACHEA
MAIN BRONCHI
LUNGS

BRONCHIOLES
AND ALVEOLI
MAGNIFIED

B.P.

FIG. 37. The respiratory tree.

The Mechanics of Respiration

The mechanics of respiration is also quite simple. It is based primarily upon the increase and decrease in the size of the chest cavity brought about by the action of the great muscle (the diaphragm) which forms the floor of the chest and the ceiling of the abdomen and of the muscles in the chest walls. When the chest is expanded during inspiration, air rushes into the elastic lungs, which stretch out fanwise to occupy the extra space made available. When the capacity of the chest is made smaller during expiration, the air is literally squeezed out of the lungs by the pressure of the rising floor and inward-moving walls of the chest. The elastic alveolar walls, by recoiling during expiration, also help to drive out the air.

Nervous Control of Respiration

Breathing is essentially an involuntary act. We can hold the breath for only so long and then we are forced to resume breathing.

The respiratory center that controls the breathing muscles is a group of nerve cells located in the lowest portion of the brain (the medulla oblongata). Breathing stops automatically when the respiratory center is put out of commission as in electric shock, for example, or in bulbar poliomyelitis.

The rate of breathing is also controlled by the respiratory center. One "respiration" consists of one inbreath or inspiration and one outbreath or expiration.

The respiration rate, like the pulse rate, is subject to many different influences. Among those which speed it up are vigorous exercise, emotional excitement, and fever. An ingenious automatic arrangement makes possible faster, deeper breathing when this is called for as a result of an increased need for oxygen. When a person is not breathing fast enough and deep enough to ventilate the lungs thoroughly, the blood flows through and out of the lungs without unloading its normal quota of carbon dioxide. Arterial blood with this extra heavy load of carbon dioxide reaches the respiratory center in the course of its regular rounds. The nerve cells of this center are very sensitive to an increase in the carbon dioxide content of the blood. Instantly stronger impulses from the center go to the breathing muscles to stimulate these muscles to more vigorous action.

Topography of the Nose

"It's as plain as the nose on your face" is a saying that emphasizes the obviousness of the nose. Yet we are not so much interested in noses from the outside as in what goes on inside. The primary function of the nose is to act as an air-conditioning system. It is especially designed to warm, moisten, and filter the air in the first stage of its journey to the lungs.

The nose is designed to permit inhaled air to spread out over as large an area as possible in flowing through it. Structural features that help to increase the nasal area exposed to inhaled air include (a) the division of the nose lengthwise into two nostrils by a wall, or septum, of bone and cartilage; (b) the extension from the side walls of the nose into the nasal cavity of three shelves, or ledges, of bone called the turbinates; and (c) cavities called sinuses in the bone of the skull and face which lead into the nasal cavity through very small openings.

A Busy Traffic Circle

The pharynx, or throat, is something like a traffic circle into which several different routes open. The posterior, or back, portion of the nostrils leads into the upper part of the pharynx. This meeting place of nose and throat is called the nasopharynx. The throat openings of the eustachian tubes, which lead to the middle chambers of the ears, are located near the throat openings of the nostrils. The lower portion of the pharynx communicates with the mouth above and with the esophagus, or food pipe, and the larynx, or voice box, below.

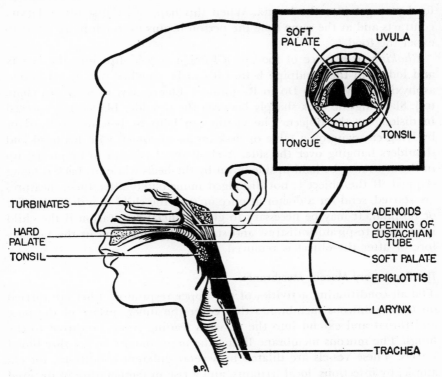

Fig. 38. Important points along the air route through the nose and pharynx, with an inset showing the location of the tonsils.

The Voice Box

The larynx, or voice box, is an oblong hollow organ composed of cartilage, muscles, and ligaments which connects the lower part of the pharynx with the trachea, or windpipe (see Fig. 38). Hence it forms an integral part of the passage through which air is carried to and from the lungs. One of the cartilages of the larynx projects forward and in boys and men may be quite prominent. It is called the Adam's apple.

During the act of swallowing, a muscle raises the larynx so that its opening is brought under the shelter of the epiglottis and the root of the tongue. This keeps food from "going down the wrong way" into the larynx and on into the trachea instead of into the food pipe (esophagus). It was once believed that the epiglottis snapped down to make a sloping lid for the larynx when food and drink were being swallowed. However, this structure stands erect, like a screen, and the food slides over its back surface into the food pipe. If the larynx is not lifted quickly enough during swallowing to bring its opening under the shelter of the epiglottis, food may get into the larynx. When this happens, the sensitive larynx contracts and at the same time the person begins to cough in an effort to expel the food.

Choking. If a piece of food or a foreign object slips into the larynx and lodges in the windpipe before it can be coughed out, it may cause asphyxia (see What to Do in Respiratory Emergency, later in this chapter). Slapping the back sharply between the shoulder blades may succeed in dislodging the object. The victim can help by bending forward or by lying crosswise on a table or desk on his abdomen with his head and shoulders hanging over the side. A child small enough to be picked up in the arms may be held upside down by the heels while his back is being slapped. If the object is not dislodged immediately after these measures are started, send for a doctor at once or rush the child to a doctor's office or hospital. It may be necessary to give artificial respiration if the child is in great respiratory distress and starts to become blue in the face before or after the object is removed.

The Respiratory Mucous Membranes

The air-conditioning activities of the upper respiratory tract are carried on by the mucous membranes that cover the inner surface of the nose and throat and extend into the passages leading from the throat to the lungs. The mucous membrane lining the nose contains many tiny blood vessels. These vessels are dilated by several different conditions, for example, by infections, local irritants, and a rise in temperature of inspired air. As a result, the mucous membrane swells and the air passages are narrowed. Cool air and certain drugs (adrenaline and ephedrine) contract the blood vessels.

Normally the respiratory mucous membranes are covered with a blanket of mucus—a sticky, slightly antiseptic fluid secreted by mucous glands—which warms, moistens, and cleans air entering the nose. Tiny whiplike extensions of special cells in the membranes, called cilia, keep this mucous blanket on the move from the back of the nose downward to the throat and from the windpipe and bronchial tubes in the lungs upward to the throat.

The Cilial Escalator. The moving mucous blanket with its propulsive force supplied by the cilia has often been called the "cilial escalator." Always riding on the escalator down to the throat from the nose and up to the throat from the lungs are the stray germs, dirt, and other foreign particles inhaled at every breath and normally caught and held in the sticky mucous blanket. Those which fall off in the throat are disposed of by being swallowed or coughed out.

The respiratory mucous membranes play a most important part in both the background and the foreground of the respiratory-infection picture. In the transfer of airborne infections they act as the reservoirs from which the causative agents are expelled into the air. And they provide a formidable barrier against the invasion of the tissues by virulent invading bacteria and viruses. The mucous membrane of the nasopharynx is never sterile. Whatever visitors from outside come to rest in the nose, the windpipe, or the bronchial tubes are eventually passed by the cilial escalator to the nasopharynx.

RESPIRATORY INFECTIONS IN GENERAL

Many different kinds of bacteria find the moist, warm, dark nasopharynx a congenial place in which to settle down. They make up the normal but constantly changing flora of the nasopharynx. Ordinarily, they do not cause trouble. But into this innocuous bacterial garden—or culture medium—come the virulent transient visitors—the pneumococci, streptococci, bacilli, and viruses. Their fate depends upon their numbers and the conditions they find. They may be disposed of before they penetrate the mucous-membrane barrier by being swallowed or by being sent forth in coughing, sneezing, talking, and laughing on aerial expeditions to other throats. Or they may be able to stage a successful invasion, that is, to produce the disease of which they are the causative agents.

The Causative Agents of Respiratory Infections

Viruses. Viruses are responsible for the most common diseases which are spread by discharges from the mouth and nose—notably the common cold, influenza, virus pneumonia, measles, German measles, chickenpox, and mumps.

All viruses are the most simply constructed of living things. They are so simple, in fact, that they lack wholly or in part the facilities for making the substances essential to their continued existence from the raw materials provided by their hosts. As a result, viruses must live right inside the cells of the host so that they can extract these substances from the cells which have the facilities for their manufacture.

One particular advantage possessed by viruses, which is extremely disadvantageous for us, is their relative immunity from attack by chemicals and antibiotics.[1] The sulfa drugs and penicillin, for example, destroy bacteria and spirochetes by making it impossible for these parasites to obtain from their hosts, or to utilize, one or more of the materials essen-

[1] An antibiotic is a specific product of one microorganism which has an injurious effect upon another microorganism. Penicillin, for example, is a product of a mold (*Penicillium notatum*) which has an injurious effect upon a wide variety of bacteria and other infective agents. Other well-known antibiotics are Aureomycin, streptomycin, polymyxin, Chloromycetin, and Terramycin.

tial to life and growth. But a virus cannot make use of these materials, even when they are available, without the help of the cells. This means that it cannot be attacked by depriving it of powers it never had. Therefore, it is the cells themselves that must be acted on in such a way as to keep them from working to synthesize certain essential substances for the virus.

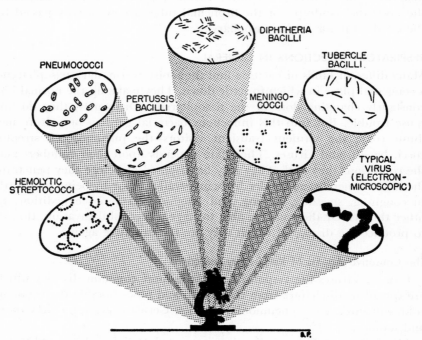

FIG. 39. Microscopic pictures of the principal causative agents of respiratory infections.

Very little success has been obtained so far in attempts to find specific remedies for virus infections. However, chemotherapy (treatment of a disease by chemicals) is in a boom period, and there is reason to believe that substances may shortly be found that will prove as effective in fighting viruses as are the sulfa drugs and certain antibiotics in fighting bacteria and protozoa. Aureomycin was the first drug of promise to be discovered. This antibiotic and one or two others are proving to be helpful in the treatment of several virus or viruslike infections, including "virus" pneumonia.

Pneumococci. Pneumococci (Greek *pneumon,* meaning "lung," plus *coccos,* meaning "berry") are lancet-shaped bacteria which usually occur in pairs and are surrounded by definite capsules. They get their name from the fact that they are responsible for about 90 per cent of all cases of lobar pneumonia. A great many specific types, or strains, of pneumococci have been discovered. Type-specific pneumococci are frequently found in the nasopharynx of healthy persons. They cause pneumonia only when certain conditions permit them to increase in numbers and invade the lungs (see Pneumonia, further on). In addition to pneumonia, pneumococci may produce other infections, particularly sinus infections and middle-ear infections.

Streptococci. Streptococci (Greek *streptos,* meaning "twisted," plus *coccos,* meaning "berry") are spherical bacteria that occur in chains like strings of beads. They belong to one of the largest families of disease-causing bacteria. In addition to an innumerable variety of local lesions, including boils (see Skin Infections, in Chap. 7) and wound infections, they are responsible for epidemic diseases such as scarlet fever, streptococcal sore throat, and erysipelas, and important infections such as blood poisoning and puerperal fever. Doctors look upon the streptococcus as a potential Jack-of-all-trades, capable of attacking in many different ways.

The grave systemic symptoms that so often accompany streptococcal infections, even mild local lesions, are produced by powerful poisons. The two in which we are most interested here are (*a*) hemolysins, which partly or completely hemolyze red blood corpuscles (that is, set free their hemoglobin), and (*b*) erythrogenic toxins, which produce a red skin rash. The term "erythrogenic" is built up of two Greek words meaning "red" and "to originate."

Streptococci that produce complete hemolysis of blood cells belong to the species known as *Streptococcus hemolyticus.* These streptococci are the chief offenders in acute streptococcal infections of the respiratory tract.

Bacilli. Bacilli are bacteria shaped like little rods. The most common respiratory infections caused by bacilli are diphtheria, whooping cough, and pulmonary tuberculosis. Diphtheria bacilli lodge and multiply in the nasopharynx, but the powerful toxin that they produce is absorbed by the body and causes systemic intoxication, or general poisoning. Whooping-cough bacilli grow in and on the mucous membranes of the respiratory tract, where they do their chief damage.

The tubercle bacillus (*Mycobacterium tuberculosis*) is the specific cause of all forms of tuberculosis. There are several individual types of tubercle bacilli, but the only two that are important from the human point of view are the human type and the bovine type. Human-type tubercle bacilli are responsible for the vast majority of all cases of the disease of the lungs known as pulmonary tuberculosis.

Resistance to Respiratory Infection

The strong local resistance of the respiratory mucous membranes and good general physiological resistance constitute our best defense against many germ invaders of the nose and throat. Other things being equal, children in good health stand a better chance of resisting colds and other respiratory infections than do children whose natural defense forces have been weakened by substandard health. There are several ways in which the local resistance of the mucous membranes may be upset.

Fatigue. Various experimenters have shown that physical exhaustion may render an experimental animal susceptible to disease-causing (pathogenic) germs to which it is ordinarily highly resistant. Similarly, studies on human beings have shown that fatigue may make a person temporarily susceptible to colds. Exactly what combination of causative factors makes it possible for fatigue to lower resistance to infection is not known.

Malnutrition. It is not yet known just how malnutrition in general lowers resistance, although there is no doubt that it does. Many studies have been made on the role of specific nutrients in maintaining good resistance. It has been demonstrated that vitamin A, for example, is required for upholding the integrity of the mucous membranes of the body, which are our first line of defense against bacterial invasion. Recently it has been shown that adequate protein is essential in maintaining the mechanism of resistance because this nutritional element is necessary for building up the protein substance (gamma globulin) in the blood plasma which carries the antibodies developed to fight disease-causing germs.

Chilling. The local cellular resistance of the respiratory mucous membranes may be temporarily upset by the adjustments associated with abrupt changes in temperature and perhaps with other atmospheric changes, such as those of humidity or air pressure. The fact that these adjustments are most frequently made necessary in the colder seasons and coincide with the congregation of large groups of people indoors (thus increasing chances of exposure to airborne germs) accounts for the marked seasonal fluctuation in the prevalence of respiratory infections.

A "cold" (in England, called a "chill") gets its name from the fact that chilling of the body has long been associated with catching cold. Chilling may be brought on by sitting around with wet feet, exposure to drafts, cooling off too quickly when overheated, or wearing unsuitable clothing in cold or wet weather.

So far as the nasal mucous membranes are concerned, chilling causes reactions which change the consistency of this important barrier to infection. Cold makes the surface of the blood vessels shrink, thus reducing the blood supply to these membranes. And cold also slows down or stops the action of the cilia responsible for keeping the mucous blanket with its freight of germs on the move toward its dumping ground in the nasopharynx. Normally, the healthy nose has a new mucous blanket about once every 10 minutes over its posterior, or back, portion and once every hour or two over its anterior, or front, portion. Halting the cilial escalator makes it more difficult to dispose of stray organisms. Hence, they may accumulate and be given an opportunity to multiply and mobilize. Since the resistance of the mucous membranes depends upon their ability to prevent the massing and combining of hostile germs, it is easy to see that any chance for team play on the part of the invaders tends to interfere with the resistance of the mucous membranes and to break it down.

Virus Activity. Another way in which the resistance of the mucous membranes may be lowered is by the activity of viruses. The nature of this activity is not known with certainty. However, it is logical to suppose that theft of essential vital materials from the cells of the mucous membranes by the robber viruses may impair, if not actually destroy, the cells. The depletion of the cells may make them a better culture medium for pathogenic bacteria. Whether this is the true explanation or not, it is an established clinical fact that an initial virus invasion sets up a beachhead for a secondary bacterial invasion of the respiratory tract.

Mechanism of Signs and Symptoms

The extreme sensitivity of the respiratory mucous membranes to the activity of viruses and bacteria readily accounts for the early signs and symptoms characteristic of the most common respiratory infections. In an acute cold, for example, the blood vessels of the nose swell to accommodate extra blood. As a result, the air passages are obstructed, the normal drainage openings are swollen shut, and the nose feels stuffed up. Also the irritated membranes of the nose and throat feel sore and scratchy. To get rid of the virus both the flushing action of mucus and the mechanical action of coughing and sneezing are employed. It is the greatly increased secretion of mucus that makes the nose (and sometimes the eyes) water. The irritation of the sensitive nose lining is responsible for the sneezing. And the tickling of the throat and windpipe linings by the activities of the virus and by the postnasal drippings of excess mucus causes the coughing.

RESPIRATORY INFECTIONS IN PARTICULAR

The bare facts about common respiratory diseases and other diseases spread by discharges from the respiratory tract are given in Tables 7A

	Chickenpox (varicella)	German measles (rubella)	Measles (rubeola)
Cause.......	A virus; present in discharges from the mouth and nose and in discharges from vesicles on the skin.	A virus; present in discharges from the mouth and possibly the nose.	A virus; present in discharges from the mouth and nose.
How spread...	By direct and indirect contact.* Very contagious.	By direct and indirect contact.* Very contagious.	By direct and indirect contact.* Very contagious.
Incubation period	From 14 to 16 days (occasionally as long as 21 days).	From 10 to 21 days; usually about 18 days.	About 10 days to onset of fever, 13 to 15 days to appearance of rash.
Onset........	Mild constitutional symptoms, slight fever, loss of appetite.	Symptoms of mild cold; slight fever; sore throat.	Slight fever; red, watery, puffy eyes; signs of cold with tight hacking cough.
Site of eruption	Scalp and trunk; less abundant on arms and legs.	Scalp, sides of face, arms and hands, spreading rapidly over entire body.	Behind ears, on forehead or cheeks, then downward over body and limbs.
Character of eruption	Begins to appear about 24 hours after early signs. Successive crops of rose-pink spots which change into vesicles and finally to crusts. Each crop completes its course in from 2 to 4 days.	Minute, rosy, itching papules giving appearance of rose-colored rash. Lasts for about 1 to 3 days.	Begins to appear 3 or 4 days after onset. Red spots which collect in large red blotches and usually itch. Ordinarily lasts about 5 days. Peeling in the form of fine, branlike flakes.
Period of communicability	From 1 day before onset to about 6 days after appearance of first crop of blisters.	From onset of symptoms of a cold to from 4 to 7 days. Exact period uncertain.	About 9 days (from 4 days before rash appears to 5 days afterwards).
Ages and seasons of greatest prevalence	Most common among children less than 15 years. Winter and spring.	Most common among children but fairly frequent in adults. Winter and spring.	Chiefly children from 5 to 14 years but common also in those less than 5. Winter and spring.
Methods of control	No specific preventive. Exclusion from school during period of communicability. Immunity usual after one attack.	No specific preventive. Immunity usual after one attack.	Gamma globulin obtained from pooled adult blood plasma may be given within 3 days after exposure to give temporary protection or to make the attack less severe. Isolation during period of communicability. Immunity usual after one attack.

Source: principally "Control of Communicable Diseases in Man," 8th ed., American Public Health Association, New York, 1955, and "Common Childhood Diseases," rev. ed., Metropolitan Life Insurance Company, New York, 1954.

* Direct contact means directly from person to person. Indirect contact means indirectly through handling, eating, or drinking anything soiled by discharges from the sick person or carrier.

Meningococcal meningitis	Scarlet fever (scarlatina)	Smallpox (variola)
The meningococcus (Neisseria meningitidis); present in discharges from the mouth and nose.	Group A hemolytic streptococci of several strains; † present in discharges from the mouth and nose and from ears, lymph nodes, etc., if affected.	A virus; present in the sores (pocks) on the skin and mucous membranes lining body openings (and so in discharges from the mouth, nose, bowels, and bladder).
By direct and indirect contact.* Carriers are important sources of infection during epidemics. Attack rate very low in those exposed.	By direct and indirect contact.* Floor dust, lint from bedding or clothing, and contaminated milk or other food may be important sources of infection.	By direct and indirect contact.* (Except for short distances, transmission through the air unlikely.) Very contagious.
From 2 to 10 days; usually 7 days.	From 2 to 5 days.	From 7 to 16 days, commonly 12, rarely 21.
Usually sudden in severe cases with chills, fever, malaise, muscle pains, intense headache, and often vomiting.	Lassitude, restlessness, followed by sore throat and fever.	Chills, intense headache, severe pains in back, vomiting, rapid pulse, quick rise in temperature.
When present, scattered over body.	Neck and chest, then over most of the body.	Face and limbs; less abundant on trunk.
Purpuric spots on skin in a small percentage of sporadic cases and in the majority of cases during epidemics. The purpuric spots are followed by small, bright red spots, which in 12 to 24 hours become successively dark red, purple, and finally blue black.	Little flat red points, close together. Under white coating on tongue red spots appear, and gradually tongue assumes a bright red color (strawberry tongue). Usually peeling begins in second week and lasts 2 or 3 weeks.	Begins to appear from 1 to 5 days after early signs. Red spots on skin which change first to blisters and then to typical smallpox pustules. Crusts form over the pustules and fall off in from 10 to 40 days. In severe cases, pitted scars, or pock marks, are left after the crusts fall off.
For as long as meningococci are present in the nasopharynx.	Uncertain. Usually from first symptoms to complete recovery (about 14 days) or until all discharges have ceased.	From first symptoms until all scabs and crusts have disappeared. Most contagious in early stages.
Between epidemics, cases most common in children; during epidemics, severe cases most common in young adults.	Children and adults; children less than 10 years, especially less than 5, most susceptible.	Children and adults, especially adult males. Occurs in epidemics where vaccination is not enforced.
Winter and spring.	Late winter and spring.	Winter.
Administration of sulfadiazine eliminates meningococci from nasopharynx of convalescents and carriers.

Isolation for 14 days or until nasopharynx is free of meningococci.

Duration of immunity after an attack, unknown. | Under certain conditions, sulfa drugs or penicillin to protect exposed persons (see Scarlet Fever, further on).

Penicillin may be used to shorten the attack and reduce the period of communicability.

Isolation during period of communicability (usually 2 weeks).

Boiling or pasteurization of milk.

Immunity to rash-producing toxin usually after one attack.‡ | Active immunization with smallpox vaccine (see Immunization Timetable, in Chap. 3).

Isolation during period of communicability.

Immunity usual after one attack. |

† Some of these strains produce a toxin which causes scarlatina (scarlet fever with rash) or scarlet fever without a rash. Other strains produce only infections of the nose and throat (streptococcal sore throat). See Acute Streptococcal Infections of the Respiratory Tract, further on, and Table 7B.

‡ In some cases rheumatic fever or acute glomerular nephritis develops after recovery from the acute attack.

Table 7B. COMMUNICABLE DISEASES SPREAD BY DISCHARGES FROM THE RESPIRATORY TRACT, NOT CHARACTERIZED BY A SKIN ERUPTION

	Diphtheria	Mumps (infectious parotitis)	Streptococcal sore throat †	Whooping cough (pertussis)
Cause.........	The diphtheria bacillus (Corynebacterium diphtheriae) present in discharges from the nose and throat, open wounds, etc.	A virus; present in the saliva of an infected person.	Several strains of Group A hemolytic streptococci; present in discharges from the nose and throat, and from ears, lymph nodes, etc., if affected.	Pertussis bacillus; present in discharges from the nose and mouth.
How spread....	By direct and indirect contact.* Contaminated milk or milk products and healthy carriers of the bacillus are important sources of infection.	By direct and indirect contact.* Less contagious than other common communicable diseases of childhood.	By direct and indirect contact.* Explosive milk-borne epidemics are usually called "septic sore throat." Carriers are important sources of infection.	By direct and indirect contact.*
Incubation period	Usually from 2 to 5 days, but occasionally longer.	From 12 to 26 days; average 18 days.	From 2 to 5 days.	From 7 to 10 days; not more than 21 days.
Onset.........	Sore throat and slight fever; possibly mild constitutional symptoms.	Moderate fever and congestion of upper respiratory tract followed by swelling of the salivary glands.	Sudden, with sore throat and fever, accompanied by muscle soreness, headache, and nausea.	Slow with catarrhal symptoms and tight dry cough. Cough becomes paroxysmal within 1 to 2 weeks after onset.
Period of communicability	For as long as the bacilli are present in the throat; usually for 2 weeks or less, rarely for more than 4 weeks.	Uncertain. Probably from 1 or 2 days before onset of symptoms until swelling of affected salivary glands subsides.	Uncertain. Usually from first symptoms to complete recovery (about 14 days) or until all discharges have ceased.	From early catarrhal stage to about 3 weeks after onset of typical spasmodic cough.
Character of the infection	The bacilli grow on the mucous membranes of the nose and throat and produce a powerful toxin which is absorbed by the	The virus attacks the salivary glands, especially the parotids, causing swelling and tenderness of the glands and mild constitu-	The streptococci grow on the mucous membranes of the tonsils and pharynx and produce a toxin which is absorbed by the	The bacilli grow on the mucous membranes of the respiratory tract and produce thick, ropy, sticky bronchial secretions which

body, resulting in systemic poisoning. Often a dirty white false membrane is formed locally by the action of the bacilli; this may block the breathing passages and cause suffocation.	tional symptoms. After puberty the testes (in boys) and the ovaries (in girls) may become involved.	body and causes constitutional symptoms.	are expelled with great difficulty. The violent repetitive coughing is characterized by a sudden inspiratory "crow" or "whoop."
Ages and seasons of greatest prevalence Most common among children less than 10 years of age. Fall and winter.	Chiefly children and young adults; less prevalent than other common childhood diseases. Winter and spring.	Children and adults. Late winter and spring.	Chiefly children less than 7 years of age. Variable but mostly in spring.
Methods of control Active immunization with diphtheria toxoid (see Immunization Timetable in Chap. 3). Passive (temporary) immunization with an antibiotic or diphtheria antitoxin for exposed children who have not been actively immunized. Isolation required until 2 cultures obtained from nose and throat at intervals of 24 hours show that no diphtheria bacilli are present. Immunity often, but not always, develops after one attack.	Gamma globulin from mumps convalescent serum or diethylstilbestrol reduces chances of sex-gland involvement after puberty. Isolation until the swelling of the salivary glands has disappeared. Immunity usual after one attack, but second attacks are not rare.	Sulfa drugs or antibiotics may be used to shorten the attack and reduce the period of communicability. Isolation required during period of communicability (usually 2 weeks). Boiling or pasteurization of milk. Immunity from infecting strain of streptococcus may develop but not from other strains.	Active immunization with whooping cough vaccine (see Immunization Timetable, in Chap. 3). Immune serums are available for giving passive (temporary) immunity to exposed susceptible children and for making cases lighter. Separation of infected child from other children (especially those under 5), and exclusion from school and public places. Immunity usual after one attack.

Source: principally "Control of Communicable Diseases in Man," 8th ed., American Public Health Association, New York, 1955, and "Common Childhood Diseases," rev. ed., Metropolitan Life Insurance Company, New York, 1954.

* Direct contact means directly from person to person. Indirect contact means indirectly through handling, eating, or drinking anything soiled by discharges from the sick person or carrier.

† See also footnotes under scarlet fever, Table 7A, and Acute Streptococcal Infections of the Respiratory Tract, further on.

and 7B. In addition, teachers may find it helpful to have fuller information about several of the more important current respiratory-disease problems and the progress now being made in solving them.

The Common Cold and Its Hangers-on

Its Virus Cause. There seems to be little doubt now that the cause of a plain cold in the head is a virus. Although it is possible to see some viruses with the help of the electron microscope, the cold virus has never yet "had its picture taken." Also, because all viruses lack the metabolic machinery to make them self-sustaining, it has not been possible to cultivate cold virus on ordinary culture media. To grow it, it must be inoculated within living animals or on living tissue. Current research on colds is being carried forward with the help of human volunteers. In one series of experiments conducted by investigators of the National Institutes of Health (United States Public Health Service), the nasal washings of persons infected with the common cold were collected within 24 hours of the first appearance of symptoms. These washings were treated chemically in such a way as to remove bacteria without destroying any virus that might be present. The washings were then sprayed into the noses of human volunteers. When they came down with colds, certain strains of the virus recovered from their nasal washings produced less severe symptoms than those obtained from the original contributors. The results of these experiments indicate either that there is a difference in susceptibility to the cold virus or that the virus under certain conditions becomes weakened. If it proves possible to weaken the virus in laboratory experiments, then effective vaccination against colds may become a reality.

Progress in Treatment. Although no drug of any kind has been found which attacks the cold virus itself, there is no doubt that chemotherapeutic agents are of great value in preventing or curing the secondary infections that so often follow in the wake of colds. As we have seen, the activity of viruses weakens the defense mechanisms of healthy mucous membrane, thereby setting up favorable conditions for the moving in and multiplication of a wide variety of bacteria. Many of these secondary bacterial invaders are highly susceptible to the action of the sulfonamides and penicillin. For that reason the worst depredation of the bacterial allies of a cold can often be avoided, or at least checked before much harm is done, by the prophylactic or therapeutic use of these drugs.

Chronic Colds (Catarrh). A common secondary infection is the cold that "hangs on." An ordinary viral cold clears up in a few days. Long-continued colds are characterized by the secretion of a thick yellowish mixture of mucus from the mucous glands and pus produced in the fight with bacteria that are ordinarily present in too small numbers to cause trouble. They are often accompanied by a persistent cough, which is caused by the continual or frequent dripping of mucopus from the back of the nose into the throat.

Sinusitis. A sinus infection in acute or chronic form is usually characterized by pain or soreness in the cheeks or over the eyes. Sometimes the teeth may ache. The severe pain of acute sinusitis is caused by the pressure of pus which accumulates in one or more of the sinuses, when these air-containing spaces are invaded by pus-producing germs from the nasal

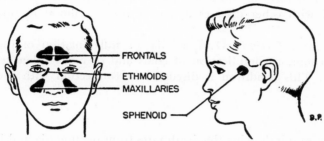

FRONTALS
ETHMOIDS
MAXILLARIES
SPHENOID

FIG. 40. The nasal sinuses.

cavity. The sinuses most often affected are the frontals above the eyes and the maxillaries on each side of the nose in the upper jawbone.

As the openings leading from the sinuses into the nose are very narrow, they frequently swell shut when the mucous membranes lining the sinuses are inflamed. The pain and soreness persist until drainage is reestablished either by natural subsidence of the infection or by medical treatment.

A child who complains of headache, pain or soreness in the cheeks or above or behind the eyes, or of aching teeth when he has a cold should always be referred to the physician or nurse, as neglect of acute sinusitis may lead to chronic sinusitis. A head cold that "hangs on" or repeated attacks of head colds, particularly when they are accompanied by a dull headache or pain or soreness over the affected sinus, are signs that chronic sinus disease may be present.

Bronchitis. Acute bronchitis is an inflammation of the bronchial tubes. It may develop independently, but usually it extends from an upper-respiratory-tract infection, such as a head cold or influenza. Acute bronchitis most commonly starts with laryngitis, that is, inflammation of the larynx, or voice box, which is located near the top of the windpipe. The chief characteristic of laryngitis is hoarseness. As the infection progresses downward into the bronchial tubes there is usually a feeling of tightness and heaviness in the chest, accompanied by wheezing and a dry cough which later becomes loose.

Acute bronchitis is commonly referred to as a "chest cold" or a "cold in the chest." In the beginning it may or may not be accompanied by fever. If the temperature is normal, the child may not feel ill. Yet it is extremely important to see that a child gets medical attention at the first signs of a chest cold, as the bronchial infection may prepare the way for pneumonia.

Chronic bronchitis may follow repeated attacks of acute bronchitis. However, this form of bronchitis affects old people chiefly, and is often associated with other diseases and conditions common in middle and old age.

Middle-ear Infections. Otitis media, or inflammation of the middle ear, is a common complication of colds and of many other respiratory infections. This condition is discussed in connection with the ear (in Chap. 8).

Influenza

In any line graph showing the death rates from pneumonia and influenza, during the first half of the twentieth century, the observer is struck by a sharp peak which abruptly rises and as abruptly drops within the short period of 3 years (from 1917 to 1919). This is the indelible imprint of the influenza pandemic of that period. A pandemic is a world-wide epidemic. Influenza is an interesting disease historically, because it made such a deep and lasting impression upon the generations of mankind whom it visited that we have the records of pandemics as far back as 1580.

Since the 1918–1919 pandemic, the long-term trend of the death rate from influenza has been sharply downward (see Fig. 41). Although fluctuations in mortality have continued to occur, the peaks have definitely become lower. However, this virus disease continues to be an important medical and public health problem. It still causes widespread illness and heavy loss of time from school and work, particularly in years when epidemics occur.

The Search for a Vaccine. Continuous and extensive research is being conducted on influenza, mainly with the object of developing an effective vaccine. It is now known that this disease is caused by a family of viruses which are more or less closely related. This relationship presumably goes back to a common virus ancestor which in the course of successive generations has given rise to two distinct types of influenza virus (type A and type B) with several different strains within each type.

The body when invaded by the virus of one strain produces antibodies to fight it. These antibodies remain in the blood for varying lengths of time, but they cannot prevent infections caused by the viruses of other strains. Consequently, the immunity conferred by the presence in the blood of antibodies produced by infection with, or vaccination against,

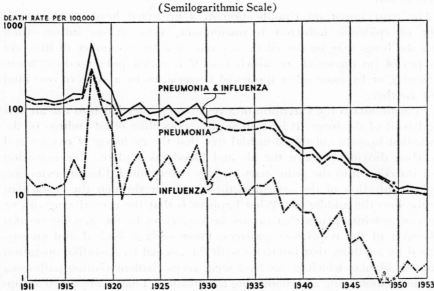

FIG. 41. Mortality from pneumonia and influenza, 1911 to 1953, ages one to seventy-four. (*From Metropolitan Life Insurance Company, Industrial Department.*)

some members of the influenza family of viruses is no guarantee of protection against infection with other members of the family.

The complete control of influenza by vaccination entails the capture of all the different varieties of influenza virus and including them in a vaccine. That is the goal toward which investigators are working. In the meantime the new and improved vaccines now available are giving good results in reducing the incidence of influenza during epidemic seasons. These vaccines are used before an expected epidemic or at once if an epidemic occurs suddenly.

Signs and Symptoms. The symptoms of influenza generally develop within 1 to 3 days following exposure. They include fever, marked tiredness, and aching, especially in the back and limbs. The disease is likely to be accompanied by signs of a cold, sore throat, and bronchitis, and may be complicated with pneumonia. The acute stage lasts, on an average, for from 1 to 5 days, but it may be followed by a period of severe exhaustion. Staying in bed until the doctor says that the danger of complications has passed is exceedingly important.

Pneumonia

The most important complication of a neglected head or chest cold or of epidemic influenza is pneumonia. This serious inflammation of the lungs may be caused by any one of a large number of different types of pneumococci (in which case it is called pneumococcal pneumonia), or by some other species of bacteria, or by a virus of one kind or another.

Pneumonia is the extension of a respiratory infection into the air sacs (alveoli) of the lungs. It is in these tiny, pouchlike blind endings of the smallest branches of the bronchial tree that the exchange of oxygen and carbon dioxide between the air and blood takes place. The extension of infection into the pulmonary air sacs is very much like the extension of an infection of the nose into the sinuses or through the eustachian tube into the middle ear. What happens is that the causative agents, or germs, get into places that cannot be kept clean by the moving mucous blanket of the respiratory passages. Pneumonia is invited and encouraged by anything that interferes with the normal escalatorlike operation of this blanket which, as we have seen, keeps virulent visiting pathogens from accumulating and mobilizing for invasion. That is why the development of pneumonia is so often associated with chilling of the body following exposure to cold and wet, with exhaustion from any cause, or, more especially, with a forerunning attack by the virus of the common cold or influenza virus.

Attack by a virus may prepare the way for bacterial invasion of the lungs, the most common being that staged by the pneumococci. Or the virus itself may extend to the alveoli of the lungs and set up an inflammation in its own right, that is, a lung infection which in recent years has become recognized as virus pneumonia.

Pneumococcal Pneumonia. The classic signs and symptoms of pneumococcal pneumonia are a shaking chill, followed by high fever; sharp pain in the side, chest, or shoulder; cough; difficult breathing; and the raising of sticky, rust-colored sputum.

In recent years sulfa drugs and antibiotics have greatly reduced the death rate from pneumococcal pneumonia (see Fig. 41). Also, combined vaccines are now available for giving a considerable degree of active immunity from the most common types of pneumococcal pneumonia (but not from other forms of pneumonia). The immunity lasts for at least 6 months and probably longer. Immunization may be advisable for groups or individuals for whom pneumonia may be especially serious (the aged and the very young) and for those most in danger of exposure to extremes of temperature, for example, foundry workers and firemen.

Virus Pneumonia. Also called primary atypical pneumonia, this is generally a mild disease, but it can be severe. It develops slowly, beginning in some persons with headache, fever, chilliness, fatigue, and malaise. In other persons it may begin with a cough and sore, dry throat. The principal symptoms are fever and a dry, hacking cough which causes soreness in the chest and abdominal muscles. Later there may be bouts of coughing, and frequently sputum is raised. The acute stage lasts, on an average, from 5 to 7 days, although the fever sometimes continues for several weeks. Recently antibiotics have been used in treatment with encouraging results.

Recurrences of Colds, Influenza, and Pneumonia

One of the conspicuous features of colds, influenza, and pneumonia is their tendency to recur in the same individual. Unlike many other diseases caused by bacteria or viruses, one attack does not confer immunity from further attacks. Vaccines for these diseases cannot be depended on to give protection for more than 6 months at best.

Any child who has more colds than most children do (the average person has at least one or two colds per year) should be brought especially to the attention of the physician who examines the child periodically. Also, a child who is subject to repeated colds or who has once had pneumonia or rheumatic fever should be given the benefit of whatever measures we now possess for controlling respiratory infections. Such measures include education regarding the things the child can do to build up good general health and to keep the respiratory mucous membranes in good condition. In some cases the doctor may prescribe one of the drugs that act to suppress secondary bacterial invaders when the child has a cold.

Acute Streptococcal Infections of the Respiratory Tract

Scarlet Fever and Streptococcal Sore Throat. Numerous strains of Group A hemolytic streptococci produce the erythrogenic toxin which causes a diffuse red skin rash (see The Causative Agents of Respiratory Infections, earlier in this chapter). A person infected with one of these strains who has no immunity to the erythrogenic toxin comes down with scarlet fever. If he possesses immunity to the toxin, but not to the infecting streptococci, he gets streptococcal sore throat without a skin rash. To catch scarlet fever, therefore, it is necessary to be susceptible both to the infecting streptococci and to their erythrogenic toxin.

Immunity to erythrogenic toxin develops within 1 week of the onset of scarlet fever. However, many persons acquire immunity to this toxin without having scarlet fever. Many strains of streptococci produce such small amounts of erythrogenic toxin that they do not cause a skin rash. A person infected with one of these strains has streptococcal sore throat without a skin rash but may—and often does—acquire immunity to the erythrogenic toxin responsible for the rash of scarlet fever. This accounts for the fact that cases of streptococcal sore throat and scarlet fever frequently occur during the same epidemic. Immunity to the infecting type of streptococcus develops, but its duration is unknown. In untreated cases streptococci may be present in the nose and throat discharges for months after recovery. Nasal carriers are particularly likely to contaminate their environment.

For each case of scarlet fever in an epidemic there may be several cases of streptococcal sore throat without a skin rash. If a group of children is exposed to a person with scarlet fever, or a carrier, some will not be affected, some will develop scarlet fever, and others may develop no more than an acute pharyngitis and yet transmit scarlet fever to other susceptible children. Susceptibility to scarlet fever is greatest among children (particularly in the five- to nine-year-old age group) and young adults.

During epidemics of scarlet fever and streptococcal sore throat penicillin may be used to protect intimate contacts and household contacts of a case, those known to have been exposed to contaminated milk or other food, or the whole population group. It is especially important to protect persons in whom recurrent streptococcal infections provide a special risk, such as individuals who have had rheumatic fever or chorea within 5 years or who are under eighteen years of age. When a streptococcal infection occurs in a household which includes someone who has rheumatic fever or who has had rheumatic fever, all members of the family should receive a course of penicillin treatment.

Even in mild cases, scarlet fever and streptococcal sore throat may have serious complications, of which cervical adenitis, otitis media, rheumatic fever, and acute glomerular nephritis are the most common. Various forms of penicillin are used in the treatment of persons sick with scarlet fever or streptococcal sore throat. This treatment serves to lighten the illness, reduce the frequency of complications, and prevent the development of rheumatic fever or acute glomerular nephritis. Adequate treatment with penicillin also eliminates within 24 hours the probability of transmission of the disease from patients or carriers.

Mild Streptococcal Infections of the Nose and Throat. In addition to the epidemic form of streptococcal sore throat, which often occurs concurrently with scarlet fever, relatively mild streptococcal infections of the throat, frequently referred to as tonsillitis or pharyngitis, are common in the winter and spring months in temperate climates. Only the common cold is more common, and sometimes sore throats accompanied by nasal inflammation are loosely called colds. In addition to the actual victims of these nose and throat infections, there are numerous carriers, who have the organisms in their nasopharynges and can spread them but do not themselves become ill. This state of affairs emphasizes the fact that the main reservoir for hemolytic streptococci is the nasopharynx.

The chief danger of mild streptococcal infections of the nose and throat lies in the chance of spreading the infection to children who are particularly sensitive to hemolytic streptococci (see Rheumatic Fever, in Chap. 4) and in the possibility of complications such as middle-ear infection, sinusitis, or adenitis. Children complaining of sore throat with or without cold in the head or other respiratory symptoms should be referred to the nurse or physician serving the school, or sent home by the principal or teacher with an explanatory note to the parents.

Septic Sore Throat. This term is used to describe epidemics of streptococcal sore throat of explosive onset. Generally, such epidemics are caused by the consumption of unpasteurized milk or milk products which have been contaminated with hemolytic streptococci either from the infected udder of a cow or from an infected milk handler. The signs and symptoms resemble those of acute streptococcal sore throat except that the disease is often more virulent and is accompanied by various manifestations of a systemic infection such as high fever and prostration. A scarlatinal rash may or may not be present.

Tuberculosis

Largely owing to the education of the people in ways of preventing the spread of tuberculosis, effective case-finding programs, and the isolation of active cases in special tuberculosis hospitals, pulmonary tuberculosis is much less common than it was at the beginning of the twentieth century. Yet tuberculosis is still causing the death of many school-age children.

In general there are two fundamental types of pulmonary tuberculosis, (a) the primary, or first-infection, type, and (b) the reinfection type.

First-infection Tuberculosis. First-infection tuberculosis takes place when tubercle bacilli invade the body of a person who has never before been infected.

A first infection is most dangerous for babies and young children up to five years of age. The relative frequency of miliary tuberculosis and

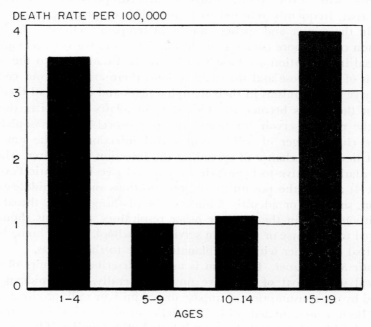

Fig. 42. Mortality from tuberculosis, all forms, total persons, ages one to nineteen (over a 4-year period, 1950 to 1953). Note that the death rate is lowest in the elementary school ages. (*From Metropolitan Life Insurance Company, Industrial Department.*)

tuberculous meningitis in young children is a well-established fact. These two serious forms of tuberculosis occur most often soon after a first infection in infancy and early childhood.

In children of elementary school age, however, first-infection tuberculosis is usually a benign disease (see Fig. 42). Many children with first-infection tuberculosis show no outward signs and symptoms whatever. Others who were formerly alert and active may act tired and listless until the infection is arrested. Tubercle bacilli are extremely difficult to find in simple primary tuberculosis. On this account it is not considered to be a contagious disease or a menace to persons coming in contact with it.

As a rule there is complete healing of the lesions [2] of first-infection tuberculosis in 1 to 2 years. It often happens that evidence of a first infection is not discovered until the child is given a tuberculin test.

The great majority of individuals with healed primary lesions will live out the rest of their lives without any further trouble from tuberculosis. A very small proportion (about 1 per cent), however, will develop fresh lesions and the signs and symptoms of reinfection tuberculosis— the chronic, destructive type of this disease.

Reinfection Tuberculosis. As the result of a first infection the body becomes highly sensitive—"allergic"—to tubercle bacilli. If tubercle bacilli should again enter the body, or escape alive from healed primary lesions, the defense forces of the body sensitized by their former encounter are mobilized much more quickly and effectively. As a result, the same sort of defense reactions take place as in a first, or primary, infection, but they happen much more quickly and vigorously.

This hair-trigger response of the sensitized tissues gives some protection from subsequent infections. However, if the reinfecting doses are very large or are repeated frequently, or if the body's defense forces have been broken down by poor nutrition or fatigue or some other condition that lowers resistance, the defense forces are overwhelmed and reinfection tuberculosis becomes established. This type of tuberculosis is most likely to develop during puberty and early maturity, but it may develop earlier or later. Pubescence seems to exert an unfavorable influence on the ability of the body to resist attacks by tubercle bacilli. This means that young people should learn not only how the spread of infection may be blocked, but also how to build up good physiological resistance to infection, especially during puberty when the body must endure greater strain.

The lesions of reinfection tuberculosis may begin to form without producing any signs and symptoms whatever. Among the earliest noticeable danger signals that the observant teacher or parent may detect are persistent fatigue, loss of weight, chronic cough with or without expectoration, flushed face in the afternoon indicating fever, night sweats, poor appetite, and digestive upsets. The sooner such signs and symptoms are brought to a physician's attention, a diagnosis made, and, if the verdict is tuberculosis, proper treatment begun, the better are the chances of a satisfactory cure. The medical diagnosis of pulmonary tuberculosis is made by means of the tuberculin test, x-ray examination of the chest,

---

[2] The lesions of pulmonary tuberculosis are formed by the destructive action of the bacilli at the points where they lodge in the lung. In healed lesions the destroyed areas are walled off from the surrounding healthy tissue by fibrous capsules or by nodules called tubercles which in time may become calcified. Living bacilli may be imprisoned within the capsules or tubercles, but they can do no harm unless the walls break down and let them out.

sputum testing, and chest sounds and other physical signs determined by the physician.

The Tuberculin Test. Tuberculin is the filtered, sterilized fluid medium in which tubercle bacilli have grown, or the protein of the tubercle bacillus extracted from it. If the tested person has been infected with tubercle bacilli, redness and swelling of the skin develop within 2 days around the place where tuberculin was injected or applied by means of a patch. This is the so-called positive reaction. If no infection has taken place, there will be no significant redness or swelling of the skin. This is the so-called nonreaction. Positive reaction to the tuberculin test *does not* show whether the disease is active or inactive. That is why a positive reaction must be followed up by x-ray examination to determine whether or not pulmonary tuberculosis is present and whether it is active or inactive. A child with only a positive reaction to the tuberculin test or with x-ray evidence of a healed tuberculous lesion may engage in the normal activities of children of his age without danger. However, he should have periodic x-ray examinations, especially before and during puberty.

Case-finding Programs. The tuberculin test is used in conjunction with chest x-rays in cooperative programs for finding unsuspected cases of tuberculosis in children. These case-finding procedures are made available to the schools through local public health units—city or county— and local tuberculosis associations.

Since very little significant tuberculosis is found in the elementary school-age group, routine case-finding programs in schools are not conducted below the high school level in many communities. In the high school and college ages the tuberculosis sickness and death rates rise sharply. Routine case finding in these age groups may uncover early cases that might otherwise be missed.

Authorities in tuberculosis control also feel that it is important for teachers and other school personnel to be routinely examined for signs of active tuberculosis. The measures recommended are the requirement of a negative x-ray of the chest as a condition for the employment of any school employee who comes in direct contact with the students and of subsequent periodic chest x-rays to find cases in employees who may later develop tuberculosis. These measures are now in effect, wholly or in part, in many cities and towns and in some states. Not only do they protect school children from infection through day-by-day close contact with unsuspected active cases of tuberculosis, but also they are proving instrumental in the saving of useful productive lives with a minimum of time lost from work. It is well to remember that at present the incidence of tuberculosis is highest in the age group twenty to forty-five.

Recovery and Rehabilitation. A child found to have active tuberculosis will require medical care and bed rest, preferably in a tuberculosis hospital where everything possible is done to bring about recovery and eventual rehabilitation. During the recovery period it is important to provide opportunities for continuing the child's education as soon as the physician permits. This is being done through educational programs in tuberculosis hospitals and through visiting teachers and other specialized workers if the child is being cared for at home.

When the child is permitted to return to regular school his teachers may be called upon to help with the plans for his scholastic and recreational activities. Over a period determined by the physician it may be necessary to adjust his curriculum to a shorter school day and to provide recreational occupations that do not require strenuous physical effort.

In helping the student to make the transition from invalidism to a normal school life, it is an advantage to know that exaggerated personality traits, such as overaggressiveness or withdrawal, are not uncommon after a long illness. As a rule, such manifestations will be temporary if they are understood and accepted by his teachers, and other adults as a natural reaction to the prolonged thwarting of his normal desires for fun and companionship. Interest in the student as a person will do much to enable him to make a satisfactory adjustment to everyday school routine.

Progress in the Prevention and Treatment of Tuberculosis. Ever since Robert Koch discovered the cause of tuberculosis in 1882, research workers have been trying to develop a vaccine to protect people against tubercle bacilli and to find a drug to cure people who have active tuberculosis. So far no such vaccine or wonder-working drug has been found. However, some encouraging results have been obtained in the use of BCG vaccination and of streptomycin and other drugs in treatment.

BCG vaccination against tuberculosis is based upon the quickened response of a body sensitized to tubercle bacilli as a result of a first infection. BCG is the abbreviation for "bacillus Calmette-Guérin." This strain of tubercle bacillus was developed by two French scientists, Calmette and Guérin, and their fellow workers. It is so weak that it cannot cause active tuberculosis. However, it is strong enough to make the body allergic to tubercle bacilli and hence heightens resistance against those bacteria. The protection given is only partial—not complete. BCG vaccination is being tried experimentally in many places in our country to find out how effective it is in protecting persons not previously infected (nonreactors to the tuberculin test) who are subject to frequent exposure, for example, certain school children and students of medicine and nursing.

The first drug found to be capable of altering the course of human tuberculosis is streptomycin. This antibiotic has given good results in the treatment of certain forms of tuberculosis, especially in combination with another drug known as paraaminosalicylic acid (PAS). The most recently discovered antituberculosis drugs are isoniazid and cycloserine. Isoniazid is a chemical compound the effectiveness of which seems to be enhanced when it is given in combination with streptomycin or PAS or both. In clinical tests cycloserine, a new antibiotic, has produced impressive improvements in severe pulmonary tuberculosis. Although there is as yet no single specific remedy for tuberculosis, there is increasing hope that a drug will be found which will combat this ancient disease with complete success.

Great strides in the surgical treatment of tuberculosis have also been made in recent years. In addition to operations for temporarily or permanently collapsing the sick lung so as to give it complete rest, surgical procedures have been perfected for the partial or complete removal of a tuberculous lung.

RESPIRATORY ALLERGIES

Children who show signs of a respiratory allergy usually come from allergic families (see Defense Reactions of Physical Origin, in Chap. 3). Specialists both in allergy and in child care emphasize the importance of early recognition of such conditions in children. Prompt diagnosis and early treatment will not only make a big difference in the child's day-by-day comfort and happiness but also will help to prevent complications which are difficult to cure and which may seriously interfere with the child's health, growth, and personality development. For example, an untreated nasal allergy, such as hay fever, may result in deformities of the face or teeth, or the development of nasal polyps or a chronic nasal infection, or chronic bronchial asthma.

Nasal Allergy

Nasal allergy may be either seasonal or nonseasonal. The seasonal type occurs in persons who are sensitive to the pollen of various trees, grasses, and weeds when the offending pollen (or pollens) is in the air. This type of nasal allergy is called hay fever. The allergens most commonly responsible for the nonseasonal type are various inhalants such as dust, orris root, and animal danders. A less common cause is sensitivity to other substances such as certain foods or drugs.

Hay Fever. The symptoms of pollen allergy are similar to those of a cold in the head, that is, obstruction of nasal breathing, sneezing, watering of the eyes, and itching of the roof of the mouth, the eyes, and the nose. When the lungs become involved, a form of bronchial asthma (see below) called pollen asthma is set up.

Tree pollens are the allergens responsible for hay fever in spring, and the pollens of grasses and weeds, in the summer and fall. The worst offender in most places in the late summer and fall is ragweed pollen. For this reason an effort is being made in some communities to stamp out ragweed either by spraying the weeds with a chemical plant killer or by cutting them down and burning them before they mature.

Helping Children with Nasal Allergies. It is now easy for doctors to diagnose hay fever. The appearance of the nasal mucous membranes is typically allergic, and the exact pollens responsible can be detected by sensitization tests of the skin (intradermal or patch tests) or of the mucous membrane (nasal sniff test and eye test).

However, a child suffering from a nasal allergy sometimes fails to get medical attention because he is considered merely to be subject to frequent head or chest colds. Or a child may be kept home from school for a cold when the condition is allergic. This is one more important reason for referring for medical check-up any child who seems to have one cold after another. Also certain mannerisms that may pass simply as bad habits are characteristic of children suffering from hay fever or allergic rhinitis. Among them are rubbing or wrinkling the nose and frequent sniffing. Using the fingers to push the tip of the nose upward and inward, both to relieve itching and to spread the walls apart in an effort to improve ventilation, is such a common mannerism that it has been called "the allergic salute." [3]

There is as yet no cure for hay fever. Specific treatment only relieves the symptoms. The most generally used treatment consists in giving subcutaneously at weekly intervals increasing doses of an extract of the offending pollen or pollens. This treatment is begun early so that the patient reaches the maximum dose at the beginning of the hay-fever season. The maximum dose is then given at weekly intervals through the season.

Several of the new antihistamine drugs are also proving very helpful for lessening the discomforts of the hay-fever victim. The physician also may prescribe drops or sprays for the eyes or nose.

Bronchial Asthma

This allergic disorder is marked by recurrent attacks of paroxysmal difficulty in breathing, wheezing, and a cough. These attacks frequently occur in the early morning hours. In children the only warning may be a persistent unexplained cough, coming on in paroxysms with little or no wheezing and without difficulty in breathing. There may be other causes of asthmatic symptoms besides allergy. Only after careful medical study of the individual is it possible to arrive at the correct diagnosis.

[3] CRIEP, LEO H., "Essentials of Allergy," pp. 334–335, Lippincott, Philadelphia, 1945.

The manifestations of bronchial asthma are caused by swelling of the mucous membrane that lines the bronchial tubes and by spasms of the muscles in their walls. The allergens responsible may be pollens and other inhalants, foods, drugs, substances handled in the course of one's work, and so on. The common cold and other acute infections of the respiratory tract often precipitate asthmatic attacks or increase their severity. For this reason the asthmatic patient is usually worse in the fall and winter, when respiratory infections are common. Emotional disturbances, exertion, and sudden temperature changes likewise play an important part in precipitating or contributing to the severity of an asthmatic attack. In children, particularly, untreated hay fever may lead to development of asthmatic symptoms toward the end of the pollen season.

THE SCHOOL AND RESPIRATORY-DISEASE CONTROL

Most of the communicable diseases with which a school may have to contend are spread by discharges from the respiratory tract. Many cases of such diseases are discovered in school, where the threshold of suspicion is lower than in the home. Cooperation with other community agencies in the education of parents and other adults in the measures required to protect children from respiratory and other infections is an important part of the school's responsibility in communicable-disease control. These measures include (a) the immunization of children from diseases for which immunization procedures are available (see Table 4, Immunization Timetable); (b) seeing that children do not come to school when they show early signs and symptoms of illness; (c) sending children home with an escort when they become ill in school; (d) protecting children as far as possible from exposure to infection while in school; and (e) notifying parents when a serious communicable disease breaks out in school, so that children who show early signs and symptoms of the disease may be kept at home.

Observing Children for Signs of Infection

Every teacher should know how to detect early indications of communicable disease, and when any of the danger signals appear, she should refer the child to the physician or nurse serving the school. If professional assistance is not available, she should isolate the child from the other pupils and arrange to have him taken home. Information about the common respiratory diseases of childhood is given in Tables 7A and 7B. In addition to information about specific diseases, the teacher should have a general picture of the symptom complex—set of symptoms—that indicates the possible onset of one of the contagions most commonly suffered in childhood. The following signs and symptoms, whether occurring singly or in combination, should be looked on with suspicion:

A chill or chilliness	Tight, dry cough
Fever (flushed face, lassitude, malaise)	Sneezing
	Headache, earache, or aching
Sore or scratchy throat	in back of legs
Red, watery eyes	Nausea or vomiting
Watery nasal discharge	

It will be noted that several of the signs and symptoms resemble those of the common cold. The characteristic signs of a particular communicable disease rarely appear at onset. For example, the eruption of vesicles characteristic of chickenpox, the typical rashes of measles and scarlet fever, the swelling of the salivary glands in mumps, and the spasmodic cough of whooping cough usually do not appear for one or more days after onset (Tables 7A and 7B).

Procedures during Epidemics

Dealing with epidemics of communicable disease in a community is the responsibility of the local public health unit. School officials should follow the recommendations of public health officials regarding special precautions, such as regular daily inspection and continuing observation of school children, when a communicable disease is especially prevalent.

It is not considered advisable, in communities that have well-organized public health facilities, to close schools during epidemics (of scarlet fever, for example, or of polio in urban centers). Unless the medical and nursing staffs are inadequate to exercise proper supervision, children are usually better off in school, where they are under constant, experienced observation. The alert teacher can play an invaluable part in limiting the spread of infection by reporting immediately any children who show signs and symptoms of illness.

Protecting School Children from Airborne Infections

The avoidance of exposure to respiratory infections is at the present time impossible. With regard to the common cold, for example, many of us have good reason to know that careful observance of all the classic hygienic rules, such as washing our hands before eating and giving careless coughers and sneezers a wide berth, does not keep us from catching cold once or twice a year. Also, the extreme contagiousness of influenza, measles, and chickenpox has made it practically impossible to control these and other easily transmitted airborne diseases by erecting the barrier of isolation.

A better understanding of what we have to contend with in attempts to control airborne infection has been reached in recent years by the discovery that droplets sprayed from the mouth and nose evaporate faster than they fall, leaving small residues called droplet nuclei. These tiny germ-laden particles may float about for long periods of time in the air of enclosed spaces in much the same manner as particles of tobacco smoke. It doesn't take much imagination to think of indoor atmosphere during late fall, winter, and early spring as being pervaded by a sort of invisible miasma, or fog, arising from the mucous membranes of those present. This picture gives us some idea of the way in which we are almost continually exposed to the respiratory flora of other people by the simple act of breathing air that contains their exhalations.

With the knowledge that the air of enclosed spaces often contains a sort of miasma consisting of contaminated dust and exhalations from the respiratory mucous membranes of those breathing it, it was natural to investigate ways of destroying airborne germs without making the air unbreathable for human beings. Experiments with ultraviolet irradiation and with aerosols, such as glycol vapors, have been carried out in many schoolrooms, barracks, offices, and hospitals as a means of evaluating their efficiency in controlling airborne infections. In hospitals ultraviolet irradiation has proved useful in operating rooms and in contagious-disease wards and children's wards. Some success has also been obtained in checking the spread of measles and chickenpox through the use of ultraviolet irradiation in classrooms and other indoor gathering places of children. However, much further study is needed before the general use of ultraviolet light or disinfectant vapors in schools can be approved.

Although there are as yet no specific practical measures available for protecting school children completely from airborne infection, the following general preventive measures may have some value.

Correction of Mouth Breathing. Since the nose is especially designed to act as an air conditioner, children should be encouraged to breathe through it. Those who are consistent mouth breathers should be referred to the nurse or the physician serving the school. The habit of mouth breathing nearly always indicates that some sort of obstacle is interfering with nasal breathing. In children, as we have seen, the chief cause usually is overgrowth of the pharyngeal tonsil (see Tonsils and Adenoids, under Tissue Fluid, in Chap. 4). Blocking of the nasal passages may also be caused by any one of several different anatomical abnormalities—for example, a deviated nasal septum or enlarged turbinates. Malocclusion, too, may favor mouth breathing, if it is difficult or uncomfortable to keep the lips closed over protruding teeth.

Mouth breathing has many disadvantages. An open mouth with droopy lower jaw gives the face a dull vacuous expression, and many a bright child looks stupid if he is obliged to breathe through his mouth. The passage of air over the tongue has a drying effect and the sense of taste may be blunted. Also interference with the aeration of the nose and sinuses may favor the development of infection.

Coughing and Sneezing. The proper technique of coughing and sneezing is a form of good manners as well as a means of avoiding the broadcasting of infection. Children should be trained in this technique until it becomes habitual. The first requirement is the possession of a handkerchief (preferably a supply of disposable paper handkerchiefs). In blowing the nose children should learn to blow gently, leaving both nostrils open so as to avoid the risk of driving the infection into the sinuses or middle ear.

In coughing, the handkerchief should be held so that it completely covers both mouth and nose. In sneezing, it is best to sneeze naturally through the mouth, with the handkerchief held as in coughing, rather than politely through the nose. Also, children should learn not to pull out used handkerchiefs with a flourish or to shake them. Experiments have shown that the shaking of dry used handkerchiefs releases thousands of germs into the surrounding air.

Seating. Children should be seated as far apart as possible. During epidemics advantage should be taken of empty seats to increase the spacing. To prevent the exposure of large numbers of children to the early or missed case of an airborne disease or to a carrier, it is considered best to preserve the same relative position of children to one another in class and to avoid the mingling of classes so far as possible. If this cannot be done ordinarily, children should be "frozen" at once if a case of infectious disease occurs.

Ventilation. Whatever the heating and ventilating arrangements of the school are, provision should be made to keep the air of occupied classrooms constantly in motion. Moving air helps to break up concentrations of airborne germs. Also, fresh outdoor air, or air properly cleaned, moistened, and warmed (as in an air-conditioning system) helps to keep the mucous membranes of the nose and throat in a healthy condition. The classroom should be neither too hot nor too cold. For moderately active children wearing ordinary indoor clothing, a room temperature of about 70°F., with 50 per cent relative humidity, is considered to be about right in cold weather.

Hand-washing Facilities. Although hand washing may not materially affect the spread of airborne infection, it is a good hygienic habit for children to form. Always washing the hands with soap and water before eating or handling food and after every visit to the toilet is an important factor in the control of diseases that are spread sometimes or usually by indirect contact, that is, by handling, eating, or drinking anything soiled with the body discharges of a sick person or carrier. The facilities required to make hand washing effective are warm water (preferably running water from a tap), soap, and individual cloth or paper towels.

Dry Clothing. There will be fewer colds caught in school if provision is made for the children to dry wet clothing and to change into dry footwear on rainy or snowy days. Children should learn to remove rubbers or overshoes and outdoor wraps when they come indoors. The moisture from perspiring bodies is as effective in making clothing and footwear damp as are rain and snow!

School Cleaning. Airborne germs in droplet nuclei or on dust particles eventually settle on the floor and on furniture. They are given a second chance to find victims if they are stirred into the atmosphere during cleaning. The floor and furniture finishes and the methods of cleaning in modern schools reduce the raising of dust to a minimum. In schools without these improvements, the use of damp sweeping and damp dusting is recommended as a means of reducing the contamination of air by germs.

Staying Home from School. In some schools so much emphasis is placed on good attendance records that many children come to school who ought to stay at home. Certainly children should be encouraged to stay home when they have early signs of respiratory infection, such as the sniffles or sore throats. Talks with parents by nurses or physicians serving the school, or by teachers, will help to emphasize the need for keeping children home and consulting a physician when the children do not seem to be in their usual good health.

WHAT TO DO IN RESPIRATORY EMERGENCY

A respiratory emergency is any condition that interferes with breathing. The body has in storage enough food to last, in a pinch, for weeks and enough water to last for several days, but no provision has been made for the storage of oxygen. In the hemoglobin of the red blood corpuscles, there is available at any one time only enough oxygen to keep us alive for two or three minutes. When suddenly it becomes impossible for the body to get oxygen from the outside world, survival is a matter of moments only. In the ordinary course of events this is not likely to happen. We are surrounded by an ocean of air which contains about 21 per cent oxygen. It is necessary only to be able to breathe to get all we need.

Under certain circumstances, however, that is just what it is impossible to do. Any accident that results in interference with the delivery of oxygen to the body cells causes asphyxia.

Asphyxia

The following are the most common causes of asphyxia:

1. Obstruction of the air passages to the lungs, either from without, as in smothering and strangulation, or from within, as in choking and submersion
2. Paralysis of the respiratory center of the brain, as in electric shock, so that the breathing muscles cannot work
3. Interference with the oxygen-carrying function of the red blood cells, as in the inhalation of carbon monoxide, which combines more rapidly, easily, and firmly with hemoglobin than oxygen can
4. Lack of oxygen in the air breathed in, as in old wells, storage bins, or airtight vaults, where oxygen has been replaced by carbon dioxide through the process of oxidation

An asphyxiated person is not breathing or breathes only with great difficulty. Even after breathing ceases, the heart usually continues to beat for a few minutes, and in this time the person's life may be saved by prompt action. To restore natural breathing, artificial respiration must be administered *immediately after rescue,* combined with the administration of oxygen, if available.

Artificial Respiration

Proficiency in administering artificial respiration is a very useful accomplishment both for teachers and for older boys and girls. Instruction and practice in giving artificial respiration are often included in high school first-aid classes.

Until recently the method recommended was the prone-pressure method. However, many studies have indicated that the back-pressure, arm-lift method worked out by Holger Nielsen of Denmark makes possible much greater ventilation of the lungs and is, in addition, easy to learn and to perform. This method, which is described on the following pages, consists of a push-pull movement producing both inspiration and expiration. It has been officially recommended by the National Research Council, the American National Red Cross, the United States Armed Forces, the United States Public Health Service, the American Medical Association, and other national organizations. Two other push-pull

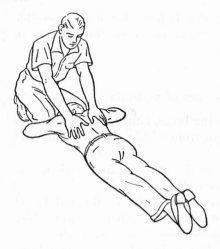

FIG. 43. Position 1. Kneel on either your right or left knee, or on both, in front of the victim's head. Place your hands, with thumbs almost touching and fingers spread out, on the victim's back just below his shoulder blades.

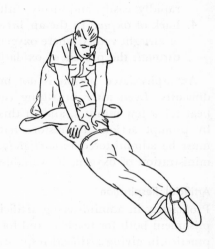

FIG. 44. Position 2. Rock forward, keeping your elbows straight. Press, with the weight of the upper part of your body, slowly and evenly downward on the victim's back. This empties the lungs.

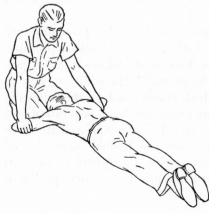

FIG. 45. Position 3. Rock back slowly, releasing the pressure easily. As you do so, grasp the victim's arms just above the elbows.

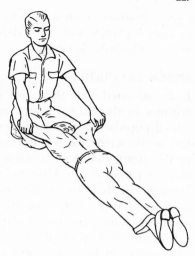

Fig. 46. Position 4. Draw the victim's arms upward and toward you until you feel a slight resistance at his shoulders. Do not bend your elbows. Lifting the arms expands the chest so that air can get into the lungs. Drop the arms.

methods, which are also efficient, are the hip-lift, back-pressure method and the arm-lift, chest-pressure method (Silvester).

The Holger Nielsen Back-pressure—Arm-lift Method.[4] Lay the victim on his stomach with his cheek resting on his hands to keep dirt out of his mouth. Examine his mouth quickly for any obstruction and pull his tongue forward. Then take Position 1 (Fig. 43).

Repeat the rhythm described in Figures 44 through 46 steadily from 10 to 12 times a minute. Each phase should take about $1\frac{1}{2}$ seconds. The release periods should be minimal.

A brief return of natural breathing is not a certain indication for stopping artificial respiration. Often the victim, after a temporary recovery, stops breathing again. He must be watched, and if natural breathing stops, artificial respiration must be begun again at once.

Resuscitation should be carried on at the nearest possible point to the place where the victim was rescued or found. He should not be moved from this place until he is breathing regularly, and then he should be moved only in a reclining position. Should it be necessary, because of weather conditions or for any other reason, to move the victim before he is breathing normally, artificial respiration must be kept up during the time that he is being moved.

To avoid strain on the heart when the victim revives, he should be kept lying down and not allowed to stand or sit up. If the doctor has not arrived by the time the victim has revived, the latter should be given

[4] Description and Figures 43 through 46 from "First Aid," Metropolitan Life Insurance Company, 1953.

some stimulant, such as 1 teaspoonful of aromatic spirits of ammonia in a small glass of water or a drink of sweetened hot coffee or tea. Do not give an alcoholic beverage.

SPEECH DIFFICULTIES

It is estimated that there are more than 12,000,000 speech and voice cripples in the United States, upward of 1,000,000 of whom are in the school population. Generally speaking, speech is considered to be defective or distorted "when it deviates so far from the speech of other people in the group that it calls attention to itself, interferes with communication, or causes its possessor to be maladjusted." [5]

Since speech is by far our most important means of communication with our fellow men, difficulty in speaking is a serious impediment in social, academic, and work relationships. Even if the difficulty is a physical abnormality, psychological aspects are bound to complicate the picture sooner or later. If young children are permitted to go along with any form of distorted speech, with the idea that they will later outgrow it, not only will the disorder or defect itself be far more difficult to cure but also the child's personality may be warped permanently.

Ideally, children entering school for the first time should have a speech examination by a trained examiner to screen out those with speech difficulties. Not many schools have this service. Authorities agree that the next-best procedure is to have the classroom teachers report speech difficulties to the nurse or physician serving the school. For this reason it is recommended that teachers, as part of their training, learn to recognize speech disorders. The procedure after recognition involves examination by a speech clinician or trained speech correctionist for diagnosis and the planning of treatment. In some cases surgical or psychiatric treatment may be required before voice and speech training are started. In school systems in which speech correctionists or specially trained teachers are not employed, this training may be carried on by the parents or teachers under the supervision of the specialist responsible for the diagnosis and treatment. In some communities speech clinics which offer diagnosis and treatment of speech disorders may be available for the individual or group treatment of children who need it.

Varieties of Speech Disorders

Speech disorders differ widely as to cause, kind, and degree of handicapping. Roughly they may be classified as follows:

[5] VAN RIPER, C., "Speech Correction—Principles and Methods," 3d ed., p. 19, Prentice-Hall, New York, 1954.

1. Speech difficulties caused by some structural defect in one or more of the organs involved in speech. Examples of such defects are cleft palate; harelip; protruding upper or lower front teeth and missing front teeth; nasal obstructions; and any abnormality in the larynx.
2. Weakness or sluggishness of the soft palate, tongue, and lips, which results in a distortion of speech because more effort is required in speaking than is normally put forth. Examples are lisping and nasality.
3. Complete or partial loss of the power to speak or to write (motor aphasia) or of the ability to understand spoken or written language (sensory aphasia) because of injury or disease of the speech centers in the brain.
4. A disturbance of the rhythm of speech, usually symptomatic of a personality maladjustment. The outstanding example of such a so-called "emotional disorder of speech" is stuttering or stammering.
5. Poor quality of voice, which may be due to a structural or functional cause. Voices of poor quality may be husky, weak, nasal, shrill, breathy, or monotonous. Excessive loss of hearing or nerve deafness (due to a lesion of the auditory nerve) is quite likely to result in monotonous phonation. Learning to speak is an imitative process. Children cannot learn to speak well if they cannot hear well.
6. Substitution of one speech sound for another beyond the period at which correctness of speech is usually acquired. The popular term for this difficulty is "baby talk." It may be due to a slight temporary interruption of the growth process, or to a home environment in which baby talk is encouraged, or to some emotional blocking.
7. A noticeable unusual accent caused by the influence on English speech of a foreign language, local dialect, or family peculiarities of utterance. Since speech (as we have noted above) is largely imitative, children cannot learn to speak English correctly if they constantly hear English spoken poorly.

The Organ of Speech

In the upper part of the larynx, directly below the epiglottis, is an aperture, or chink, shaped like an isosceles triangle. This is the glottis. The two equal sides of the glottis are formed by the vocal cords. The vocal cords themselves are strands of yellow elastic tissue which run from the front to the rear of the larynx. They are attached at the rear to two small cartilaginous bodies (the arytenoid cartilages) and are fixed to the wall of the larynx in front. The vocal cords are swung outward against the walls of the larynx or inward toward each other by small muscles which rotate the arytenoid cartilages. Ordinarily the vocal cords lie against the walls of the larynx, leaving the glottis wide open for breathing. In speaking or singing they are brought toward each other until the glottis shrinks to a small chink. The flow of air expelled from the lungs sets the edges of these tautened cords into vibration, thus producing the voice. Slender muscles in the cords themselves make it possible to tighten or slacken them so as to change the frequency of their vibration and thus

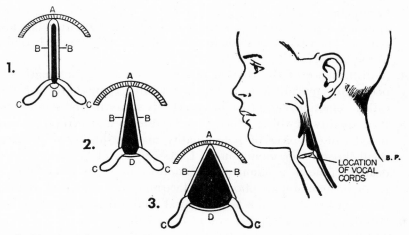

FIG. 47. Vocal cords as seen from above. 1, cords brought closely together as in singing a high note. 2, cords brought toward each other as in speaking. 3, cords swung out against wall of larynx as in breathing. *A*, front of the larynx. *B–B*, the vocal cords. *C–C*, the arytenoid cartilages. *D*, back of larynx.

vary the pitch of the voice. In children and women, the vocal cords are short and high-pitched. In men they are longer and the voice is deeper.

The timbre or quality of the voice is produced by numerous resonating spaces, just as the vibrations of violin strings or the reeds of an organ are transformed into a complex tissue of tones by the sounding board of the violin or the pipes of the organ. The resonating spaces of the human vocal instrument include the chest, the throat, the mouth and nose, and the nasal sinuses.

Voice is not speech, but rather a series of musical tones and overtones. To produce the sounds of speech, the sound waves sent forth by the vibrating vocal cords are modified by other structures—the nose, lips, teeth, and tongue. Broadly speaking, there are vowel and consonant sounds. Vowel sounds are formed by the passage of air through the mouth, which assumes characteristic positions for each vowel. Consonants are produced by the blocking or interruption of the passage of

Table 8. HOW CONSONANT SOUNDS ARE PRODUCED

Lip sounds........	P, as in pet, pull, apple, pipe, stop, pie, help B, as in boy, baby, butter, box, boat, able	The lips are closed, blocking the air, and then suddenly opened, allowing it to escape with a "puff"
	WH, as in white, which, when, whither, where	The lips are rounded (pursed); in the sound as properly made the H comes first (HW) *
	M, as in man, room, summer, moon, from, limb, lame, slim	The lips are closed, forcing air through the nose; this is a nasal sound
Lip-teeth sounds....	F, as in feet, after, calf, fair, feel, roof	The lower lip is raised gently against the cutting edges of the upper teeth and then lowered just as the air is forced through
Tongue-teeth sounds	TH (silent) as in thank, thick, thin, south, earth TH (sounded) as in this, those, other, father, brother	The tip of the tongue is placed between the teeth lightly touching the cutting edges of the upper ones, and the air forced through
Front tongue sounds	T, as in table, tell, talk, take, butter, star D, as in day, deed, did, dinner, candy, glad	The tip of the tongue is placed broadly against the roof of the mouth (just above the upper gums) and then suddenly removed, releasing the air in a burst
	N, as in night, now, noise, pony, man	The tip of the tongue is placed against the upper gums, blocking the air so that it passes out through the nose; this is a nasal sound
	S, as in see, so, class, ice, house, asleep Z, as in zoo, zebra, because, scissors, zinc, those	The tongue is hollowed (made narrower) by raising it on both sides and is pointed at the nearly closed front teeth without touching them; the hissing sound is produced by the forcing of air against the cutting edges of the teeth
	SH, as in sheep, shine, she, dish, wash, show ZH, as in leisure, pleasure, azure	As in S, but the tongue is made slightly flatter (broader) and the lips are slightly protruded and rounded
	CH, as in chair, teacher, child, watch, each, picture	A combination of T and SH: the tongue is placed as in T and then suddenly lowered so that the air is discharged as in SH (a similar combination sound (TSH) accompanies a sneeze)

* The H sound is the whispered beginning to any vowel at the beginning or in the middle of a word, as in house, behind, and perhaps. The W sound is a glide (that is, two vowel sounds produced in quick succession) as oo to e, in we, and oo to il in will.

Table 8 (Cont.). HOW CONSONANT SOUNDS ARE PRODUCED

Front tongue sounds (cont.)	J, as in jump, judge, jumble, pigeon, ginger, bridge	A combination of D and ZH: produced in a manner similar to CH but with a slightly different manipulation of the tongue
	L, as in live, lay, low, balloon, full, animal	The tip of the tongue is lifted to the gums just behind and above the upper teeth while the air passes out along the sides of the tongue
	R, as in rabbit, race, rain, red, former, door	The tip of the tongue is pointed toward the roof of the mouth, with its base depressed; the air passes out while the tongue tip moves upward or downward
Back tongue sounds	K and hard C, as in kitten, coat, cat, book, snake, make, stick, school G, as in good, great, game, garden, dog, pig	The back of the tongue is raised against the soft palate and then lowered so that the air is suddenly released through the mouth
	NG, as in bang, tangle, finger, angry, morning, wrong	Similar to N except that the back of the tongue is raised against the soft palate to block the passage of air through the mouth and allow it to pass through the nose

expired air in various parts of the vocal pathway by the tongue, teeth, lips, or soft palate.

You can learn a great deal about the production of individual sounds by pronouncing the letters of the alphabet and observing in a mirror the positions assumed by the various structures involved.

The voice change from childish soprano to baritone or bass in adolescent boys is caused by the descent of the larynx to a lower position in the throat. The cracks or breaks in the voice so characteristic of boys in this transition period are due to the fact that the larynx does not immediately become accustomed to its new position and occasionally moves up to the old.

Falsetto Voice. In some boys the shift in position of the larynx does not take place, with the result that they retain the high soprano of childhood. A soprano voice in a man is called falsetto (Italian for false) because of its unnaturalness. The failure of the larynx to descend may be caused by psychic factors, by bad habits of speaking contracted during the change in voice, or by an endocrine disturbance.

An example of a psychic cause is an unconscious fear of assuming the responsibilities of adult life. The resulting anxiety may inhibit the voice

Table 9. HOW VOWEL SOUNDS ARE PRODUCED

ā (long a) as in ale	The lips and teeth are held well apart and the sides of the tongue lightly touch the back upper teeth
ă (short a) as in at, add	The mouth is opened wider than for long ā
ä (ah) as in arm, mama	The mouth is opened still wider, with the tongue relaxed
a (aw) as in all, saw (represented in pho- netic spelling as ô)	The lips are pursed with the tip of the tongue lowered and its base somewhat raised
ē (long e) as in be, eel	The lips and teeth are held about as far apart as for long ā (as in ale) and the tongue is raised and tense
ĕ (short e) as in pet, net, end	As long ē, but the mouth is opened wider
ī (long i) as in mile, child	As long ē, but with the mouth wide open
ĭ (short i) as in ill, it	As long ē, but with the tongue slightly lower and less tense
i before r as in bird, fir (represented in pho- netic spelling as û)	The teeth are brought closer together than for long ī, and the lips are slightly protruded and the tongue flat
ō (long o) as in old, over	The lips are rounded, with the tongue held low but with its back part raised toward the soft palate
ŏ (short o) as in not, stop, and o as in or, order, saw (represented in phonetic spell- ing as ô)	The lips are rounded slightly and the back of the tongue is raised but not so high as in long ō
oo̅ (long oo) as in food, do, moon, rude, rule	The lips are closely rounded and the back of the tongue is raised close to the soft palate
oŏ (short oo) as in foot, good	As in oo̅ but with the tongue a little lower and less tense
ū (long u) as in use, music	As in oo̅ (food) preceded by the sound of y as in yes
ŭ (short u) as in up, cup	The teeth are wide apart and the tongue flat
u before r as in her, bird, burn, word (repre- sented in phonetic spelling as û)	As in i before r

change which proclaims to the world that the boy is becoming a man. In that case the muscles that keep the larynx raised (elevator muscles) may retain their dominance over those which lower it (depressor muscles), and the larynx remains high in the throat. If this condition is allowed to persist, the continued psychic blows to the personality may have serious consequences. Fortunately, the larynx may be lowered by manipulation, but this procedure must be reinforced by psychotherapy to remove the basic feeling of inadequacy and by voice training. If the condition is caused by an endocrine disturbance, glandular treatment will be necessary. Whatever the cause, persistent falsetto voice in a boy who in other respects is close to manhood indicates that the assistance of a competent medical specialist is necessary.

The Tongue in Speech

From time immemorial the tongue has been intimately associated with speech. *Lingua,* in Latin, means both "tongue" and "language." In the Old Testament we find Moses complaining to the Lord that he was "slow of speech and of a slow tongue" and Isaiah prophesying that on the day of judgment "the tongue of stammerers shall be ready to speak plainly." At one time it was thought that moistness of the tongue caused stammering, and attempts were made to dry the tongue by blistering it. A more modern version of loosing the "string of the tongue," which is how St. Mark described Christ's cure of a speech sufferer, was the actual cutting of the lingual nerves in attempts to cure stuttering. Thousands of tongues were cut and mutilated until it became evident that operative measures were entirely useless as means of curing stammerers.

The tongue participates in the production of a great variety of speech sounds, although it is not the all-important organ of speech it is popularly supposed to be. It is the only muscle in the body that is attached only at one end. This arrangement makes it especially mobile and flexible. In producing individual sounds it assumes a great many different forms and positions, as you can see for yourself by looking in a mirror while talking.

Tongue-tie. Teachers or parents have often remarked carelessly, "Oh, he is tongue-tied," to explain an otherwise inexplicable speech impediment in a child. As a matter of fact, very few speech difficulties are caused by defects of the tongue, and true tongue-tie is a rare condition.

Normally, the fold of membrane that attaches the undersurface of the tongue to the floor of the mouth is located at some distance back from the tongue tip. You can see this membrane by protruding and lifting your tongue while looking into a mirror. In tongue-tie the membrane is attached close to, or right at, the tip of the tongue. As a result, the tongue literally is tied down.

It is easy for teachers or parents to find out whether a child is truly tongue-tied. If the child can stick out his tongue and curve it upward to touch the groove in the middle of his upper lip; or if he can run the tip of his tongue along the roof of his mouth, with his lips and teeth slightly open, he is not tongue-tied. The operation to correct tongue-tie is a simple one. Of course it should be performed only by a surgeon and only when he says there is need for it.

The Lips in Speech

Several sounds in English speech are primarily lip sounds or lip-teeth sounds. It is impossible, for example, to make the sound of P or B, or to say "which" or "what," without moving the lips. A common fault in speaking is a failure to use the lips enough in forming consonant sounds.

Harelip is the defect most commonly involved in speech disorders that are due to structural malformation of the lips. This is a congenital cleft of one or both lips, but usually of the upper lip only. It can be corrected by surgery, the earlier the better for the child born with it. As in cleft palate (see under The Palate in Speech, further on) voice and speech training are required after the defect has been repaired.

The Teeth in Speech

The forcing of air against or between the cutting edges of the front teeth is responsible for several consonant sounds. If the teeth of the upper and lower jaws do not come together (occlude) or if any front teeth are missing, some of these sounds may be made incorrectly.

Lisping. The speech disorder most commonly connected with defective or missing teeth is lisping. In lisping, the sounds for S, Z, Sh, and Zh are made incorrectly or the Th sound is substituted for them. It is easy to understand why a child who is losing his deciduous front teeth may say "ith" for is, "clath" for class, "horth" for horse, "thithers" for scissors, and so on, when we realize that the hissing sound of S and Z is produced by forcing air from behind against the nearly closed cutting edges of the front teeth, whereas in pronouncing Th, the tip of the tongue protrudes from between the teeth.

Sluggishness or wrong manipulation of the tongue may also produce lisping. Some lispers protrude the tongue in pronouncing words in which S or Z sounds are required instead of pointing it at the teeth from behind (lingual lisp); others fail to raise the tongue on both sides, with the result that air slides over the sides instead of through a channel in the middle (lateral lisp). By asking children who lisp for no obvious cause (such as missing teeth or malocclusion) to pronounce such words as sleep, slide, see, shine, wish, show, zoo, zebra, pleasure, and please, and watching their tongues meanwhile, the teacher may be able to observe the trouble in managing the tongue which is responsible. Gymnastic exercises for the tongue which are helpful in efforts to overcome lisp are given in books or manuals on the correction of speech disorders.

The Nose in Speech

The nasal cavities and nasal sinuses are part of the resonating apparatus in the production of voice. Also a few of the sounds of speech normally are produced by blocking the passage of air through the mouth and allowing it to pass out through the nose. These nasal sounds of speech are M, N, and Ng.

The familiar speech distortions often caused by the temporary congestion of the nose during a bad cold in the head illustrate what may happen to the voice as a result of an obstruction due to some structural defect of the nose or throat. The diagnosis and treatment of such defects naturally are the responsibility of the physician.

Nasality. Talking through the nose, or nasal intonation, is one of the most common faults involved in voices that are unpleasant to hear. The nasal voice is a whining voice, and the whine, which literally is the low plaintive nasal sound evoked in complaint or distress, is associated with a complaining, nagging personality. Actually a cheerful, happy person may be the unfortunate possessor of a "whining voice."

Nasal intonation is produced by the escape of air into the nose while the person is speaking. The reason that some people talk through their noses can best be explained by describing the structure and functions of the normal palate.

The Palate in Speech

The palate forms the roof of the mouth and the floor of the nose. It has two parts, one hard, one soft (see Fig. 38). The function of the palate is to separate the nose from the mouth so that they can work separately.

If you will run your tongue over the roof of your mouth, you will feel a hard bony structure covered with membrane. This is the hard palate. Now look into the back of your mouth in a mirror. You will see a flap of soft muscular tissue which moves as you say "Ah." This is the soft palate. You will also notice that the soft palate hangs down into a fingerlike bulge. This is called the uvula.

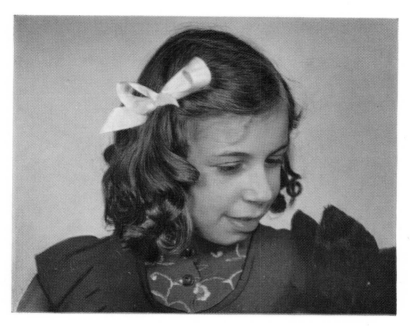

PLATE 1. This is a picture of Jane as her teacher sees her when she is healthy and happy.

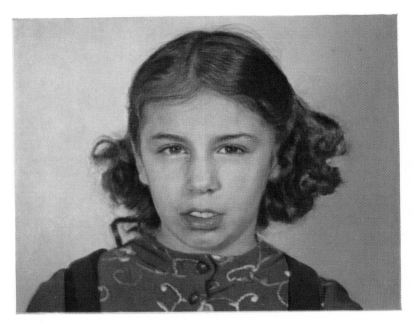

PLATE 2. This is a picture of Jane as her teacher saw her when she returned to school after an illness.

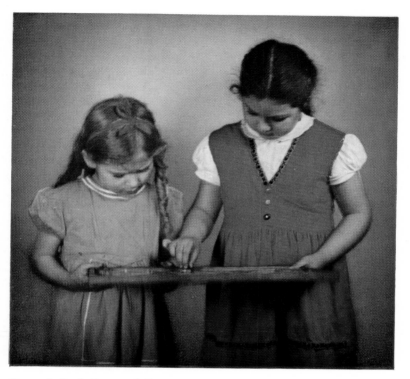

Plate 3. Both Jean and Frances are six years old. This is a good illustration of the fact that each healthy child develops along his or her own pathway.

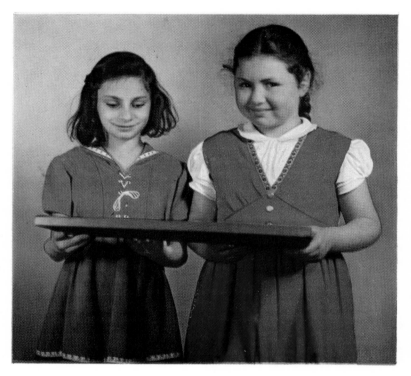

PLATE 4. In this picture ten-year-old Rosalie is compared with six-year-old Jean. Rosalie is definitely undersized for her age and shows other signs that made her teacher suspect malnutrition.

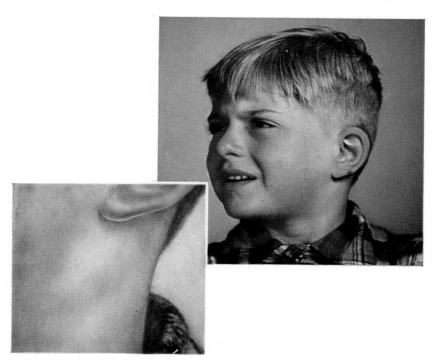

PLATE 5. The small lump below the lobe of Tommy's left ear indicates a swollen gland. The swelling is barely noticeable because Tommy is almost well now, and his physician has given him permission to return to school.

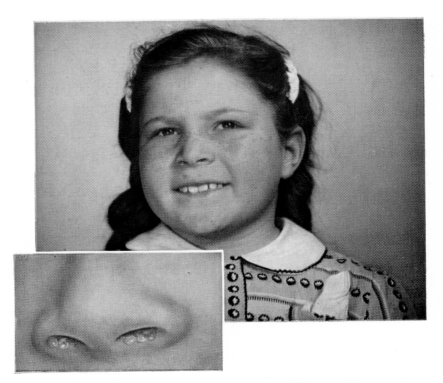

PLATE 6. If you will look closely, as her teacher did, you will notice that Lois has a slightly running nose.

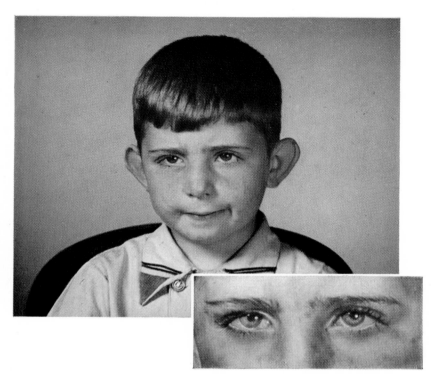

PLATE 7. Johnny is not very happy today. His eyes are red and watery, with puffiness of the lower lids. He is just coming down with the measles.

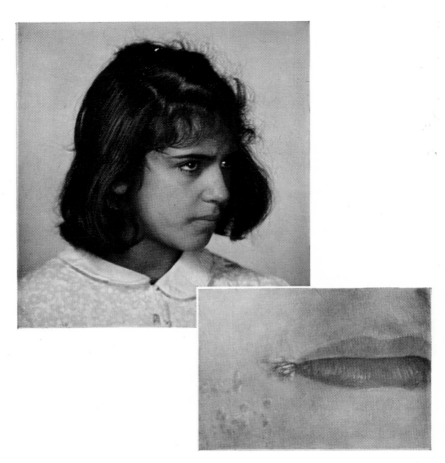

Plate 8. Anne was referred by her teacher for a medical examination because her general appearance and posture indicated fatigue. Also, the teacher had noticed a persistent cracking and slight redness at the corner of Anne's mouth. The physician discovered that Anne was suffering from inadequate nutrition, and more particularly from a B-vitamin deficiency.

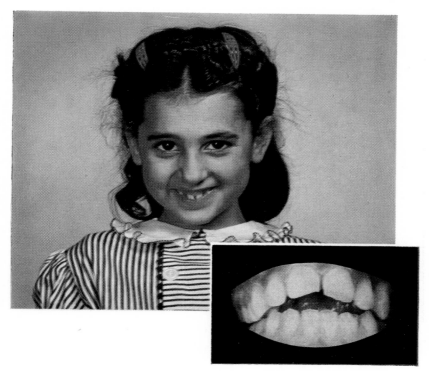

PLATE 9. The only thing that keeps Evelyn from being a pretty little girl is the possession of teeth that do not come together properly. Malocclusion may spoil a child's looks and interfere with happy adjustment to life.

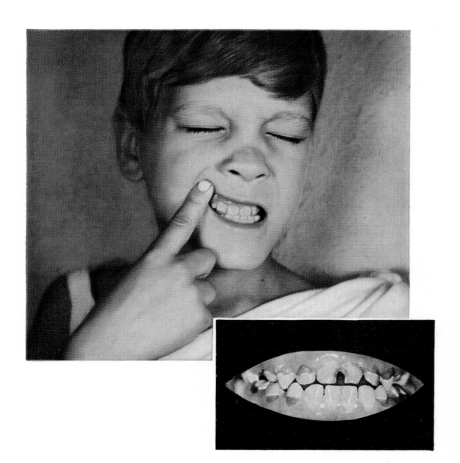

PLATE 10. A slight dental defect, like the one to which George is pointing, may not be visible to his teacher. On the other hand, no one can miss obviously decayed teeth like those shown at the right.

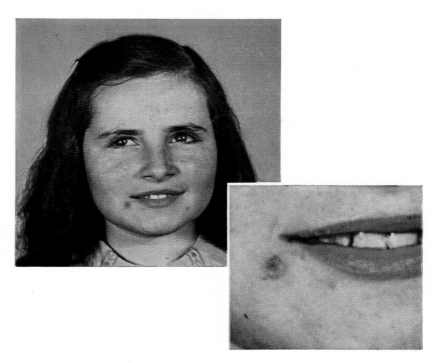

PLATE 11. The small red spot near the right corner of Peggy's mouth is impetigo. This very contagious skin infection is marked by groups of little blisters, which later turn to crusty sores.

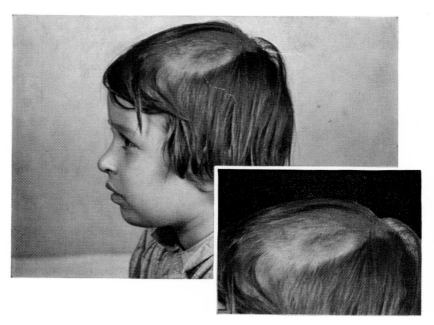

PLATE 12. Dorothy has an advanced case of ringworm of the scalp. The affected hairs become dull and brittle and snap off near the root, leaving bald spots on which raised gray scaly patches appear.

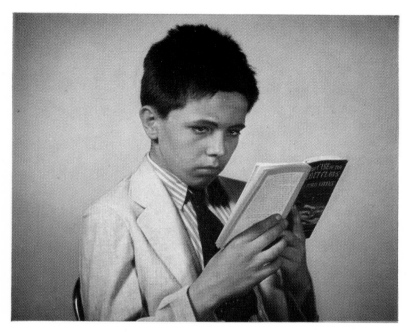

PLATE 13. Both in appearance and in behavior, Kenneth shows the signs that signal "nearsightedness" to a keen observer. In this picture he is holding his book too close to his eyes.

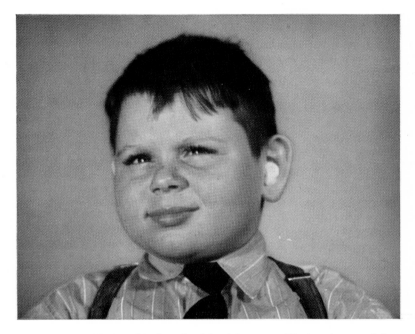

PLATE 14. Teddy is a big boy for his eight years. He is robust and has good color, but the piece of cotton in his ear indicates that his ear is draining. Teddy's look of watchful waiting is typical of children who do not hear well.

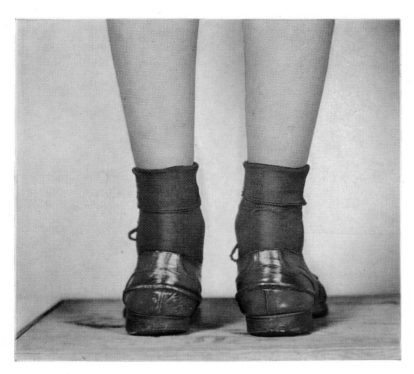

PLATE 15. Nina's teacher has observed that Nina wears down the heels of her shoes toward the inside in a short time. Besides indicating something wrong that needs correction, run-down heels are hard on the feet and are frequently the cause of bad falls and "turned" ankles.

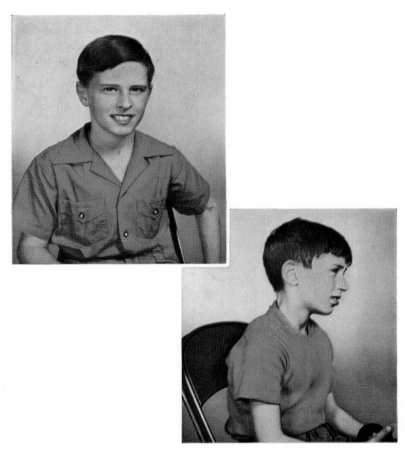

PLATE 16. By comparing postures and expressions it is easy to tell which of these two boys is suffering from chronic fatigue. Charlie, at the left, is a healthy alert youngster, whereas poor Freddie cannot enter whole-heartedly into any activity. Freddie's teacher referred him for a special medical check-up, and a physician found that he had large adenoids, which were interfering with his breathing and lowering his vitality.

Between the soft palate and the back of the throat there is a small space called the "postnasal space" which permits air to flow from the throat into the nose in breathing out. During speech this space is closed off by the soft palate and muscles at the top of the throat in much the same manner as a drawstring is used to close a tobacco pouch or old-fashioned purse. The effect is to raise the soft palate and bring it in contact with the back of the throat so as to keep the vocalized air from escaping into the nose, thereby compelling it to flow out through the mouth.

Generally speaking, the larger the postnasal space, the greater the chance of nasality, since a large space is harder to close off than a smaller one. A weakness of the soft palate, requiring more effort than is usually put forth in speaking, also may result in nasality. Functional nasality, that is, nasality without any discoverable defect or weakness of structure, may be present in children who have fallen into poor habits of speech.

Voice exercises are of great help in correcting nasality, whether of structural or functional origin. Preferably they should be carried on under the supervision of a speech correctionist. Blowing games are excellent for increasing the mobility of the soft palate and for teaching the child to direct the current of inspired air through the mouth instead of allowing it to escape through the postnasal space into the nose. Such play exercises include blowing bubbles into water through a straw, blowing a small celluloid ball across a flat surface, blowing soap bubbles, and blowing up balloons. For older children, learning to play musical instruments that require blowing, such as the mouth organ or the clarinet, will make the exercises interesting.

Cleft-palate Speech. This term is applied to the speech of a person who has a cleft, or opening, in the roof of the mouth. Although it is comparatively rare, it is one of the most distressing of all speech defects. Cleft palate is a congenital defect, that is, the child is born with it. No matter what may be the size or shape of the cleft, the child has great difficulty in speaking and eating. Speech, as might be expected with a hole through the roof of the mouth, is nasal in character.

Fortunately the cleft can often be closed if the operation is done in time by a surgeon specializing in the repair of such defects. The operation is most successful if it is performed before the child's third or fourth year. Even after a successful operation, however, massage and exercise are needed to make the soft palate move correctly, because a repaired palate is not so flexible and mobile as is a completely normal palate. Postoperative massage, exercises, and speech training are best carried on under the supervision of the trained speech correctionist, but parents or teachers can learn how to give them if a specialist's services are not available.[6]

The Brain in Speech

The mechanics of speech are the functions of the larynx and its assistants, the tongue, teeth, nose, lips, and palate. The ability to speak, however, is located in the brain. In learning to speak the little child first associates the sounds (words) he hears with the sensations aroused by the objects he sees, touches, or otherwise apprehends. These associations are stored in his brain as memories. When definite meanings have become attached to certain words, pathways are established between the auditory center of the brain (the area where sounds are recognized and interpreted) and the motor area for speech (the area from which impulses are sent to the muscles involved in speech). The child then tries to form and utter the words that he has heard. As we have seen, this marvelous act of speaking depends upon the coordinated movements of a large group of muscles— the respiratory muscles, and the muscles of the larynx, pharynx, tongue, and lips.

Later on, as the child learns to read, he associates auditory speech with visual symbols of speech, that is, printed words. Finally association is established between the visual symbols of speech and the motor area that directs the movements of the hand. Then the child is able to express in writing both his auditory impressions (what he hears) and his visual impressions (what he sees).

Handedness. In most children the areas involved in speaking, reading, and writing are more highly developed in the left hemisphere of the cerebrum than they are in the right. Since the left half of the brain controls the right half of the body, most children are right-handed, "right-speaking," and "right-reading."

About 4 per cent of children, however, are left-handed. Babies begin to show their preference for the right or left hand when they are about six months old. As we live in a right-handed world, parents and teachers may try to correct left-handedness. This is a mistake. There is nothing wrong in being left-handed. Of course the child must put up with the inconvenience of living in a world in which the buttons on his clothes, the knobs on doors, and many other contrivances are designed for right-handed people. However, left-handed children seem to take such inconveniences in their stride. It is only when they are made to feel conscious

[6] An excellent manual giving instructions for working with a child who has had a cleft-palate operation is "Has Your Child a Cleft Palate?", rev. ed., State of Illinois, Commission for Handicapped Children, 1949.

of their difference from other children by being heckled or ridiculed that speech difficulties or other forms of maladjustment may develop.

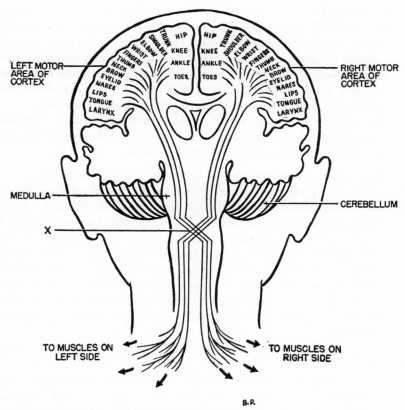

B.P.

FIG. 48. Motor nerves from one half of the brain cross with those descending from the other half at the spot marked X. Hence the left motor area of the brain controls the muscles in the right side of the body and vice versa.

Aphasia. If the auditory, visual, or motor speech areas of the brain are injured or diseased, a condition called aphasia is the result. Aphasia may be characterized by any one of four different speech defects:

1. The power to express ideas in words may be almost completely lost. If the defect is less severe, words may be mispronounced, but the ability to construct sentences is not impaired. Persons with this type of aphasia have related difficulties in reading and writing.
2. The ability to speak is not lost, but the words come out in a jargon, or jumble, which is difficult to understand. Sometimes the speech

is slurred or resembles baby talk. A person with this type of aphasia may be able to write but not to read coherently what he has written.

3. The ability to speak is not lost, but there is great difficulty in finding the right words to express meanings or to name objects. Persons with this type of aphasia often substitute a descriptive phrase for the word they cannot recall. Best and Taylor give this example: "A painter when asked to name a series of colors could not say 'violet' but instead explained that 'it was made with black, red and a bit of blue.' " [7] It is difficult for these people to write coherently and carry out simple mathematical calculations.

4. The ability to speak, name objects, and understand individual words, or the details in pictures, is not lost, but the general meaning of what is said or seen is not comprehended.

Aphasia occurs most frequently in adults as a result of disease or injury, but many children show a form of it. Such children may be very slow in learning to talk, although they are mentally alert. Or they may have great difficulty in acquiring any of the language skills. Of course, there are many possible causes for slowness in learning to speak, read, and write, but there is at least the possibility that a child who has this difficulty may have been born with some weakness in the language sphere. Since there are remedial measures that are helpful in many cases, a child who seems more than usually slow in acquiring the language skills should be referred to a physician, who may advise examination by a specialist.

Stuttering

Stuttering is a common speech disorder in children. A distinction used to be made between the intermittent blocking of speech called "stammering" and the repetition or prolongation of syllables and words or phrases called "stuttering." Now, "stuttering" is generally used in referring to both conditions.

A distinction should be made between persistent stuttering and the sporadic hesitations and repetitions of which practically all of us are guilty on occasion. We may be speechless, or more or less incoherent, or needlessly repeat certain words or phrases—that is, stutter—when we are nervous or tired or frightened or angry or excited or speak too hurriedly or forget what we started out to say. In children of two or three who are beginning to talk, the speech mechanism often does not work fast enough to allow them to express what they have in mind, and they stutter.

[7] BEST, CHARLES HERBERT, and NORMAN BURKE TAYLOR, "The Physiological Basis of Medical Practice," 6th ed., p. 1048, Williams & Wilkins, Baltimore, 1955.

Primary Stuttering. The stuttering of young children is called primary stuttering. Usually it disappears in a few months. In some children, however, normal hesitations in speech are turned into a real speech disorder. Usually the disorder develops so gradually that it is difficult for the parents or speech correctionist to discover exactly why and when a particular child began to show an excessive amount of halting or hesitating in his speech or pronounced repetitions or prolongations of verbal sounds.

It may be found that the child belongs to the small group of children who have difficulty in coordinating the muscles involved in speech. A child with this difficulty will be more susceptible than are most children to emotional conflicts of one kind or another.

Emotional conflicts and frustrations are often expressed in stuttering. At times most of us have been torn between conflicting desires to speak and to remain silent—before making a speech, for example—or in soliciting contributions for a cause, or in asking for a raise. Children are sometimes placed in such situations. We have seen that children may be torn between love and hate. Yet the child who feels deep-seated resentment is required to express his love verbally. The naughty child who doesn't feel sorry at all inside must say "I'm sorry." Frustration may be experienced merely by interruptions or a show of impatience on the part of parents or teachers who do not realize how long it takes for little children to become fluent in expressing themselves. To be commanded in the middle of a sentence to stop and begin over again, or to be ignored or diverted before one is able to get out what one is trying to say, is bound to be frustrating. Occasionally a particular experience may precipitate stuttering. Here are two examples:

By the time Marilyn was halfway through the fourth grade, her family had moved so many times that she had been in four different schools. Then she began to stutter. When the doctor told her parents that the many school changes were probably the precipitating cause, they pointed out that Marilyn was a bright child who had never had trouble keeping up in her classwork. They failed to understand that a child who enters a new school from an old one is an outsider who has to be tried and tested by other children before being accepted or rejected. An unusually sensitive child, like Marilyn, may be able to weather this ordeal once or twice, but cannot go through it repeatedly without ill effects.

Another child—Dan—started to stutter when he tried unsuccessfully to keep up with an older boy who was visiting in his home. The visitor escaped punishment because he *was* a visitor. All the spankings and scoldings for their misdeeds fell upon Dan. As a result, Dan felt that he was losing his parents' favor and love. He had begun to stutter and was well on the way toward developing deep-seated feelings of inferiority and hostility until the situation was explained to the parents. When the visitor left and peace and harmony were restored, the stuttering disappeared.[8]

Often primary stuttering grows less and less frequent and periods of fluency become longer and longer if no attention is paid to it. Eventually the stuttering may disappear altogether. The speech correctionist called in by anxious parents or the nursery school usually explains that the best treatment is no treatment. There must be no interruptions of speech, no rewards or punishment, no expressions of concern that the child can hear. Situations in which fluency in speech is made easy or in which attention is distracted from speech, such as partly verbal games, are suggested. Also adults who are with the child are asked to speak more slowly, more simply, and more calmly. The speech of adults is often too fast or too complicated for children to imitate, and it is imitation that lies at the root of speech development.

Secondary Stuttering. In primary stuttering the child is usually not aware of his difficulty. He prattles along repeating, pausing, prolonging certain syllables without the slightest concern. It is only when he becomes conscious that his speech is unpleasant or funny to others that he is on the way to becoming a secondary or confirmed stutterer.

Although confirmed stuttering is not a disease, it is a very serious affliction because of the social taboo on lack of fluency in speech and on the strange twitches and contortions, especially of the face and lips, which stutterers employ in their effort to force out words.

Many youngsters who stutter form the habit of side-stepping pitfalls in the way of words that are especially difficult for them to pronounce (fear words), with the result that they talk so incoherently that they are looked upon as dumb or silly by their contemporaries. Eventually they may dodge situations in which it is difficult to talk (fear situations) or may greatly limit their conversation. It is easy to see how such "silent stutterers," as they have been called, may grow up to be unhappy, repressed individuals.

When the primary stutterer first notices that his speech is not socially acceptable—perhaps as a result of ridicule from playmates or expressions of concern or even punishment from adults—he first shows signs of bewilderment and then of tension and struggle. Having recognized that the stuttering is an obstacle, he tries to overcome it by force. He attacks words as if they were concrete objects to be forced past his tense tongue

[8] Reported in *Talk*, Vol. 25, No. 9 (September), 1944 (published by the National Hospital for Speech Disorders, New York).

or lips by pressing or squeezing harder than usual with his abdominal muscles. Of course, this only makes the tightness worse. Then he may stamp his foot, or beat his side with his fist, or toss his head, or jerk his jaw as if the word could be jarred out with sudden movements. As he does eventually succeed in saying the word, he associates these queer gyrations with his success. Thenceforth whatever forcing device he has employed becomes an established part of his particular stuttering complex until the device no longer works and he has to invent some other trick.

In studying large numbers of stutterers, psychiatric specialists frequently find tension states, anxiety reactions, emotional immaturity, and feelings of insecurity and apprehensiveness. Unfortunately, the stutterer is usually unaware of what is making him stutter until the psychiatrist is able to discover the underlying cause or causes of his anxiety.

Underneath the anxiety and tension the psychiatrist usually finds resentment or hostility toward parents, teachers, or people in general. This is not surprising if we remember that a child begins to be a confirmed stutterer when he realizes that his speech is displeasing to others. It is easy then to take the next step and feel that he himself is displeasing. Without knowing it, the stutterer may "project" his injured feelings on the world at large. Particular people or perhaps all people are potential enemies lying in wait to take advantage of his weakness. That is why many stutterers are able to talk without difficulty when they believe themselves to be alone. Others will stutter only when in the presence of superiors—parents, teachers, employers—or only when in the classroom surrounded by classmates presumably waiting to laugh. In general, any situations that are anticipated with anxiety—for example, reciting, making a speech, apologizing, explaining a poor report card to parents— will invariably bring on or accentuate the stuttering. On the other hand, situations in which attention is diverted from the stutterer, such as reciting in unison or singing in a group, favor comparatively easy and smooth-flowing speech.

Means of overcoming stuttering have been sought all through history. Engraved on a clay tablet excavated from the ruins of the Biblical town of Beth Shemish was this prayer: "Oh God, cut through the backbone of my stammering. I desire that Thou shalt remove the spring of my impediment." Two of the various cures suggested were running uphill with pebbles in one's mouth reciting as one ran, and chewing pungent substances such as mustard, garlic, and onion. Presumably these practices were designed to take the stutterer's mind off his speech. There have been many modern versions of such distractions, but they have seldom worked a permanent cure because they do nothing to influence the underlying causes.

A stuttering child should have expert attention as early as possible. In some schools, speech correctionists or speech correction teachers and psychologists and psychiatrists are available for helping children with this form of crippling. In schools without these services, the child should be referred to a speech correctionist, a speech clinician, or a speech clinic for the correction of speech disorders and defects. As there are many so-called "stammering schools" and self-styled "speech experts" who trade on the fear and anxiety associated with stuttering, the teacher or nurse serving the school should get reliable information for the child's parents by consulting the school physician or the local medical society or public health unit.

It is important that a child who is learning to speak correctly, no matter what his defect or disorder, should not be made unduly speech-conscious. In school his teachers should not notice and attempt to correct each mistake as it occurs during ordinary conversations or recitations. It will help the child to realize that he is not the only one who has trouble in speaking—that hesitations and repetitions in speech are not uncommon and that other children in the class may stutter or stammer when called on to recite if they are unprepared or talk too fast. And it should be explained to the other children, without the stutterer's knowledge, that stuttering is not done on purpose and cannot be overcome at once. They can help their friend to overcome it if they will overlook his handicap and not laugh at or make fun of him.

DO YOU KNOW?

1. In the following mix-up, words and terms have become separated from their definitions; bring them together again: alveoli; the great muscle responsible for changes in the size of the chest cavity during respiration; respiratory center; air passages in the lungs; sinuses; shelves of bone extending from the side walls of the nose into the nasal cavity; larynx; the air sacs in the lungs where the exchange of respiratory gases takes place; nasopharynx; the group of nerve cells that controls the rate of breathing; diaphragm; the meeting place of nose and throat; bronchial tubes; cavities in the bone of the skull and face; epiglottis; the hollow organ connecting the lower part of the pharynx with the windpipe; turbinates; the structure that keeps food out of the air passages during swallowing.

2. In the following groupings of infections there is one in each group that does not belong. Select the one that is out of place and tell why.

   a. Influenza, measles, pneumococcal pneumonia, chickenpox
   b. Scarlet fever, streptococcal sore throat, blood poisoning, the com-
      mon cold
   c. Mumps, diphtheria, whooping cough, tuberculosis

3. What specific contribution to the present or future well-being of
   children as individuals or in groups may be made by the teacher who

   a. Refers for medical attention a child who is subject to frequent
      head or chest colds? a child who complains of a sore throat? a child
      who persistently breathes through the mouth? a child who has a
      speech difficulty?
   b. Encourages parents to keep children at home when they show early
      signs and symptoms of illness?
   c. Is familiar with the early signs and symptoms of the common
      respiratory infections of childhood?
   d. Trains children in the proper use of handkerchiefs?
   e. Can give artificial respiration?
   f. Has periodic chest x-rays?

4. Tell the difference between

   a. First-infection tuberculosis and reinfection tuberculosis
   b. Tuberculin test and BCG vaccination
   c. Lisping and nasality
   d. Hard palate and soft palate
   e. Primary stuttering and secondary stuttering
   f. Asphyxia and aphasia
   g. Epidemic and pandemic

SUGGESTED ACTIVITIES

1. Count the respirations per minute of a child who is sitting quietly.
   (Do not let the child know that you are doing it. Why?) Count the
   respirations per minute of the same child immediately after he has
   jumped rope twenty times. What is the physiological explanation for
   the difference between the resting rate and the rate after vigorous
   exercise?
2. As a class activity keep a record of the colds suffered by members of
   the group over a specified period of time. Have each victim tell why
   he thinks he caught cold, what the earliest signs and symptoms were,
   how long the cold lasted, what he did for it, and what inconvenience
   it caused him. On the basis of the students' reports and the results of
   research on the transmission of colds, plan a unit for an elementary

or high school class with the object of motivating the children to follow the procedures recommended for preventing the spread of colds and other respiratory infections and for building up good resistance to infection.

3. Have different students prepare and give talks suitable for a meeting of the parent-teacher association, or some other group composed wholly or partly of parents, on the importance of keeping children home from school when they show early indications of illness. Have the rest of the class criticize each talk as to clarity and convincingness.

4. Suppose that a tuberculosis case-finding program is to be launched in a high school. Plan an educational program for the students and their parents designed to win their wholehearted cooperation.

5. Have a member, or committee, of the class prepare a report on the rehabilitation of the tuberculous patient after his disease has been arrested. Suppose that a child is about to return to school after a long stay in a tuberculosis sanatorium. Make up a set of restrictions placed by the physician on the child's study and play activities. Predicate certain emotional problems. Then draw up a plan for helping the child to make a satisfactory adjustment to school life.

6. If possible, arrange to have a member, or committee, of the class visit

   a. The tuberculosis clinic and laboratory of the health department, to obtain data for a report on the official tuberculosis control work of the community

   b. The local tuberculosis and health association, to obtain information for a report on the tuberculosis control work of voluntary agencies in the community

   After hearing the report, the class may conduct a panel discussion on the importance to teachers of knowing what facilities are available in the community for fighting tuberculosis and other menaces to the health of school children.

7. Obtain from the local or state department of health or education a copy of the official regulations regarding the control of communicable diseases in the schools of the community or state. After studying the regulations, have a discussion in class on ways in which teachers can help to increase their effectiveness.

8. Observe the speech of several children whose speech is considered normal. Count the repetitions of single sounds, syllables, words, and phrases and other forms of interruptions (such as prolongation of sounds and excessive use of "uh" or "ah") heard in 5 or 10 minutes. Also observe signs of nonfluency in the normal extemporaneous

speech of fellow students and other adults. How would you use the results of your observations to allay the fears of the parents of a young child who have labeled the child a "stutterer" although his repetitions are characteristic of the speech of all young children?

9. Have panel discussions on what the teacher can do to help

   a. A child who has returned to school after a long illness
   b. A child in the class who stutters
   c. A child who is subject to frequent colds or sore throats
   d. During an epidemic of respiratory disease
   e. In preparing for the tuberculin testing of school children

10. Arrange with a local Red Cross chapter or Boy Scout troop to have a demonstration in class of the back-pressure, arm-lift method of artificial respiration, using a child as the subject.

11. Make a survey of the measures taken to ensure adequate ventilation in the classrooms of your school. As a preliminary to making the survey, you may construct a questionnaire for collecting data on the room temperature found to be most comfortable by each individual. If there is no air-conditioning system, make a plan which will, in the opinion of the class, secure the best atmospheric conditions (temperature, air movement, and humidity) for the comfort of the majority of students in the classrooms.

SELECTED REFERENCES

American Medical Association: *Wonder Stories of the Human Machine: The Breather Pipes and Thermostatic Control (Lungs and Skin)*, Chicago, 1948. (Pamphlet 3 in a series explaining how the principal systems of the body work.)

Anderson, Virgil Antris: *Improving the Child's Speech*, New York, Oxford University Press, 1953.

Chapin, Amy Bishop, and Ruth Lundin: *Your Child's Speech and How to Improve It*, Cleveland, Ohio, Western Reserve University Press, 1949.

Fabricant, Noah D.: *The Common Cold and How to Fight It*, Chicago, Ziff-Davis Publishing Company, 1945.

Johnson, Wendell, ed.: *Speech Problems of Children; A Guide to Care and Correction*, New York, Grune & Stratton, Inc., 1950.

McCall, Marie: *The Long Adventure: Chapters in the Story of Tuberculosis Control*, New York, National Tuberculosis Association, 1946.

PERKINS, JAMES E., and FLOYD M. FELDMANN: *You and Tuberculosis,* New York, Alfred A. Knopf, Inc., 1952.

VAN RIPER, CHARLES: *Case Book in Speech Therapy,* New York, Prentice-Hall, Inc., 1953.

WASSERSUG, JOSEPH D.: *Your Coughs, Colds and Wheezes,* New York, Wilfred Funk, Inc., 1949.

Organizations

American Speech and Hearing Association
National Tuberculosis Association

Chapter 6   ALONG THE ALIMENTARY ROUTE

Preparation of Food for the Body's Use
Signs and Symptoms of Gastrointestinal Disorders
Gastrointestinal Infections
Observations about the Mouth
Observations about the Teeth
How the Body Uses Food Materials
Meeting the Food Needs of School-age Children
The Kidneys and Their Work

PREPARATION OF FOOD FOR THE BODY'S USE

Health is profoundly influenced by the adequacy with which the food needs of the body are met and the efficiency with which the food eaten is digested and utilized. Many of the physical distress signals and complaints of school children are related to minor or major disturbances in the big businesses of digestion, metabolism, nutrition, and excretion. As an aid to understanding why such disturbances may occur, some information is given in various parts of this chapter regarding the normal set-up and operation of these businesses.

Food Patterns

Foods are complex substances made up of many different kinds of raw materials. We may think of any food—meat, potatoes, milk, or bread, for example, as if it were a complicated design built up of blocks of several different compositions and shapes. The blocks, then, would be the foodstuffs of which that particular food is synthesized or built. If we had a whole box of such blocks and could use them to synthesize a food, as actually we cannot do, we should first have to separate them into six groups, or classes, of foodstuffs: (a) carbohydrates, (b) fats, (c) proteins, (d) vitamins, (e) mineral salts, and (f) water. If we wished to go further into the matter, we should find that these raw materials are in turn built up of much simpler elements.

Assuming that it were humanly possible to arrange these simple food elements into the multifarious patterns characteristic of the different foodstuffs, and then to combine the foodstuffs into the great variety of foods with which we are familiar, we should have to turn right around and break them all down again before they could even get into our bodies. As a matter of fact, we do this every time we eat. It is the function of digestion.

Digestion

Digestion takes place in a long tube of varying diameters, open at both ends to the outside world. This tube is called the alimentary canal. In it complex foodstuffs are broken down into simple molecules and dissolved in water so that they can pass into the blood stream and eventually into the cells.

It is illuminating to think of the alimentary canal as being outside the body in the sense that food, while it is in it, is not actually in the body. A potato as eaten, for example, could not get through the intestinal and capillary walls into the blood stream, but a watery solution of glucose (the simple sugar into which all carbohydrates are changed during digestion) can. Similarly, fats like butter and oil, and the proteins of meat, eggs, milk, and so on must be broken down chemically into their soluble constituents before they can pass into the blood stream.

Mechanical Digestion. Before solid foods can be acted upon by the enzymes, or digestive ferments, which change them chemically, they must be broken down mechanically and thoroughly saturated with water. The mechanical part of digestion consists (a) in breaking up the food into small pieces by the teeth and kneading it into a swallowable bolus by the tongue; (b) in mixing the food with digestive ferments, or enzymes, in the mouth, stomach, and small intestine; and (c) in moving the food along in the direction away from the mouth toward the anal canal.

The passage of food through the four large divisions of the alimentary canal—the mouth and esophagus; the stomach; the small intestine; and the large intestine—is regulated by ringlike bands of muscle called sphincters. When a sphincter contracts, it closes the tube at that point so that the food cannot pass onward. One of these sphincters is located at the place where the esophagus leads into the upper end of the stomach. Another guards the opening from the lower end of the stomach into the upper part of the small intestine (duodenum). Still another is placed at the point where the lower end of the small intestine (ileum) leads obliquely into the cecum, or blind beginning of the large intestine (colon). The vermiform appendix projects from the cecum (see Appendicitis, further on). Last of all come the anal sphincters, which guard the beginning and end of the short anal canal leading back from the lowest portion of the large intestine (rectum). Only the external anal sphincter is under voluntary control. It opens when we obey the urge to defecate, or "move the bowels."

All the other sphincters open and close automatically in response to stimuli which indicate that the food is ready to pass from one division of the alimentary canal into the next. The orifice leading from the

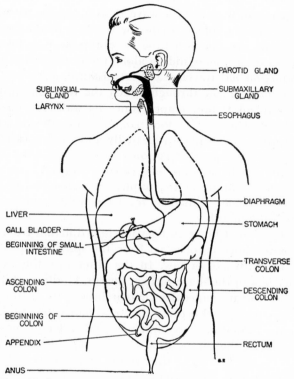

FIG. 49. Important points along the alimentary route.

esophagus to the stomach, for example, opens at the gentle tapping, or pressure, of a well-chewed food bolus after each swallow. Sometimes it stays open for two or three swallows when fluid is being drunk. The sphincter between the stomach and the small intestine opens at the touch of an acid morsel, that is, a morsel thoroughly saturated with the acid gastric juice on the stomach side, and closes behind it as the acid morsel comes in contact with the alkaline mucous membrane on the intestinal side.

Peristalsis. From the lower end of the esophagus to the anal canal, the kind of muscle responsible for moving the contents of the alimentary canal along is smooth muscle. This kind of muscle is involuntary, that is, it is controlled only by the autonomic nervous system. The smooth muscle of the alimentary canal is arranged in two layers—an inner circular layer and an outer longitudinal layer.

The pressure of food against the muscular walls of that part of the tube through which the food is passing is responsible for setting up the wavelike motions of the walls which force the food along. These waves are called peristaltic waves. As a wave of contraction passes along the intestinal tube, for example, it strips the contents of the tube before it, in much the same manner as a tube of toothpaste may be stripped by the strong pressure of fingers sliding along the outside surface. After the wave of contraction has traveled a short distance, a wave of relaxation spreads along the segment through which the food has just been propelled. This segment is now empty. Since its walls are relaxed, it can be filled with another load of food coming from the direction of the mouth. This process takes place repeatedly and rhythmically.

Normally peristaltic waves travel only in one direction, that is, away from the mouth and toward the anal canal. However, reverse peristalsis can and does occur. Many of the unpleasant sensations resulting from digestive misbehavior are caused by reverse wavelets and ripples passing upward toward the mouth.

Chemical Digestion. Chemical digestion is as different from mechanical digestion as is the burning of wood from the splitting up of wood into small fragments with axe or saw. In the latter case the wood remains wood, whether it is in the shape of logs, boards, kindling, chips, shavings, or sawdust, because its molecules remain intact. In burning, however, the wood ceases to be wood because the wood molecules are dismembered and their atoms recombined to form new and different molecules. The wood is gone—into the air as CO_2 (carbon dioxide) and H_2O (water vapor), and onto the hearth or the ground as the noncombustible minerals of which ashes are composed.

In essence, the purpose of chemical digestion is the taking apart of food so that it can get through openings otherwise too small for it. After the food mass has been ground into fine pieces mechanically, its large molecules must be chemically taken apart so that the simpler molecules can pass by the process of osmosis through semipermeable membranes from the small intestine into the blood and lymph streams and on into the cells.

Enzymes. We know that food substances are in themselves more or less stable compounds. That is, they will keep for a long time when dried or frozen or sterilized in cans. A lump of sugar (if protected from moisture) can be kept for centuries without undergoing any appreciable change. If a chemist wanted to split starch molecules into the small soluble sugar molecules of which they are composed, he would have to boil the starch for many hours and add certain acids besides. But we change starch to sugar in a few minutes whenever we eat bread or potatoes or any other starchy food. We can do this because saliva—the digestive juice in the mouth—contains a powerful reagent which can quickly and expertly

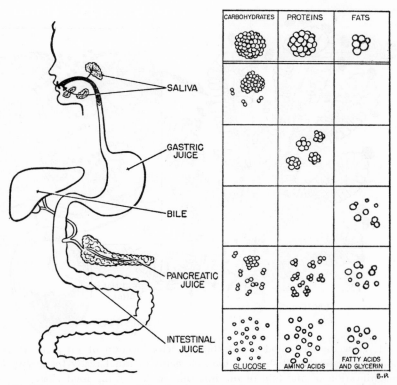

Fig. 50. Chemical digestion. The foodstuffs in the top row are broken down by enzymes in the digestive juices into the simple elements in the bottom row.

change starch into sugar. This reagent is ptyalin, a member of a large class of substances called enzymes. These extraordinary agents participate in practically all chemical wrecking and building operations that take place in living tissues.

Enzymes, like hormones, belong to the family of chemical substances known as catalysts. These substances, as we have learned, change the speed of a reaction by their mere presence without taking part in it.

In the mouth, the salivary enzyme begins the splitting up of starch molecules into sugar molecules. In the stomach, enzymes in gastric juice begin splitting up the giant protein molecules into smaller molecules.

In the duodenum, or upper part of the small intestine, bile from the liver divides the large fat droplets into very fine droplets, that is, emulsifies them. Here, too, pancreatic juice and intestinal juice, each of which contains three different enzymes or ferments, finish up the splitting of all higher starches and sugars into simple grape sugar (glucose), all the

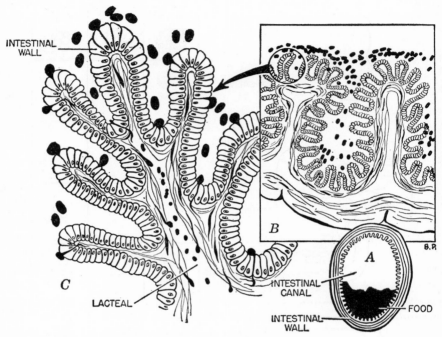

FIG. 51. How digested food is absorbed. *A,* cross section of intestine. *B,* cross section of intestinal wall showing food elements in canal ready for absorption. *C,* magnification of one fold of the intestinal wall showing food elements passing through intercellular spaces into the lacteals (lymph vessels).

larger protein molecules into their constituent amino acids; and all the fats into fatty acid and glycerin. These three groups of substances are the products of digestion, that is, they are the digestible portions of food as chemically split up into soluble particles that can be absorbed into the blood and lymph streams.

Removing the Waste Products of Digestion

After most of the good, except water, has been absorbed from food in the small intestine, what remains passes onward into the large intestine for elimination from the body. Other names for the large intestine are the colon and the bowel.

The colon is shaped somewhat like the small letter n. It begins in the lower right segment of the abdomen, ascends to a point just below the stomach, crosses over to the left side, and descends to the rectum. Many of the feelings of fullness (distention) and rumblings of various kinds blamed on the stomach actually arise from the transverse colon.

The Make-up of Feces. Food residues as they pass into the ascending colon are in almost a liquid state. A little more than 13 ounces of this liquid material passes into the colon in 24 hours; about 5 ounces are evacuated in the same length of time. The difference is made up mostly of water which is absorbed during the progress of the food residues through the colon to the rectum. The evacuated material is called feces.

The bulk of the feces is composed of a much smaller proportion of cellulose and other indigestible materials in food than is popularly supposed. About 9 per cent of the solids in feces is made up of bacteria; in addition there are materials secreted through the walls of the intestine and in the bile, connective-tissue cells, and leukocytes.

Bacterial Decomposition. The bacterial flora of the colon is very luxuriant. The bacteria decompose cellulose (the woody, or fibrous, parts of vegetables, fruits, and grains) and other materials. The color of the feces normally comes from a substance produced by the action of bacteria on bile pigment. The odor of feces is due to the breakdown by bacteria of amino acids (proteins) into various aromatic substances. Some of these substances are highly toxic. It was once thought that their absorption into the blood stream from the large intestine was responsible for many of the ills of mankind. It has been determined, however, that only insignificant amounts of such toxic products get through the intestinal wall into the blood stream and those that do are detoxified in the liver. There is no truth in the idea that constipation (see further on) "poisons the system."

Defecation. Defecation (a bowel movement) is initiated by the propulsion of the feces into the rectum by peristaltic waves traveling across the transverse colon and down the descending colon. When the pressure of the feces on the wall of the rectum reaches a certain height, the defecation reflex, consisting of a strong peristaltic contraction of the colon, occurs. The movements of the bowel wall are accompanied and helped by voluntary contractions of the diaphragm and the abdominal muscles. Relaxation of the sphincters at the beginning and end of the short anal canal permits defecation to take place. The external anal sphincter is under voluntary control. That is, under ordinary circumstances we can obey or disobey the urge to have a bowel movement.

The defecation reflex has a center of its own in the medulla oblongata not far from the respiratory and vomiting centers and a subsidiary center in the spinal cord. As we have seen, pressure on the rectal wall pushes the button, so to speak, which sets off this reflex. However, the rectum adjusts its capacity to the bulk of the feces, and when that happens the pressure stimulus is abolished (see Constipation, further on).

Nervous Control of Digestion

Throughout practically the entire length of the alimentary canal, networks of nerve cells in the walls act as local stations for the autonomic nervous system. One important service made possible by this innervation is the conducting of messages from one part of the digestive tract to another by way of local hookups. Thus widely separated portions can act together for the good of the whole. For example, the exit of food from the stomach into the duodenum signals the colon to get rid of its contents to make room for new waste material coming along. This signal stimulates peristalsis in the colon and explains the call to defecation following a meal.

The tone and motility of gastrointestinal muscle and the secretion of the digestive juices are controlled by impulses from the autonomic nervous system. Many of these impulses are psychic. That is, they are aroused by our feelings about food. If these feelings are pleasant, psychic impulses help to make the digestive mechanism ready for work. They increase muscular tone before or while eating food that is pleasant in odor and taste and start the secretion of the digestive juices. Almost everyone has experienced the watering of the mouth due to the psychic secretion of saliva at the smell, sight, or even thought of appetizing food. Psychic influences also start the secretion of gastric juice and pancreatic juice when we start to eat food that is palatable.

It has long been known that the stomach and intestines are extremely sensitive to intense or prolonged emotions such as fear, anger, and resentment. These emotions use the autonomic nervous system (predominantly the sympathetic division) to achieve their physical effects. Their influence is inhibitory, that is, they stop operations instead of starting them, as the pleasant impulses do. We have all experienced the disagreeable feelings that occur when the movements of the stomach and intestines and the secretion of the digestive juices have been brought to a standstill. They include the "all gone" feeling in the pit of the stomach at moments of impending disaster, the dryness of the mouth in moments of fear, the indigestion following intense excitement or worry or fatigue.

The moral of all this, of course, is that many of the digestive disturbances of childhood—and maturity, too—can be avoided by taking advantage of the beneficent influence of pleasant psychic impulses. That is why doctors tell us that it is important to have food pleasant in taste and smell at regular times each day, to eat with relish and enjoyment, to have cheerful, or at least interesting, table talk, and to avoid excessive exertion before or after a meal. If anything has made us angry or scared or excited, we should calm down before eating.

SIGNS AND SYMPTOMS OF GASTROINTESTINAL DISORDERS

The term gastrointestinal is a combination of a Greek word meaning "stomach" and a Latin word meaning "intestine." Gastrointestinal upsets are extremely common in children, partly because the stomach and intestines are so sensitive both to psychic and to physical stimuli.

Indigestion is practically the generic name for a set of symptoms which varies according to the ways in which digestion fails to proceed in a calm and orderly manner in different individuals. There are many different causes of gastric indigestion, or dyspepsia, which range all the way from hurried eating, indiscretion in eating, or eating when nervous or tired, to allergic sensitivity to certain foods or organic disease of one kind or another.

The mechanism of the more common signs and symptoms associated with gastrointestinal disorders is described here.

Furred Tongue

"Stick out your tongue" is a command with which most youngsters are familiar. Furring of the back of the tongue, accompanied by bad breath and perhaps with loss of appetite and regurgitation of fluid into the mouth, is a common indication of an upset stomach or constipation. It is believed that reverse peristaltic wavelets or ripples are responsible for coated tongue and its accompanying signs. In constipation, according to this explanation, small waves of contraction originating in the loaded bowel travel in a reverse direction over the small intestine, stomach, and esophagus.

Halitosis

The disagreeableness to others of bad breath is a potent argument for the advertisers of products designed to sweeten the breath. It is possible to have bad breath without knowing it, because expired air flows along the floor of the nose, where there are no endings of the olfactory nerve (nerve of smell).

Halitosis may have any one of a number of causes, including stomach or intestinal trouble of one kind or another; infections of the sinuses, tonsils, and gums; and extensive decay or uncleanliness of the teeth. Malodorous breath also may be caused by the odors of incompletely digested fats and of volatile substances like garlic which have been absorbed from the large intestine by the blood and carried to the lungs where they are thrown off in expiration. Medical attention should be secured for a child who continues to have this affliction in spite of faithful brushing of the teeth after each meal and the use of a mouthwash.

Heartburn

A burning sensation in the esophagus which is often felt in the heart region is a common complaint. It is caused by the regurgitation of acid fluid from the stomach. The mucous membrane of the esophagus is very sensitive to acid but the gastric mucosa (mucous membrane lining the stomach) is not. Gastric juice contains hydrochloric acid, which is necessary for the activation of pepsin, one of its ferments, or enzymes. Hence, anything regurgitated from the stomach after it has been mixed with gastric juice will have a sour acid taste and cause an unpleasant burning sensation in the esophagus.

So-called "acid indigestion," which is associated with excessive secretion of hydrochloric acid, may or may not be accompanied by heartburn.

Belching

Many healthy individuals have a tendency after a meal to expel small amounts of gas from the stomach by way of the esophagus and mouth. Normal belching has become associated with hearty eating and was once more polite than it is now when large meals are not in fashion. Among the Chinese, belching to this day is said to be a means of expressing appreciation for a good meal. Belching is brought about by peristaltic waves operating in reverse from the upper end of the stomach.

Although occasional belching after a meal is normal, the repeated belching of gas is considered to be abnormal. In repeated belching, the gas expelled is not produced by the fermentation of food in the process of digestion; rather, it is swallowed air, most of which collects at the lower end of the esophagus. We all know that babies swallow air in nursing and have to be "burped" or "bubbled." In older individuals the swallowing of air seems to be a trick to induce belching in order to gain relief from the sensation of "gas on the stomach." As a matter of fact this feeling is not accompanied by increased pressure within the stomach, and the pressure within the stomach is not lowered after belching.

Children who belch repeatedly are likely to be of the nervous type. They may do it deliberately to attract attention, or they may actually have some gastric discomfort. In any event they need medical attention.

Lump in the Throat

The sphincter guarding the entrance to the stomach from the esophagus is sensitive to anything swallowed which might damage the stomach. If something large or hard like an unchewed piece of meat or a tablet is swallowed, the sphincter may not relax and open up until the substance has had a chance to dissolve or disintegrate.[1]

In hurried eating, food may pile up in the esophagus waiting its turn to go through the sphincter as it contracts and relaxes to let the food descend gradually into the stomach. As a result a feeling of fullness, or heaviness, of the throat or chest may persist for some time after eating.

Very rarely the sensation of "something sticking in the throat" is caused by the failure of the sphincter in the esophagus to relax properly during swallowing. Only a physician can detect and treat this condition.

The feeling of having a lump in the throat is quite often a psychogenic symptom. Probably most of us have experienced this sensation when we felt like weeping. The sensitivity of the throat to psychic influences has been celebrated by some of our greatest poets. The fear-ridden, conscience-stricken Macbeth complains:

> But wherefore could not I pronounce
> "Amen"?
> I had most need of blessing, and "Amen"
> sticks in my throat.

And Browning in "Prospice," imagining the onset of death, cries

> Fear death?—to feel the fog in my throat,
> The mist in my face.

Vomiting

Vomiting is a reversal of the normal movement of food away from the mouth toward the stomach and intestine. A common prelude to vomiting is nausea or "feeling sick to the stomach" (see further on).

In order to vomit, the muscles of the stomach, esophagus, and abdominal wall must work together. This muscular mechanism is governed by a vomiting center located in the medulla oblongata close to the respiratory center. The vomiting center may be influenced by impulses coming in from the stomach and other organs in the abdomen or from practically any region of the body. Consequently, almost any disorder may result in upheaval of the stomach's contents.

The act of vomiting is essentially a reflex act. Various mechanical and chemical irritants acting on the gastric mucosa may be responsible for pulling the trigger, so to speak. Among them are toxic substances in food

[1] If a child swallows a foreign body such as a piece of broken glass or a pin or a coin, the physician should be consulted at once. A laxative should not be given. (See under Choking, in Chap. 5, for any object lodged in the windpipe.) What to do when poisons are swallowed is not described in this book because poisoning accidents very rarely occur in school.

or toxic products formed in the process of digestion. Certain chemical substances are very irritating to the endings of nerves running to the vomiting center. These substances are called emetics. Those most commonly used to induce vomiting are ipecac, mustard water, and salt water.

Impulses coming from structures other than the stomach also excite the vomiting center. It is well known that tickling the throat with a feather or pushing a finger into the throat will induce vomiting. Any inflammation or obstruction in the intestine, appendicitis, for example, may cause violent vomiting. Also irritation of any other organ, such as the heart, kidneys, urinary bladder, or gall bladder, may initiate vomiting when nothing whatever is irritating the stomach.

Severe pain anywhere in the body; strong emotions such as disgust, fear, or anxiety; and unpleasant stimulation of the sense organs of sight, taste, or smell by greatly disliked or unappetizing foods may set off the vomiting reflex. Physical fatigue and mental stress may have the same effect. Also vomiting may be a neurotic sign if it recurs frequently for no apparent reason.

The motions of the stomach in vomiting are very interesting. In human beings, except babies, there are usually no reverse peristaltic movements of the stomach walls. However, there may be violent churning movements. Just before vomiting there is a sudden reduction in the tone of the stomach walls and the lower part of the stomach drops a couple of inches. This coincides with the sensation of nausea. That sinking feeling in the stomach has a sound physiological basis. Sharp pressure on the relaxed stomach by contractions of the diaphragm and abdominal muscles ejects the stomach's contents.

Nausea

Nausea may precede vomiting or occur alone. It is usually associated with pallor and sweating. The actual sinking of the stomach that takes place when a nauseous odor or some other stimulus is applied stretches the esophagus and stomach walls. It is thought that this movement exerts tension on the nerve endings and so induces nausea.[2] The sensations experienced in the changes of speed of an elevator, or in the rolling of a ship at sea or in an airplane, or while riding in an automobile or train are probably the result of tension on the esophagus and stomach walls. However, the most powerful factor in the production of motion sickness, or "seasickness," as this sensation is popularly called, is the stimulation of nerve endings in the semicircular canals near the ears (see Observa-

[2] BEST, CHARLES HERBERT, and NORMAN BURKE TAYLOR, "The Physiological Basis of Medical Practice," 6th ed., p. 602, Williams & Wilkins, Baltimore, 1955.

tions about the Ears, in Chap. 8). Dramamine or some other recently introduced drug is used in its prevention.

Loss of Appetite

Appetite and hunger are different sensations, although they often occur together. In hunger a hollow or empty feeling in the stomach and contractions of the walls of the empty stomach (sometimes called "hunger pains") direct us to eat in order to "keep the home fires burning." Few persons in lands of peace and plenty experience the pangs of hunger caused by dire need for food. Usually there is plenty of unabsorbed food in the intestine when an empty stomach causes the sensation of hunger.

It is common knowledge that the more active a child is the hungrier he is at mealtime. An active child eats more than the child who is temperamentally inclined to lead a quiet existence, because he spends more energy which must be replenished by food. Eating meals at the same time each day tends to establish the periods at which a child begins to feel hungry. Appetite is connected with pleasure in eating. It may coincide with hunger, but also may exist independently. The habit of "nibbling" or consuming sweet foods or drinks between meals, which most children fall into if they are allowed to, is one of the chief causes of lack of appetite at mealtimes in healthy children.

Happy memories of the taste of certain foods, appetizing odors, and foods pleasing to the eye normally stimulate appetite; fatigue and emotions like worry, fright, and sorrow normally banish it (see Psychogenic Reactions, in Chap. 3). The smell or even the thought of disgusting or unpleasing food will, as we have seen, cause nausea, which is the exact opposite of appetite.

Poor appetite or loss of appetite (anorexia) may be associated with lowered tone in the stomach walls. As gastric tone is low in various disorders, poor appetite or loss of appetite in children whose appetite has hitherto been good may indicate the onset of illness.

In some cases lack or loss of appetite is an expression of resentment caused by adverse attitudes of the parents toward the child or toward each other or by some psychological shock connected with food or with the mouth. Very often the child gets extra and gratifying attention from his parents because of his lack of appetite, and this so-called "secondary gain" must be removed before steps can be taken to find and remove the underlying cause through psychiatric treatment.

Pain

Several different types of pain are among the most common symptoms of gastrointestinal disturbances and diseases. Yet the organs of the abdomen (and of the chest, also) are not sensitive to the various stimuli that arouse the sensation of pain in the skin, muscles, and other superficial structures of the body. The stomach, intestine, and heart, for example, can be touched, cut, pinched, or burned without immediately causing pain. Food or drink would have to be very hot or very cold indeed before the stomach would "feel" it. The sensations of heat and cold aroused by the temperature of what we eat and drink originate for the most part in the lower portion of the esophagus. The stomach, as we have seen, is also insensitive to acid.

What then does give us a stomach-ache or some other kind of abdominal distress? The answer to this question is highly controversial. It is safe to say, however, that the pain felt as a result of a disease process or disturbance in any organ of the chest or the abdomen may be referred pain (see Referred Pain, in Chap. 3) or pain localized in or near the organ itself. In the case of stomach-ache, for example, the pain is usually referred to the superficial structures overlying the stomach; in coronary heart disease, to the left arm; in gall-bladder disease, to the right shoulder. If the pain is localized in the organ itself, the stimulus is thought to be tension.[3] Pain may be felt in any hollow organ if it is distended by its contents (an overstuffed stomach or too-full bladder, for example) or by inflammation or obstruction of any part. The pain impulses arise in response to the stretch stimulus acting on the nerve endings in the organ's walls.

Jaundice

The yellowish tinge of the skin which goes by the name of jaundice is caused by the presence in the blood of an excess amount of bile pigment. The pigment escapes from the blood into the skin, mucous membranes, and conjunctivae of the eyes, which then become stained a yellow tint.

The chief bile pigment is bilirubin, the iron-free fraction of the red-blood-cell pigment, hemoglobin. When the red cells fall apart as a result of bumping around at great speed through the blood vessels, their hemoglobin is set free. This liberated hemoglobin is in turn broken up. Part of it is used to produce new hemoglobin and the other part—bilirubin—is carried in the blood stream to the liver, whence it is excreted in bile. Besides serving as a vehicle for the excretion of bilirubin and other waste products, bile also is essential for the efficient digestion of fat (see How the Body Uses Food Materials, further on).

In general, jaundice may be caused in three ways. In the following conditions bilirubin will accumulate in the blood and produce a yellowish skin discoloration:

[3] *Ibid.,* p. 599.

1. When red blood cells are destroyed faster than the liver can excrete bilirubin. The excess pigment then piles up in the blood. Any illness in which the destruction of red blood cells is a pronounced feature may produce this type of jaundice.
2. If the bile duct through which bile passes from the liver to the small intestine is obstructed (by a gallstone, for example).
3. If for some reason the liver itself cannot excrete bilirubin in normal amounts, as, for example, in infectious hepatitis (see Table 10).

In any given case of jaundice two or all three causative factors may, and frequently do, exist together. The important point is that a pronounced yellowish tinge of the skin and eye whites is not normal and should always be brought to the attention of the doctor or nurse. A period of observation and tests of various kinds are required to determine the cause of the jaundice.

Constipation

Constipation (from a Latin word meaning "crowding together") is the term used in referring to the retention of feces for a longer period than is normal for a particular individual. Children—and adults, too—differ from one another in their bowel habits. It may be usual for an individual to have one bowel movement in 24 hours; for another to have two or three movements in the same time; for still another to have one movement every two or every three days. The average is once or twice in 24 hours.

Occasional constipation is rarely harmful. Its worst feature is the anxiety it rouses in worried parents or in others who have been conditioned—largely by advertising—to look upon a daily bowel movement as essential. Chronic constipation, however, is difficult to correct. The habit of "cleaning out the bowels" by taking cathartics or purgatives which stimulate peristalsis penalizes the whole digestive tract for the sluggish action of only one part. It is like burning down the house to roast a pig, as Charles Lamb tells us the Chinese did before they learned a better way. Moreover, depending upon purgatives or laxatives (which are mild purgatives) is likely to make the colon lazy and hence to prolong the very condition that they are supposed to correct.

Aside from mechanical obstruction the chief causes of constipation are

1. *Irregular toilet habits.* We have seen that defecation is on the borderline between a voluntary and an involuntary act. The sensation of a full rectum automatically arouses the urge to defecate, but the act can be inhibited voluntarily. Refusal to respond to this sensation and failure to acquire the habit of clearing the bowels at a

regular time each day (for example, after breakfast) are common causes of constipation. The tone of the muscles in the colon and rectum will suffer, and the nervous impulses responsible for the call for defecation may cease to be given if it is persistently disobeyed. This means that the rectum has become resigned to the increased bulk of feces and has made the necessary adaptations. Also more fluid is absorbed from the retained feces. As a result, they become hard and dry and difficult to expel. It is very important to make it easy for youngsters to have a regular time for moving their bowels. Once the colon has established the habit, it usually continues to function automatically at that time throughout life.

2. *Too little roughage and water in the diet.* Indigestible materials, especially cellulose, increase the bulk of the feces and stimulate intestinal activity. Water is an aid to elimination, as to many other body functions.

3. *A misbehaving colon.* In some individuals the colon may be too tense (hypertonic or spastic) or too slack (atonic or weak) or too absorbent ("greedy" or "thrifty"). These conditions can be detected and treated only by a physician.

Diarrhea

In diarrhea the bowels move much more frequently than usual and the feces have a watery consistency. Feces may be hustled through the colon before the normal amount of water can be absorbed (premature evacuation) for many reasons besides the irritation of the intestinal wall by the action of transient bacteria (not normal inhabitants of the colon) or their toxic products.

Psychic influences, such as excitement or fear, may speed up peristaltic movements in some individuals, with the result that diarrhea persists until the exciting cause is removed.

In severe diarrhea caused by bacteria or their toxins, such as cholera or bacillary dysentery (see further on), water is drawn into the intestine from the tissue spaces to aid in flushing out toxic substances. As a result, dehydration of the body occurs and weight is lost.

GASTROINTESTINAL INFECTIONS

Infectious diseases of the gastrointestinal tract are much less common than formerly, chiefly owing to the successful efforts of public health officials in our country to safeguard our water, milk, and solid-food supplies and to ensure the sanitary disposal of human and animal intestinal wastes.

The average American family and its members and the American school also may take part of the credit. An important part of the health education of children and their elders has been, and still is, concerned with sanitary food handling, sanitary dishwashing, fly and rodent control, and similar measures in the home, and with personal habits, such as hand washing before eating and preparing food and after toilet, which make it difficult for germs to gain access to the body by being swallowed alive.

Take up only the ones underlined

Bacterial Infections

Typhoid Fever. The classic water-borne, milk-borne, fly-borne disease is typhoid fever. Its control in our country has been called "perhaps the greatest triumph of organized preventive medicine." Since the beginning of the twentieth century the annual death rate from this disease has been reduced by 99 per cent. Many large cities are now free of it. It occurs chiefly in outbreaks which can be traced to a single polluted well or other source of drinking water, or to a single unknown carrier concerned with milk handling or with the handling of food in a home, camp, or eating establishment. The typhoid carrier (a person who harbors and spreads the bacilli of typhoid without himself being ill) has always been a great problem in typhoid control.

The bacillus of typhoid fever has been given many names, the latest of which (1948) is *Salmonella typhosa.* There seems to be no doubt that this bacillus belongs to the genus *Salmonella,* which we shall meet later on in this chapter as the genus responsible for food infections.

It is not necessary for teachers to be on the lookout for early signs and symptoms of typhoid (see Table 10) except during an epidemic in their own locality and during floods or other disasters that threaten the purity of communal or family water supplies.

Dysentery. Dysentery is a common disease among children, especially children under the age of five. Since the decline of typhoid fever, it has assumed a greater relative importance as a cause of gastrointestinal infection. Bacilli belonging to the *Shigella* group are the most frequent cause of dysentery. Amebas (*Endamoeba histolytica*) are responsible for another fairly common form of the disease.

Bacillary dysentery (shigellosis) is spread in the same way as is typhoid fever. However, it is much more difficult to prevent by public health measures because most measures are ineffective against the direct (person-to-person) contact which plays a large part in epidemics of dysentery. Bacillary dysentery has always been the curse of armies. Hans Zinsser in his famous biography of typhus fever, "Rats, Lice, and History," pointed out that "typhus with its brothers and sisters—plague, cholera, typhoid,

Table 10. COMMUNICABLE DISEASES CONTRACTED MAINLY

	Bacillary dysentery (shigellosis)	Food infections (salmonellosis)	Food poisoning (staphylococcal intoxication)
Cause...	Bacilli of the *Shigella* group; present in intestinal discharges.	Bacteria of the *Salmonella* group; present in feces of infected persons or carriers and in feces of infected fowl, rodents, and domestic animals; in eggs of infected ducks and hens.	The toxin of certain strains of staphylococci present in contaminated foods.
How spread	By consuming milk and milk products, other foods, and water contaminated with bowel discharges of infected persons or carriers; by hand-to-mouth transfer of such discharges and by objects soiled with them. (Flies may carry bacilli on their feet.)	By consuming food or milk contaminated by feces of infected rodents or other infected animals; by feces-soiled hands of infected food handlers; also by eating insufficiently cooked foods containing dried duck eggs or hen eggs.	By consuming milk from infected cows and foods in which staphylococci have been deposited by infected food handlers. Starchy foods, such as custard-filled pastry and salad dressings, when kept at room temperature, are especially good culture media for the staphylococci.
Incubation period	From 1 to 7 days; usually less than 4.	From 6 to 48 hours; usually about 12.	From ½ hour to 4 hours; usually 2 to 4 hours.
Onset....	Usually sudden with fever, irritability or drowsiness, loss of appetite, vomiting or nausea, diarrhea, and abdominal pain.	Sudden with diarrhea, abdominal cramps, fever; occasionally nausea and vomiting.	Sudden with severe nausea, vomiting, prostration; in some cases, severe diarrhea.
Period of communicability	From onset until bowel discharges are free of bacilli.	For duration of illness; usually 3 days to 3 weeks or as long as carrier state persists.	None.
Character of the infection	The bacilli grow in the intestinal mucosa and excrete a toxin. Mild cases are characterized by abdominal discomfort, slight fever, and a few loose stools; in severe cases there are fever, nausea, vomiting, stools containing blood and pus, and colicky pains.	Salmonella grow rapidly in the intestinal tract and produce a toxin which causes the diarrhea and other signs and symptoms. Recovery is usually complete in from 2 to 4 days. Explosive outbreaks occur among large numbers of individuals who have consumed the offending food.	The toxin produced by the staphylococci in food *before it is eaten* is responsible for the signs and symptoms of acute gastrointestinal poisoning. Staphylococcal toxin is probably the principal cause of acute food poisoning.
Methods of control *	No specific preventive. Antibiotics used in treatment remove bacilli from stools in from 24 to 48 hours and bring freedom from infection within a few days. Isolation during acute illness. Relative temporary immunity after attack.	No specific preventive. Isolation not required, but adults excluded from food handling and care of children until recovery. No lasting immunity after attack.	No specific preventive. Exclusion from food handling of individuals suffering from boils and other skin infections until infection has cleared up. No immunity after attack.

Source: principally "Control of Communicable Diseases in Man," 8th ed., American Public Health Association, New York, 1955, and "Zinsser's Textbook of Bacteriology," 9th ed. (revised by David T. Smith, *et al.*), Appleton-Century-Crofts, New York, 1948.

* General preventive measures for the control of water-borne, milk-borne, and food-borne diseases include protection and purification of water supplies; pasteurization of milk supplies; sanitary disposal of excreta; prevention of fly breeding; elimination of rodents and other vermin; protection of food

Hepatitis, infectious	Typhoid fever	Undulant fever (brucellosis)
A virus; present in intestinal discharges, in blood, and possibly in nose and throat discharges of infected persons.	The typhoid bacillus (*Salmonella typhosa*); present in intestinal discharges and in urine.	Bacilli of the type species *Brucella*; present in the tissues, blood, milk, and urine of infected goats, cattle, sheep, and swine.
Uncertain; probably by direct and indirect contact; † epidemics occur most commonly in groups of children or young adults living closely together, as in camps or institutions. Transmission also occurs through transfusions of whole blood and by injection of blood serum or plasma from infected persons.	By direct and indirect contact † with sick persons and carriers. Contaminated food, milk, water, and shellfish important sources of infection. Flies may spread the bacilli from feces to food under some conditions.	By consuming raw milk or milk products from infected cows and goats and by direct contact with infected animals and the tissues of slaughtered infected animals.
Probably from 21 to 35 days.	From 1 to 3 weeks; average 2 weeks.	Usually 14 to 30 days; occasionally 3 months.
Slow or abrupt, with fever, loss of appetite, nausea, vomiting, and abdominal distress.	Slow with headache, malaise, loss of appetite, and congestion of upper respiratory passages; slight fever which steadily rises day by day.	Slow with irregular fever, sweating, chills or chilliness, and muscle and joint pains.
Unknown; virus persists in stools for as long as 1 month after onset; may persist in blood for as long as a year.	For as long as typhoid bacilli appear in the excreta. Usually from onset throughout illness until all symptoms cease.	Practically not communicable from person to person, but bacilli may be present in the urine or other discharges.
The virus causes inflammation of the liver; as a result jaundice develops in from 5 to 7 days after onset. Recovery usually takes place in 2 or more weeks. In some cases convalescence is slow, with lassitude, weakness, mental depression, and loss of appetite.	The bacilli penetrate the intestinal mucosa, thereby gaining entrance to the blood stream and causing a systemic infection. Rose spots (small hemorrhages into the skin) may appear over the chest and abdomen between the tenth and fifteenth day. Illness is protracted, convalescence slow, and relapses are common.	The bacilli enter the blood stream from the intestinal tract or skin and cause a systemic infection. Acute cases usually recover in from 1 to 3 months. Periods of apparent recovery and relapses alternate in a characteristic pattern. If allergy to the bacillus develops, subacute or chronic brucellosis (lasting for from 1 to 20 years) may follow the acute attack.
Gamma globulin obtained from pooled human blood plasma injected promptly after exposure gives passive protection lasting 6 to 8 weeks. Isolation during the first week of illness is recommended. Persons who have had the infection should not act as blood donors.	Typhoid vaccine gives active immunization for about 1 year. Chloramphenicol (an antibiotic) is effective in treatment. Isolation required in flyproof room until repeated negative cultures of stool and urine specimens, taken at 24-hour intervals, have been obtained.	Avoidance of unpasteurized milk and milk products is the best preventive for the general population. Certain antibiotics, especially a combination of Aureomycin and streptomycin, are effective in treatment. Isolation not required.
Immunity usual after attack.	Immunity usual after attack.	Duration of immunity uncertain.

from flies, rodents, and other vermin; methods of refrigeration and cooking which inhibit bacterial growth or destroy bacteria or other pathogens in possibly contaminated foods; detection and elimination of infected persons and carriers in eating establishments; sanitary dishwashing; and thorough washing of the hands with soap and water after toilet and before handling or eating food.

† Direct contact means directly from person to person. Indirect contact means indirectly through handling, eating, or drinking anything soiled by discharges from the sick person or carrier.

dysentery—has decided more campaigns than Caesar, Hannibal, Napoleon, and all the inspector generals of history."

The hallmark of dysentery is diarrhea (see Table 10 for signs and symptoms at onset). Attacks differ in severity with different individuals. Some children may have only mild discomfort with a few loose bowel movements. Others may be extremely ill with severe prostration and colic. In severe cases the diarrhea begins with a thin watery discharge, which later contains blood and pus.

Contact with a mild case of bacillary dysentery may result in severe cases in other children. All children who complain of diarrhea in school should be referred to the nurse or physician serving the school. Laboratory examination of the stools (bowel movements) is the only sure means of detecting whether a child has dysentery and, if so, what type is present.

Food Infections (Salmonellosis) and Food Poisoning (Bacterial Intoxication). "Food poisoning" is the term used generally in referring to gastrointestinal upsets caused by "something we ate." We hear of it chiefly as occurring simultaneously in large numbers of persons who have eaten the same food at a picnic or church supper or school cafeteria or some other eating establishment. Probably it is more common than reports of outbreaks of this kind lead us to believe, because many cases of "common diarrhea" or dysentery are in reality food infections or food poisonings.

Food infections are caused by members of the *Salmonella* group, of which there are 150 species. Any one of the 150 except *Salmonella typhosa* (the cause of typhoid fever) may be responsible for the intestinal upset known medically as salmonellosis. However, only three or four members of the *Salmonella* group are common in the United States.

The *Salmonella* organisms are very widely distributed in nature. They are present in the feces of infected human beings and carriers, in the meat of infected cattle and other livestock, in the eggs of infected ducks and hens, and in the intestinal droppings of infected domestic fowl, household pets, rodents, and domestic animals. Rodents are dangerous sources of infection because they often contaminate food both before and after it has been prepared for the table. Perhaps the most common source of salmonellosis, however, is the human carrier who handles food with soiled hands during its preparation or serving. Oily salad dressings and creamy cake and pastry fillings are good vehicles for transmitting the organisms from the careless carrier to his victims.

Salmonella organisms, taken into the body in food or drink, lodge in the intestinal tract, where they grow rapidly. They may produce enough poison there to cause symptoms (see Table 10) within 6 hours. The usual incubation period is 12 hours.

Intestinal food poisoning is caused by toxins preformed in food by our ubiquitous foe, the staphylococcus (see under Skin Infections, in Chap. 7). Staphylococci may be planted in food by food handlers with staphylococcal skin infections (such as boils or pimples) on the hands or wrists, or in milk from the udders of infected cows.

When the contaminated food stands at room temperature for 8 to 10 hours, the staphylococci produce enough toxin in the food to poison those who eat it. The foods in which these bacteria grow best are those which contain starch, for example, éclairs, cream puffs, cake fillings, and salad dressings.

The poison works quickly. Usually persons who have eaten food containing it become acutely ill (see Table 10) in 2 to 4 hours. Recovery usually takes place in 24 to 48 hours.

Undulant Fever (Brucellosis). Three closely related bacilli of the genus *Brucella*—one infecting goats, one infecting cows, and one infecting swine—are responsible for the animal disease known as brucellosis. The family name *Brucella* was bestowed in honor of the British army surgeon Sir David Bruce, who first isolated the goat-infecting species (1887) from British soldiers on the island of Malta. The name undulant fever was given to brucellosis in human beings because of the characteristic up-and-down—wavelike—nature of the fever.

Human beings catch undulant fever by direct contact with infected goats, cows, sheep, and swine, or their carcasses, or by consuming the raw milk or milk products of infected goats, sheep, and cows. By far the most common route of infection in our country is direct invasion of the intestinal tract by living *Brucella* bacilli present in unpasteurized cow's milk, cheese, and butter. Undulant fever is rare in cities and large towns, where most of the milk supply is pasteurized. However, these city dwellers are more susceptible to the disease than are country dwellers, who have had a chance to build up immunity by repeated slight infections. There have been many cases in which city dwellers on vacation have contracted undulant fever by drinking a single glass of raw cow's milk.

Undulant fever occurs in human beings in three typical forms—acute, subacute, and chronic. All three can be produced by any of the three species of *Brucella*.

The acute form of the disease usually begins insidiously (see Table 10). Periods of apparent recovery followed by relapse are characteristic. Usually the infection subsides spontaneously in 1 to 3 months.

The subacute form of undulant fever may follow the acute phase if the infected person becomes allergic to the infecting organisms. The chronic form may last for 1 to 20 years. The symptoms are mild but persistent and disabling. Blood tests and skin tests for allergy are essential in diagnosis and in checking up on the progress of the disease.

Vaccines are available for immunizing stockyard workers, farmers, veterinary surgeons, and laboratory workers who handle cultures of *Brucella* bacilli. As for the rest of us, the best preventive is to make sure that we and our children use only milk and milk products that have been pasteurized.

Infectious Hepatitis. This inflammation of the liver (Greek *hepar,* meaning "liver," plus "-itis") has been known for generations under the name of catarrhal jaundice. It is now known to be caused by a specific virus. The disease occurs most commonly in children and young men. It spreads in epidemic form among children who are gathered together as in schools, summer camps, and institutions. Extensive outbreaks have occurred among military forces during wars. Epidemic hepatitis was a great problem among the troops stationed in the Mediterranean area during the First and Second World Wars.

The disease appears to be spread by direct person-to-person contact, although the experimental evidence shows that the circuit consisting of intestinal discharges → to food or fingers → to mouth is the most important method of transmission. That is why it is of great importance during epidemics to emphasize personal cleanliness, especially after toilet and before eating or handling food. The onset of infectious hepatitis (see Table 10) is similar to that of many other so-called digestive upsets in children. The jaundice usually does not appear until 5 to 7 days after onset.

Appendicitis

The appendix is a small wormlike (vermiform) pouch composed of lymphoid tissue which projects from the cecum like one finger of a glove. The cecum itself is the closed lower portion of the ascending colon (see Fig. 49). This blind alley extends some $2\frac{1}{2}$ inches below the juncture of the small and large intestines, low down on the right side of the abdomen. Opening from a cul-de-sac as it does, with no outlet at its other end, the appendix has poor drainage.

The inflammation of the appendix known as appendicitis probably starts in most cases as a result of the blocking of the appendix by foreign matter entering it from the large intestine. Blockage of the appendix interferes with its drainage, injures its walls, and permits bacteria present in the intestinal tract to set up an infection.

Children and young adults are unusually susceptible to appendicitis, but it may occur at any age.

Pain in the abdomen, with nausea and vomiting, is the earliest sign of acute appendicitis. Frequently it starts with generalized pain or pain in the upper part of the abdomen which shortly becomes localized in the lower right side. The pain may be severe and cramplike, or it may be a dull ache. Occasionally it may let up, but this does not mean that the attack has passed.

Soon after the pain sets in, nausea and vomiting usually, but not always, begin. The temperature usually rises slightly above normal; and the abdomen, especially over the appendix, becomes increasingly tender and painful.

Any child who vomits and complains of pain or tenderness in the abdomen should have medical attention as quickly as possible. He should be taken home from school, not sent home by himself, and his family should be impressed with the importance of

1. Sending for a physician without delay
2. Doing *nothing* except to keep the child lying down and quiet until the doctor gets there

It is especially dangerous to give the child a laxative or an enema. The action of the laxative or enema increases the pressure in the appendix and may cause it to rupture or "blow out" and spread the infection. This may be followed by the serious condition called peritonitis. The sulfonamides and penicillin are now often used successfully in the treatment of peritonitis, but peritonitis may cause death.

Appendicitis is sometimes difficult to diagnose. The physician may need to take several blood counts and make other tests. Surgical operation after the diagnosis of appendicitis is made results in recovery of the great majority of children in whom the appendix has not ruptured.

Sometimes a child has an attack of acute appendicitis in which the inflammation subsides without an operation but never entirely clears up. Mild attacks may recur from time to time, and between attacks the child may be troubled with spells of indigestion or have rather constant pain or discomfort soon after eating. Any child complaining of such symptoms should be referred for medical attention.

Intestinal Parasites

Several species of worms are parasitic in the intestines of human beings. Three of these, the pinworm (*Enterobius vermicularis*), the roundworm (*Ascaris lumbricoides*), and the hookworm (*Necator americanus*), are the ones most likely to be found in children.

Infestation with any of these worms may not produce symptoms. In that case, the discovery that the child has "worms" may be made only by having the stools examined by a physician. Ordinarily, however, the child shows that something is wrong by losing weight, by becoming paler than usual, or by complaining of dizziness, headache, nausea, abdominal pain, diarrhea, constipation, or feeling tired all the time. He may lose his appetite or have an increased appetite. Of course this bewildering array of signs and symptoms will not occur in any one child. Moreover, any of them, either singly or in combinations of two or more, may be present in a great variety of conditions. Parents used to suspect "worms" more often than they do now when any child seemed "out of sorts" or not like his usual self.

Pinworms (Enterobiasis). Other names for these tiny, white, threadlike intestinal worms are "threadworms" and "seat worms."

Infestation occurs when pinworm eggs from the anal region are transferred directly to the mouth of the same host by way of the fingers or indirectly to the mouth of the same host or to new hosts by contaminated foods or other articles. Frequently a child with pinworms reinfests himself by scratching the anal region, thus getting eggs on his fingers, and then putting his fingers in his mouth.

After being swallowed the eggs hatch in the stomach and small intestine. The young worms reach maturity in the lower part of the small intestine, cecum, and upper part of the large intestine. They then migrate to the rectum and deposit their eggs on the skin in the anal region.

The presence of pinworms in the rectum and anus (and sometimes in the vagina and urinary bladder of girls) causes intense itching. This constant irritation makes the children restless and interferes with their sleep and appetite. Infestation with pinworms is one possibility when a child continually squirms in his seat and acts irritable and tired. Appendicitis in children is sometimes caused by pinworms which get into the appendix from the cecum.

Pinworms can usually be cured quickly by appropriate chemotherapeutic drugs given under medical direction. Improvement in the child's health after cure is often dramatic.

To prevent reinfestation and spread to new hosts, the strictest hygienic measures must be observed. Children must be impressed with the necessity for washing their hands with soap and water after going to the toilet and before eating and for not putting their fingers in their mouths (as in nail biting, for example). Toilet seats in the home and the school should be washed daily with a disinfectant. The bed linen and underclothing of members of an infested household should be changed daily and boiled to kill the eggs.

Roundworms (Ascariasis). Roundworms are large and resemble earthworms. They lead a parasitic existence in the small intestine, which they reach by a circuitous route. Eggs containing the embryos are present in soil or on various articles in and about the house which are polluted with the intestinal excreta of infested persons. When taken into the mouth, the embryonated eggs travel to the intestinal canal, where they hatch. The larvae penetrate the intestinal wall and reach the lungs by way of the blood stream. Thence they pass through the air passages into the throat and are again swallowed. Upon reaching the small intestine they settle down and develop into mature worms.

Roundworm infestation is most prevalent in families where standards of hygiene are low and essential toilet facilities are either lacking or so poorly constructed that the soil can be polluted by excreta containing the eggs. Preschool children and children of early school age are likely to be more frequently and more heavily infested with roundworms than are older children and adults.

Children infested with roundworms may show no symptoms other than vague indications of poor health. When heavily infested, however, they usually have colicky pain and diarrhea and are nervous, restless, and tired because of disturbed sleep.

Roundworms can be readily eliminated by medical treatment. To prevent infestation and reinfestation in homes and neighborhoods where ascariasis is prevalent, measures must be taken to avoid soil pollution by the construction of sanitary toilets or privies; and the children, especially, must be encouraged to use their toilet facilities and to wash their hands thoroughly before handling food and after toilet.

Hookworm (Ancylostomiasis). Full-grown hookworms are small whitish worms not quite half an inch long and as thick as an "invisible" hairpin. In most cases they enter the body in the larval stage by penetrating the skin, usually of the feet. The larvae pass by way of the lymphatics to one of the big veins leading into the right heart. Thence they travel in the blood stream to the lungs, whence they pass through the capillary walls into the alveoli. From there they pass up the bronchi and windpipe to the throat and are swallowed. Eventually they reach the small intestine, where they develop into adult worms. Infestation can take place by mouth from water, food, or fingers contaminated with larvae, but the most common avenue is through the skin.

Hookworm disease is endemic in regions where soil pollution is favored by inadequate facilities for disposing of human intestinal wastes and where the temperature does not get low enough in winter to destroy the larvae in the soil by freezing. The practice of going barefoot is an important factor in its spread. Hookworm disease is widely endemic in the Southern United States although its prevalence has been greatly decreased in recent years by determined efforts to control it.

The signs and symptoms of hookworm disease vary greatly according to the degree of infestation. Inflammation of the skin of the feet or of other parts of the skin coming in contact with polluted soil may be the first sign. The itching sore spots are called by various names—"ground itch," "dew itch," "cow itch," "foot itch," or "toe itch." If only a few worms are present, there may be no general symptoms. In mild infestations the person may seem merely listless or lazy. Moderate to severe infestations are marked by great depression, indigestion, and diarrhea or constipation. There may be severe anemia and swelling (edema) of the abdomen and legs. The skin is pasty yellow, harsh and dry, and the gums and lips pale. Children infested with hookworm may be retarded physically and mentally. They may crave unusual things to eat such as paper, chalk, dirt, or clay—hence the name "dirt-eater's disease" which is sometimes used.

All that is necessary to cure hookworm disease is to get the worms out of the small intestine. Physicians have several effective ways of doing this. In a section where hookworm is endemic, any child who shows any signs or symptoms of having the disease should be referred to a doctor, or a clinic, for a stool examination. If the child has the disease, eggs will be found in the intestinal discharges.

The prevention of hookworm disease depends primarily upon keeping human excreta containing hookworm eggs off the ground. This may be accomplished by the construction of sanitary privies in communities not served by communal sewerage systems and by teaching children—and their elders—never to defecate on the ground. Hookworm disease also may be prevented by wearing shoes so that the larvae cannot bore their way through the skin of the feet. But the most effective measure is to keep intestinal discharges off the ground.

OBSERVATIONS ABOUT THE MOUTH

The first section of the alimentary canal is the mouth. Here the food is tested by the taste buds on the tongue and the olfactory (smelling) apparatus of the nose, masticated by the teeth, mixed with saliva, and rolled into a swallowable bolus by the tongue.

The Lips

The portals of the mouth are the lips. Reference has already been made to the function of the lips in forming speech sounds (see Speech Difficulties, in Chap. 5). The lips are covered with mucous membrane which is an extension of that which lines the mouth and throat. In healthy children the lips are pink, smooth, and firm. The chief disorders of the lips are harelip, cracking at the corners, and cold sores.

Cheilosis. Scarring, cracking, or sores at the angles of the lips (cheilosis, Plate 8) should be called to the attention of the physician, as it may indicate a deficiency of riboflavin, one of the B vitamins. Cheilosis is usually associated with inflammation of the tongue (see further on).

Herpes Simplex. Practically everyone is familiar with the appearance on the lips or skin of the face of the superficial watery blisters called cold sores or fever blisters. Their scientific name is herpes simplex. Herpes simplex is an infection caused by a virus. The frequent recurrence of cold sores in persons subject to them was something of a puzzle until a satisfactory solution was proposed as a result of studies made several years ago. According to this explanation the primary infection occurs during infancy (before the age of three), and after recovery the virus remains permanently implanted in the skin. At any time thereafter the virus may be called into activity by the appropriate stimulus. This may be exposure to sunlight, weather changes, menstruation in girls and women, or a variety of conditions, including certain infectious diseases (colds, for example) which lower body resistance.

If a primary infection with the virus does not take place in infancy, the person seems to acquire a nonspecific immunity. Hence, with reference to herpes simplex, the population may be divided into two classes— the nonherpetic, those who never have cold sores—and the herpetic, those who frequently do.

Cold sores ordinarily are a minor affliction and dry up within a few days if they are let alone. Camphorated ointment or an astringent like powdered alum may be helpful. With children, the trick is to keep them from touching or picking at the sores so as to avoid secondary infection or delay in healing. The antibiotic drug aureomycin is proving to be helpful in the treatment of severe cases of herpes.

The Mouth

The mucous membrane lining the inside of the oral (mouth) cavity is pinkish in healthy children. A sore inflamed mouth may be the sign of any one of several different conditions including infections and nutritional deficiencies. Inflammation of the mouth is known medically as stomatitis (from the Greek word meaning "mouth," plus "-itis").

Canker Sores. Sometimes children are bothered with canker sores— small white spots on a red base—which appear on the inner lining of the lips or cheeks or on the tongue. If they do not clear up spontaneously within a week, or recur frequently, the child should be referred for medical attention.

Trench Mouth. Trench mouth is a fairly common contagious disease which may occur in epidemic form. Its scientific name is Vincent's angina. Although Vincent's angina may attack the mucous membrane in other parts of the body, it most commonly affects the throat and sometimes the mouth and gums. The infection is caused by a specific bacillus with which a spirillum is usually associated. These germs are spread by the use of common drinking cups, improperly washed eating utensils—in short, any articles on which they may be transmitted from one mouth to another.

When the mouth is affected in Vincent's angina, the gums become swollen, and sores covered with a whitish membrane appear. Medical attention is required for a child with this infection both for treatment (in which penicillin is proving most successful) and for the education of the child and his parents in the measures that must be taken to prevent the spread of the infection. These measures include the sterilization by boiling of all articles that have come in contact with the child's mouth. In school the child should use paper drinking cups and refrain from "swapping bites," putting his fingers in his mouth, or any other practices, like loaning his pencils or using those of others, which might lead to the spread of infection.

The Tongue

The tongue is an organ of many functions. Reference has already been made to the assistance it gives in the formation of many of the sounds of speech (see Speech Difficulties, in Chap. 5). By means of the taste buds on its surface, it cooperates with the olfactory nerve endings in the nose to give us information about each mouthful of food. What we like and what we dislike in the way of food and drink depends very largely upon whether this information is pleasing or not pleasing according to the associations connected with it. Finally, the tongue kneads food, after it has been cut and ground by the teeth, in much the same way that a baker kneads dough.

The surface of the tongue is rough, as we can easily see by inspecting it in a mirror. As the saliva-moistened food is kneaded by the tongue against the hard palate, it is pulverized, frayed, and rolled into a lump that can be swallowed.

Beefy Tongue. Redness and soreness of the tongue (glossitis) are associated with B-complex vitamin deficiencies. A beefy red or magenta tongue accompanies the dermatitis and digestive and nervous disorders of pellagra (see under How the Body Uses Vitamins, further on in this chapter). The particular nutritional deficiency or other condition responsible for a beefy red or sore tongue can be determined only by a physician.

Other conditions that require medical attention include a furred or coated tongue (see Furred Tongue, earlier in this chapter); a tongue marked by deep depressions or furrows; and a tongue with denuded patches surrounded by thickened areas in its top covering, or epithelium (geographic, or mappy, tongue).

The Salivary Glands

The parotids are the largest of the three pairs of glands which manufacture and secrete saliva into the mouth through ducts. They are situated one in front of each ear. The next largest salivary glands are the submaxillaries, located one on each side below the angle of the jaw. The smallest are the sublingual glands, one on each side beneath the tongue (Fig. 49).

The discovery of the parotid duct was made by Niels Stensen (1638–1686), a Danish physiologist, while he was still a young medical student. One morning when he was dissecting the head of a sheep, the instrument he was using was inserted by chance into the opening of the parotid duct and slipped down to strike with a sharp clink against the teeth. Stensen knew at once that he had discovered the duct of the gland.

The salivary glands, particularly the parotids, are open to attack by a specific virus. This virus is the cause of mumps, or infectious parotitis.

Mumps. Primarily, mumps is a disease of childhood. The greatest incidence is between eight and fourteen years. However, mumps is not nearly so communicable as are measles and chickenpox. As a consequence many individuals escape infection in childhood. In males who catch mumps after puberty a painful inflammation of the testes, called orchitis, frequently develops as a complication. More rarely, in adolescent girls the ovaries may be involved.

Generally, prolonged and intimate contact is required for the transmission of mumps. The virus is present in the secretions from the mouth and possibly from the nose of the infected person. Airborne droplets probably play an important part in the transmission of mumps in schools.

In children mumps is ordinarily a mild disease—so mild, in fact, that a private New York school once made the experiment of not attempting to control an epidemic, on the principle that it was far better to gain immunity from mumps in childhood than to take the risk of contracting it later, when it would be more likely to have serious consequences. The experiment was abandoned, however, when it was found that the free spread of mumps among the children resulted in the exposure of more adults than would have been the case had the usual isolation procedures been set up at the beginning of the epidemic.

Mumps is characterized by swelling and tenderness in front of the ear, extending down the neck behind the angle of the jaw. One or both parotid glands may be affected. The other two pairs of salivary glands also may become inflamed either at the same time or in rotation. Before the swelling develops the child may have slight fever and sometimes earache, sore throat, or vomiting. He may complain of pain.

For his own sake a child with mumps should stay home in bed until the swelling subsides. For the sake of adolescent boys and girls and adults, he should be isolated during the period of communicability (see Table 7B).

When boys and girls after puberty have been exposed to mumps it may seem advisable to the physician to give them temporary passive immunity by the injection of gamma globulin prepared from the pooled blood serum of persons convalescing from mumps. Convalescent serum gamma globulin also may be used early to prevent complications.

A preventive vaccine against mumps may give immunity for 1 year following two injections. The course of mumps in children who have not reached puberty is usually so mild that it is not recommended for the routine immunization of young children. Its use may be indicated, however, for children and young adults who are living in close quarters with persons who have or who are likely to have mumps, for example, children in summer camps, military personnel, college students, and hospital personnel.

The fact that mumps orchitis is almost never seen in boys before puberty suggests that the mumps virus seldom attacks the inactive testes. Acting on the knowledge that the normal functions of the testes are inhibited by high concentrations of female sex hormones (estrogens) in the body tissues, a group of physicians recently used an estrogenic substance (diethylstilbestrol) with very good results in relieving the pain of their male patients with orchitis.[4]

OBSERVATIONS ABOUT THE TEETH

Mastication involves biting off pieces of food of the right size to fit the dimensions of the mouth, tearing these pieces apart into smaller fragments, and then grinding them into bits. To perform these functions we have biting teeth (incisors), tearing teeth (cuspids and bicuspids), and grinding teeth (molars). The location of these teeth in the permanent set and the ages at which they erupt are shown in Figure 52.

How Teeth Grow

Teeth begin to develop within the jaws in little sacs which are filled with a jellylike substance composed of dentine-forming cells, enamel-forming cells, blood vessels, and nerves. Enamel (the hard substance that

4 HOYNE, A. L., J. H. DIAMOND, and J. R. CHRISTIAN, "Diethylstilbestrol in Mumps Orchitis," *J.A.M.A.*, Vol. 140 (June 25), 1949, p. 8.

covers the crown of the tooth as a thimble covers a finger tip) and dentine (the ivorylike substance that makes up the principal mass of the tooth) are deposited in layers until the crown is completed and root formation begins. As the crown grows larger, the sac in which it started shrinks to form the pulp of the tooth (see further on). After the enamel is completely formed, the enamel-making cells disappear. Hence, there is inadequate

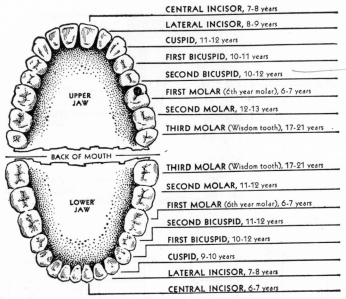

FIG. 52. The teeth of the permanent set and the ages at which they erupt. (*From "For Good Teeth," Metropolitan Life Insurance Company.*)

provision for self-repair. The margin of safety for the teeth is narrow compared with that of other body structures. However, a few dentine-forming cells remain after the dentine is completed and can deposit additional dentine as long as the tooth remains alive and healthy.

The root of each tooth is fixed in the jaw in its own individual socket. It is coated with cementum, a slightly less hard substance than the enamel which coats the crown. An outer sheath called the periodontal membrane, or dental periosteum, cushions the tooth root in its socket. The neck of the tooth is at the gum line, that is, it forms the transition area between the crown above the gums and the root below.

Children from the age of six onward are shedding their first, or deciduous, teeth and acquiring the teeth of the permanent set. It is a sad fact that a very large percentage of these newly acquired teeth are doomed to early decay. Dental defects are extremely common among school-age children, even among those from high-income families (Fig. 54).

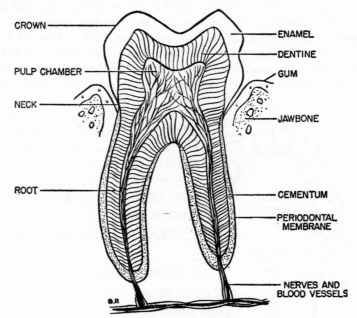

FIG. 53. Cross section of a tooth showing its structure.

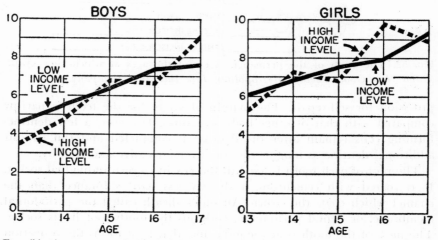

FIG. 54. Average number of defective, missing, and filled teeth per child in families of high and low income levels. New York City high school children—after Klein and Palmer. *(From "The School Child, Health Progress and Needs," Metropolitan Life Insurance Company.)*

Dental Caries

Conceivably the coating of the crowns of the teeth with enamel, the hardest substance in the body, might be sufficient protection if the teeth had nothing to contend with except the wearing down of the enamel over a lifetime of chewing or the accidental cracking or chipping of the crowns. Unfortunately, however, teeth are subject to a very common disease which attacks the enamel. This disease is dental caries. The damage done by dental caries steadily mounts through the entire period of youth and early maturity. In middle age the pace of the caries process slackens and, for this reason, prevention during youth is of particular value.

The discovery of the precipitating cause of dental caries was made in 1882 by W. E. Miller, an American dentist. Dr. Miller found that tooth enamel is readily dissolved (decalcified) by acids produced in the fermentation of carbohydrates by bacteria (notably the lactobacilli) present in saliva. Decalcification of the calcified tissues by these acids, accompanied or followed by disintegration of the organic substance of the tooth, is now widely accepted by dental authorities as the cause of dental caries. Enough acid to carry on the decay process is held in contact with the enamel by firmly adhering gelatinous plaques containing multitudes of acid-forming bacteria.

Although we know the cause of dental caries, several other factors enter the picture.

Susceptibility. It has long been common knowledge that some persons are more susceptible to tooth decay than are others, although very few are immune. Probably many teachers have observed that some youngsters who do not take care of their teeth have perfect ones, while others who follow the rules about diet and toothbrushing have many dental defects. Inherited differences in the ability to resist caries may account for a great many of these variations in susceptibility.

Solubility of the Enamel. At one time it was believed that a daily diet containing all the essential food elements in the right amounts would result in the development of caries-resistant enamel. It appears now, however, that nutritional status has little or no bearing on the caries process. It has been shown that well-nourished children may have as many cavities as poorly nourished children, or more. And well-calcified teeth may develop many cavities, whereas teeth with gross defects in the structure of the enamel may not develop any cavities at all. It appears that differences in the solubility of the enamel account largely for variations in the number of cavities in different individuals. Recent studies indicate that it may be possible to change the surface of the enamel so as to make it less soluble in weak organic acids.

The Oral Environment. Individual differences in the environment of the mouth seem to account for many variations in susceptibility to dental caries. One of the most important factors is the number of acid-forming bacteria, particularly lactobacilli, present in the saliva. Persons highly susceptible to tooth decay have a high lactobacillus count, but persons in whom caries is inactive or absent have few or no lactobacilli.

The Role of Saliva. Another factor in the oral environment, besides the bacterial count, is the biochemical nature of saliva. It has been shown that in persons with rampant caries the composition of the saliva differs from that of persons free of caries. This becomes understandable when we realize that 12 or 13 enzymes and coenzymes are essential to the production of lactic acid from sugar (sucrose) and that the presence or lack of certain substances in the saliva seems to inhibit or encourage the action of one or more of these ferments. A number of investigators are engaged in attacking the caries problem from this angle, but the results of such research so far are inconclusive.

Some persons are immune from dental caries because they have the ability to develop ammonia compound naturally in their mouths. Not only does the ammonia interfere with the production of lactic acid by the lactobacilli, but also it serves to neutralize the acids produced.

Our National Sweet Tooth. Since lactobacilli produce acids by the fermentation of carbohydrates, especially sugar, most dental authorities now believe that our national "sweet tooth" is very largely responsible for our high caries attack rate. Indeed, controlled experiments have shown that lactobacilli have been eliminated (literally starved to death) from the mouths of children by removing readily fermentable carbohydrates from their diets. This drastic measure is possible in experiments with cooperative children as subjects, or in the dental treatment of individual children with rampant caries. However, it would hardly be possible to cut down refined-sugar consumption in a whole population that is said to consume in a year approximately its own weight in sugar.

Can Toothbrushing Be the Answer? It would seem that the removal of tough patches of mucin, mouth debris, and bacteria (bacterial plaques) which readily form on the surface of tooth enamel and provide feeding grounds for lactobacilli and other acid-forming and acid-tolerating bacteria would be an important factor in preventing tooth decay. However, these plaques adhere firmly, especially on surfaces that cannot be reached by toothbrush bristles or even by the instruments used in prophylactic cleansings. It has been shown that within a few minutes of being bathed in a sugar solution (as happens in eating candy or drinking highly sweetened beverages, for example) the acidity of dental plaques in caries-susceptible mouths becomes high enough to dissolve tooth enamel and remains so for 30 to 90 minutes. The feltlike consistency of the plaque keeps this acid from being neutralized by the saliva, which normally maintains a nice balance between acidity and alkalinity.

Toothbrushing and mouth rinsing, therefore, if given a sporting chance, might be of great help in reducing the caries rate by getting rid of fermentable carbohydrate residues. For these measures to be effective, the teeth would have to be brushed and the mouth thoroughly rinsed with water immediately after every meal or between-meal snack that included refined sweets.

Beneficial results have been reported in the use of "caries-inhibiting dentifrices" and mouthwashes in controlled experiments. Few if any, however, have stood the test of practical application in the practice of dentistry. It is a simple procedure for a dentist to prescribe a dentifrice, or a mouthwash, but it is almost impossible to control effectively the actual use of any of them by the individual patient.

The old admonitions regarding toothbrushing ran something like this: Brush your teeth after each meal, if possible, or at least twice a day—in the morning and before going to bed. However, the usual 30-second brush-offs the first thing in the morning and the last thing at night accomplish little except to make the mouth and teeth feel pleasantly clean. It remains to be seen whether our children can be trained to brush their teeth and rinse their mouths after every meal that includes some refined sweets (such as sugar-sweetened foods or drinks, jams, jelly, honey, and so on), and after each indulgence in lollipops, candy sticks or bars, or sweetened drinks.

Fluoride in the Prevention of Dental Caries

The most important development in preventive dentistry in recent years has resulted from the discovery that fluoride (a compound of the chemical element fluorine) is helpful in controlling dental caries. The investigation of the use of fluoride in preventing dental caries had its beginning some twenty-five years ago when the mottling of tooth enamel observed among children living in certain geographical areas was traced, first, to the drinking water and, later, to the presence in the water of unusually large amounts of fluoride. It was then learned that the prevention of tooth mottling depends upon measures taken to provide drinking water with a fluoride content below the threshold at which mottling appears. This threshold has been established as one part of fluoride to 1,000,000 parts of water (abbreviated as 1 p.p.m.).

After fluoride was recognized to be the cause of tooth mottling, a still more striking discovery was made. It was found that persons who have lived all their lives in areas in which the drinking water contains fluoride, or who have lived in such areas at least during the period of enamel formation (from birth to eight or ten years of age), experience a dental caries incidence only one-half or one-third as much as that of persons living in areas where the drinking water contains no fluoride. Whether the influence of the fluoride is helpful, in that it gives relatively high protection from caries, or harmful, in that it causes tooth mottling, depends upon the amount ingested.

Long-term controlled experiments were begun in 1944 in the United States and Canada to determine whether the fluoridation of communal water supplies in localities where the drinking water is not naturally fluoridated would result in a reduction in the incidence of dental caries. The reports from these experiments are so favorable that all dental, medical, and public health authorities have endorsed water fluoridation as a practical, economical, simple, and safe approach to the overwhelming problem of dental caries. The latest reports from the Newburgh–Kingston (New York) fluoridation experiment, for example, indicate that the number of teeth with new cavities found among Newburgh children whose drinking water is fluoridated is less by an average of two teeth per child at each year of age than among children of the control city of Kingston.

The American Dental Association has indicated that the total number of cavities resulting from dental caries in children's teeth is so high (285,000,000 is the nationwide figure) that if all the dentists practicing now were to devote all their time to children, they could not hope to be able to fill all the cavities. "From the dental public health point of view, the benefit to the community of a decrease in caries experience of two teeth per child per year is significant." [5]

An increasing number of towns and cities whose water is not naturally fluoridated are now adding fluoride to the communal drinking water supply. In communities without fluoridated water the application of a solution of sodium fluoride directly to the teeth at ages three, seven, ten, and thirteen is giving good results. This treatment will prevent nearly 40 per cent of the cavities which otherwise might be expected to occur.

Devitalized Teeth

The end result of unchecked dental caries is the death of the tooth. When alive each tooth is supplied with the necessities of life by blood vessels and nerves which run up through canals in the roots. The spongy mass of blood vessels and nerves which forms the pulp of the tooth occupies a central chamber within the tooth called the pulp chamber. Minute tubes filled with pulp material ramify into the dentine to nourish it.

As the processes of decay extend inward toward the pulp cavity, its ivory walls become so thin that heat and cold can penetrate them more

[5] *Health News,* New York State Department of Public Health, Vol. 32, No. 1 (January), 1955.

readily. Sensitivity to hot and cold foods and liquids is an alarm signal transmitted by the nerves in the pulp. Toothache may begin even before the dentine wall finally breaks down, thereby exposing the soft pulp to bacterial action. Possibly a dentist may be able to save a tooth's life after it starts to ache. But when the pulp has been invaded, the fate of the tooth is generally sealed. After the spongy pulp collapses under bacterial attacks the tooth is devitalized—dead. The pressure of the pus and gas that form during the process of destruction makes the tooth feel very sore. If at this point the dentist can successfully clean out all the infected pulp and sterilize and plug the pulp chamber and the root canals, the tooth may last for a long time without giving trouble. But if the tooth is still neglected, the tragedy may, and usually does, close with a final act that is very painful for its owner.

The infection in the pulp chamber extends down the root canals and collects at the ends of the roots. The pus may push through the jawbone and gum to form a gumboil and drain into the mouth. Or it may remain concealed as an abscess at the roots of the tooth. Sometimes a hidden abscess may not cause pain or swelling of the face. It is, however, a focus of infection which drains into the blood and lymph vessels (like chronically infected tonsils or sinuses) and may be responsible, at least in part, for lowered physical resistance to arthritis or some other condition.

Referral to a dentist for an x-ray examination of the teeth is usually included in any thorough medical check-up of a child whose health is substandard. The x-ray machine has become an indispensable instrument in dental practice because it often shows up hidden abscesses, decay under fillings, impacted teeth, and many other abnormal dental conditions that can be detected in no other way.

Malocclusion

In looking at the picture of Evelyn (Plate 9) it is easy to see that she would be a pretty little girl if only her teeth came together properly. Malocclusion—the condition in which the upper and lower teeth do not occlude, or meet, correctly—may spoil a child's looks and interfere with happy adjustment to life. Also it may make adequate chewing and proper cleansing impossible and as a result favor tooth decay and gum inflammation.

Heredity plays an important part in determining the size and shape of the jaw, which in turn may influence the size, shape, and position of the teeth, and the relation of one jaw to the other. One often hears of a certain type of jaw as "running in the family." The best known example is the famous "Hapsburg jaw." In many cases there is not enough room in the jaw to accommodate all 32 teeth of the permanent set. Hence they erupt in a crooked position or become shifted from their normal places in the jaw during the growth period. If a tooth in the lower jaw is not in its proper place, the opposing tooth in the upper jaw also gets out of line.

The conditions under which the jaws develop and the teeth erupt may also favor malocclusion. Bad influences on growing jaws and teeth include

1. Thumb sucking, or biting the tongue, lips, or cheeks, if continued during the time that the permanent teeth begin to erupt
2. Failure to take proper care of the primary teeth
3. Losing the primary teeth too soon or keeping them too long; this often results in an irregular line-up of the permanent teeth
4. Failure to replace permanent teeth that have been extracted

The teacher who notices that a child has malocclusion and encourages the parents to get dental advice may make a valuable contribution to the child's future health and happiness. Besides checking faulty habits and giving needed dental care, the dentist may advise taking the child to an orthodontist—that is, a specialist in preventing and correcting malocclusion and irregularities of the teeth. The corrections may take some time and cause some inconvenience, but they are well worth while, because they will eventually give the child a normal chewing surface and at the same time greatly improve his appearance.

Gum Inflammations

Gingivitis is the general term used in referring to an inflammation of the gums (*gingivae,* in Latin). It is characterized by tender, inflamed spongy gums that bleed easily (the "pink toothbrush" syndrome). An inflamed condition of the gums can readily be observed and ought always to be brought to the attention of a physician.

One form of gingivitis is caused by a vitamin-C deficiency. Although most dental authorities are now of the opinion that no single nutrient has more than a very small role in controlling the caries process, there is no question that ascorbic acid (vitamin C) is essential for healthy gums. Probably George (the boy shown in Plate 10) has not been getting enough vitamin C.

Tartar. Another common cause of gum irritation is a deposit of tartar around the necks of the teeth. Tartar is a brownish or greenish incrustation formed by a mixture of calcium carbonate (chalk) and organic matter derived from saliva. It most often collects on neglected teeth—that is, teeth that are not brushed daily and are not given thorough prophylactic cleansings by a dentist or dental hygienist at regular intervals. Although tartar is not known to favor tooth decay, it does affect the health of the gums.

Other possible predisposing factors in the development of gingivitis include persistent wedging of food in crevices between the teeth, poor mouth hygiene, and defective dental fillings, crowns, and bridges.

Pyorrhea. A possible complication of neglected gingivitis is pyorrhea, a much more serious condition. The word pyorrhea is derived from the Greek words for "pus" and "flow," and means literally "a discharge of pus." It is now used almost exclusively to refer to an infection of the periodontal membrane—that is, the elastic tissue that connects the roots of the teeth with their bony sockets. If not checked, the infection spreads to the sockets themselves and the teeth become loosened and finally lost.

Gingivitis favors the development of pyorrhea because any gum inflammation, if neglected, spreads deeper into the tissues, becomes chronic, and provides a fertile field for the growth of the pus-producing germs. Active pyorrhea can be checked successfully by a dentist if it has not progressed too far, but some permanent damage to the tissues will result in almost every case. That is why prevention is doubly important.

The School Dental-health Program

Dental disease is almost universal, and no infallible means of preventing it have been found. This means that regular examinations by a dentist and dental treatment of the defects found hold out the best hopes at present for the control of serious tooth decay, malocclusion, and the premature loss of teeth. Observations by teacher and nurse will aid in the detection of gross dental defects, and inspection by a physician who uses a throat-stick and flashlight in examining the mouth during a medical examination will reveal many that are less obvious. Experience has shown, however, that a high proportion of caries will be missed unless all children regularly receive a dental examination (Fig. 55) with mirror and explorer, supplemented, when advisable, by dental x-rays. The American Dental Association recommends that each child be given such an examination by a dentist at least once a year.

The dental hygienist has a strategic place in the school health program. She is trained to make preliminary inspections of the teeth which are of great value in case finding. Her work of prophylactic cleansing, although it may not have much effect in reducing the incidence of caries, does help greatly in preventing gum troubles of various kinds and in improving personal appearance. Furthermore, she acts as liaison officer between the dentist and the classroom teacher in providing the teacher with information about the condition of the teeth of individual children and with material for dental-health education.

The dental hygienist, the nurse serving the school, and the teacher working together can be of great service in promoting corrections through follow-up procedures. However, the teacher's most important job in the school dental program is that of presenting the story of what good dental

PHILADELPHIA SCHOOL CHILDREN, 1945-1946

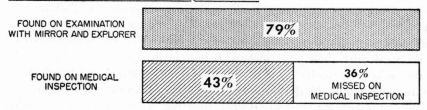

16-TO 24-YEAR-OLDS, NATIONAL YOUTH ADMINISTRATION, 1941* (CHIEFLY CARIES)

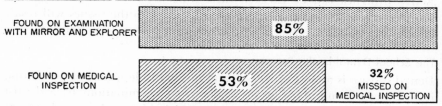

*BASED UPON NUMBERS RECOMMENDED FOR TREATMENT.

Fig. 55. Medical inspection fails to disclose a high proportion of caries. (*From "The School Child, Health Progress and Needs," Metropolitan Life Insurance Company.*)

care is and its importance in growth and development in ways that will motivate the child and his parents to go to the dentist regularly for dental examination and needed corrections.

HOW THE BODY USES FOOD MATERIALS

To the body cells the comparatively simple chemical compounds into which the various foodstuffs have been broken down by digestion are merely raw materials. The cells must smash these raw materials literally to atoms in the process of using them and discard the parts they cannot use as by-products, or wastes. Thus the changes that foodstuffs undergo in digestion are only the overture to the more dramatic changes that take place during their metabolism.

Metabolism comes from a Greek word meaning "change." It is the sum total of all the building-up and tearing-down operations involved in the utilization by living tissues of the food materials required for growth, maintenance and repair, regulation of vital functions, and heat and energy production.

How the Body Uses Carbohydrates and Fats

Carbohydrates (sugars and starches) are made up of molecules of glucose. The chemical recipe for this basic sugar molecule is 6 atoms of carbon, 12 atoms of hydrogen, and 6 atoms of oxygen ($C_6H_{12}O_6$).

Fats are formed by the union of fatty acids (which also are compounds of carbon, hydrogen, and oxygen) and glycerin.

The body uses glucose and fatty acids for the production of heat and energy and for the production of body fat (adipose tissue).

Energy Metabolism. The transformation by which energy is made available for the uses of the body is called energy metabolism. Essentially it consists in the juggling of oxygen atoms into new combinations with carbon and hydrogen atoms. As a result carbon dioxide (CO_2) and water (H_2O) are formed and heat is set free. This process is called oxidation.

About 25 per cent of the heat produced by oxidation is converted into energy for all types of muscular activity and for the maintenance of vital functions. Another portion is used to maintain body temperature (see Reactions to Internal Temperature Changes, in Chap. 3). Excess heat is lost through the skin. The other by-products of oxidation (carbon dioxide and water) are removed by way of the lungs. The heat, or fuel, value of a food is expressed in terms of calories,[6] which are heat units just as inches or feet are units of length. One gram of fat when burned or oxidized in the body yields 9.3 calories; 1 gram of carbohydrate yields 4.1 calories.

The body's favorite source of heat and energy is glucose, the sugar into which carbohydrate foods are converted by digestion. When glucose is provided abundantly through a diet rich in carbohydrates, it is preferably utilized and the oxidation of fat is almost completely stopped.

If more glucose is made available than is needed at the moment, it is put into "live storage." The readily soluble sugar is changed for storage purposes into an insoluble starch called glycogen. Glycogen is stored in the liver and muscles. When the glycogen is needed for muscular work, enzymes help to turn it back into glucose.

Production of Adipose Tissue. Fatty acids that are not oxidized and glucose that is not required for immediate use and for "live storage" are changed into fat droplets and placed in "dead storage" in the fat depots of the body. The internal fat depots form soft elastic shock absorbers

[6] One calorie is the quantity of heat required to raise the temperature of 1 liter (about 1 quart) of water 1°C.

between various organs and help to hold them in place. The fat deposits just beneath the skin (subcutaneous fat) help to cushion blows and to hold in heat.

Another important function of the fat depots is the storage of fat for nutritional purposes. The body does as Joseph advised Pharaoh to do— that is, it sets aside a store of food to be used in time of famine, so that it will not perish through the famine.

How the Body Uses Proteins

Proteins are broken down during digestion into long chains of organic compounds called amino acids. All amino acids contain a basic nitrogen group in addition to carbon, oxygen, and hydrogen groups.

The amino acids are split up by the body cells and regrouped in the most varied ways to build the protein molecules characteristic of human protoplasm. There are at least 21 different kinds of amino acids. Hence each tissue has a wide variety from which to choose the materials for building and repair which are adapted to its particular style of cell architecture. Various tissues also use amino acids in manufacturing hormones, enzymes, and other products that are used in regulating the body's work.

Recent scientific work has shown that amino acids also play a fundamental role in maintaining both natural and acquired resistance to infection. Protein is required for the formation of phagocytes (see Blood and Its Composition, in Chap. 4), and "a direct relationship exists between the amount of protein consumed and the efficiency of phagocytic activity." [7] Also the production of the globulins in blood plasma which carry bacterial antibodies (see Defense Reactions, in Chap. 3) depends upon a sufficient intake of protein.

Surplus amino acids, unlike surplus glucose and fat, are not stored in specific depots. However, the body maintains in the blood plasma and in the cells a large pool of circulating amino acids which may be drawn upon by any body cell needing protein or capable of storing surplus protein. When more protein is taken in than the body needs at the time for building and repair, manufacturing operations, and the emergency pool, most of the excess amino acids are deaminized. That is, the amino group that contains nitrogen is split off. This split-off amino group is converted by the liver to urea, which is then excreted by the kidneys in the urine (see The Kidneys, further on). The leftover nonprotein fraction is changed by the liver into carbohydrate and fat and as such is stored or burned to furnish heat and energy. One gram of protein as eaten yields 4.1 calories when burned in the body.

[7] McLester, James S., "Protein Comes into Its Own," *J.A.M.A.* (April), 1949, pp. 897–902.

How the Body Uses Minerals

Minerals are present in a wide variety of foods in the form of salts. They do not require digestion, as they are present in foods in molecules small enough to pass through the walls of the small intestine into the blood stream.

Mineral salts are used by the body (a) as building materials (for example, calcium and phosphorus for the building of bones and teeth, and iron for the manufacture of red blood cells); (b) as essential ingredients of several body secretions (for example, iodine in the thyroid secretion, thyroxine); (c) to help in making a favorable environment for the cells (for example, sodium chloride to keep the blood and tissue fluid slightly salty or brackish, and sodium bicarbonate to protect the blood and tissue fluids from any considerable change in the acid direction); and (d) to regulate many different body processes (for example, the clotting of blood, the beating of the heart, and the functioning of nerves and glands).

Some of the minerals known to be required by the body are calcium, iron, phosphorus, iodine, copper, sodium, chlorine, sulfur, magnesium, manganese, cobalt, potassium, and zinc. Many minerals are utilized better in the presence of other minerals, certain vitamins, and protein. Iron and calcium, for example, are used to greater advantage in the presence of a generous amount of ascorbic acid. Vitamin D is necessary for the absorption and deposition of calcium, especially important during growth periods. Adequate protein also promotes the utilization of calcium.

Minerals are widely distributed in different foods, which is one of the reasons for encouraging the use of varieties of food. Actually, if care is taken to select foods that contain enough calcium, iron, and protein (which contains phosphorus), it is believed that the other minerals the body needs, with the possible exception of iodine,[8] will be adequately supplied.

How the Body Uses Vitamins

Vitamins are organic compounds built up by plants and animals of carbon, oxygen, hydrogen, and in some cases of other elements. Each one has its own distinctive chemical pattern, which can now be duplicated in the laboratory. That is, the known vitamins can be synthesized outside the living plant or animal body. Some of them are dissolved in the fat (fat-soluble vitamins) and others in the water (water-soluble vitamins) of many different foods.

---

[8] Although only a very small amount of iodine is needed, it is so essential that the Food and Nutrition Board of the National Research Council recommends the use of iodized salt for everyone.

The vitamins all play essential roles in nutrition and bodily welfare. Those which are recognized as important in meal planning are A, B complex, C, and D. If one or more is lacking in the daily diet for any length of time, a characteristic disease or disorder may appear.

Vitamin A. This vitamin exists in animal food sources in the form of fat-soluble crystals which are readily destroyed by oxidation at all temperatures. In plant food sources it exists in the form of carotene which must be converted into active vitamin A in the body. When more vitamin A is consumed than is immediately required, the surplus is stored in the liver.

Vitamin A is needed by the bone-building and tooth-forming cells in childhood and youth and throughout life for keeping the skin, mucous membranes, and eyes in a healthy condition. It protects these structures through its influence on the glands which secrete substances that moisten and lubricate them. In vitamin-A deficiency the glands waste away and as a consequence the skin, hair, eyes, and mucous membrane linings of body openings and tracts become excessively dry.

The specific vitamin-A deficiency disease is xerophthalmia (from two Greek words meaning "dry" and "eyes"). The tear glands dry up, and the eyes, having lost the protective and lubricating action of tears, become the prey of invading germs.

Vitamin A also is necessary for the prevention of "night blindness," that is, inability to see in dim light. A rose-red pigment called "visual purple" in the retina of the eye is essential for normal vision in dim light. It becomes exhausted when the eyes are exposed to bright light, and vitamin A is required for its regeneration.

Vitamin-B Complex. The vitamin-B complex includes a whole family of vitamins, many of which are now known by their chemical names (for example, thiamine, riboflavin, niacin, and folic acid). The B vitamins have intimate functional relationships. They are of the highest importance for the growth and energy metabolism of all forms of life from the highest to the lowest—from microbes to mammals—presumably because they form an essential part of the enzyme systems that underlie living processes.

Thiamine in pure form consists of water-soluble white crystals which break down under prolonged heating and are destroyed in alkaline media, such as water to which bicarbonate of soda has been added. Surplus thiamine is not stored to any extent in the body and so it is needed regularly.

Thiamine is necessary for healthy nerves, for good muscle tone in the digestive tract, and for the oxidation of carbohydrates in the body. The classic thiamine deficiency disease is beriberi. Beriberi is an inflammation of the nerves (polyneuritis) resulting in progressive paralyses of the limbs. Because thiamine prevents its development, this member of the vitamin-B complex is sometimes called the antineuritic vitamin.

Riboflavin in pure form consists of water-soluble yellow crystals which are stable to heat but are destroyed by alkalis and light. It increases vigor at all ages through its influence on the nerves, digestion, the skin, and general body resistance. It also helps to prevent degenerative changes in the cornea of the eye (keratitis). Like thiamine, riboflavin is not stored in the body in appreciable amounts.

Riboflavin deficiency produces a set of symptoms which includes cheilosis (an inflammation and cracking of the lips and corners of the tongue) and glossitis (inflammation of the tongue).

Niacin in pure form consists of water-soluble white crystals. It helps to protect the health of the skin and nerves and aids digestion. There is little evidence that surplus amounts are stored in the body.

The classic niacin deficiency disease is pellagra (literally "rough skin"). Pellagra is the most common form of nutritional deficiency characterized by dermatitis. In addition, nervous and digestive disorders usually occur. Red, dry, scaly patches form upon skin surfaces exposed to the sun's rays, for example, the back of the hands, the neck, cheeks, and bridge of the nose. These patches usually appear as matched spots, as on both hands, or both cheeks. Because it prevents pellagra, niacin is frequently referred to as the pellagra-preventive (P-P) factor in the vitamin-B complex.

Vitamin C (Ascorbic Acid). Pure ascorbic acid exists in the form of water-soluble white crystals which are readily destroyed by heat, sunlight, oxidation, and alkalis. Surplus amounts consumed are not stored, and so daily supplies are needed.

Vitamin C is known as the antiscorbutic vitamin. It was a lack of this element in the diet of seafaring men that was responsible for the scurvy which was once the curse of all those who went in for long-range navigation. In the eighteenth century it was discovered that eating fresh vegetables and fruits (especially citrus fruits) would prevent scurvy.

Ascorbic acid is required for the formation of the intercellular cement which binds together the cells forming the walls of the capillaries. A lack of it makes the walls of the capillaries so weak that blood can leak through. This accounts for the hemorrhages into the gums and other tissues which are characteristic of scurvy. A very small amount of vitamin C is needed to prevent this disease. Well-defined cases have practically disappeared in lands of plenty. However, much more vitamin C is needed for health than for the prevention of frank scurvy.

Vitamin D. Vitamin D is indispensable for the normal calcification of bones and teeth. Its absence from the diet causes the disease called rickets (see Rickets, in Chap. 9). This disease is characterized by defective ossification of the bones and the development of various bone deformities. Because it prevents rickets, vitamin D is called the antirachitic vitamin.

In the search for this vitamin, the discovery that sunlight possesses antirachitic properties came first (1919). Then it was found that cod-liver oil, halibut-liver oil, and the oils of other bony fishes are potent rickets preventives.

The antirachitic power of sunshine comes from the ultraviolet rays in sunlight, which activate a fatty substance in the skin associated with a fatlike pearly substance called cholesterol. This activated substance (vitamin D_3) is the form of vitamin D present in fish-liver oils and in milk and other foods exposed to ultraviolet irradiation. In pure crystalline form vitamin D exists as calciferol. The fat-soluble crystals of calciferol (vitamin D_2) are stable to heat and oxidation.

Children need more vitamin D than grown-ups do. However, they get very little vitamin D from ordinary foods, and the antirachitic effects of sunshine are lessened during the winter months in temperate climates. Even in summer the haze hanging over most cities filters out the ultraviolet rays. Hence children's diets should be reinforced with a fish-liver oil or with some other concentrated form of vitamin D.

Cellulose

Cellulose is the woody carbohydrate substance used by plants as structural material. It contains some valuable minerals and vitamins which are released and absorbed into the blood stream during digestion, but mostly it consists of a mass of fibers that cannot be digested. This indigestible bulk, which is sometimes called "roughage," is pushed into the colon for removal from the body. As it helps to stimulate the movements of the colon, it is a valuable part of the diet. The parts of plant foods that are rich in cellulose are edible leaves, edible stems, the hulls of grains, and the edible skins of fruits and vegetables.

Water

Water is used in the body to maintain the water level of the vast inland sea in which the cells live, to keep the blood volume uniform, and to carry on most of the body's activities. It is essential to the processes of removing waste products and excess heat. Hence there is a necessarily large loss of water from the body every day via the kidneys (urine), the sweat glands (perspiration), the lungs (water-laden expired air), and the large intestines (defecation). To balance this daily loss of water, we take in already formed water in liquids and in solid foods and potential water in foodstuffs containing hydrogen which unites with oxygen to form water in the process of oxidation. The water content of food varies greatly. Green vegetables contain 90 to 95 per cent; fruits, 85 per cent; and meats, 50 to 75 per cent. An average day's meals contain about two quarts of potential and already formed water.

MEETING THE FOOD NEEDS OF SCHOOL-AGE CHILDREN

To meet all the nutritional needs of the body, it is necessary to know how much of each nutrient is required and what foods supply it in the largest amounts. In 1941 the Food and Nutrition Board of the National Research Council developed what is often called a "yardstick of good nutrition." This yardstick consists of a table of recommended daily

Table 11. RECOMMENDED DAILY DIETARY ALLOWANCES FOR SCHOOL-AGE CHILDREN *

	Calor-ies †	Pro-tein, gm.	Cal-cium, gm.	Iron, mg.	Vitamin A, I.U.‡	Thi-amine, mg.§	Ribo-flavin, mg.§	Nia-cin, mg.§	Ascorbic acid, mg.	Vitamin D, I.U.
Girls and boys ‖										
4–6 yr. (42 lb.).	1,600	50	1.0	8	2,500	0.8	1.2	8	50	400
7–9 yr. (58 lb.).	2,000	60	1.0	10	3,500	1.0	1.5	10	60	400
10–12 yr. (78 lb.).........	2,500	70	1.2	12	4,500	1.2	1.8	12	75	400
Girls ‖										
13–15 yr. (108 lb.).........	2,600	80	1.3	15	5,000	1.3	2.0	13	80	400
16–20 yr. (122 lb.).........	2,400	75	1.0	15	5,000	1.2	1.8	12	80	400
Boys ‖										
13–15 yr. (108 lb.).........	3,200	85	1.4	15	5,000	1.5	2.0	15	90	400
16–20 yr. (141 lb.).........	3,800	100	1.4	15	6,000	1.7	2.5	17	100	400

Source: Food and Nutrition Board, National Research Council (revised 1948).

* *Table of measures used.* 1 gram (gm.) equals approximately 1/30 part of an ounce. 1 milligram (mg.) equals 1/1000 part of a gram. 1 international unit (I.U.) of a vitamin is the activity of a certain specified very small amount of that vitamin. 1 milligram of thiamine equals 333 international units. 1 milligram of ascorbic acid equals 20 international units. There are no international units for riboflavin and niacin.

† Proper calorie allowance is that which maintains body weight or rate of growth at the level most conducive to well-being.

‡ About two-thirds of the vitamin-A value of the average diet is contributed by the provitamin carotene (from vegetables and fruits) which has half or less than half the value of vitamin A (from animal products, such as liver and eggs).

§ Other members of the vitamin-B complex also are required, though no values can be given. Foods supplying adequate thiamine, riboflavin, and niacin will tend to supply sufficient amounts of the remaining B vitamins.

‖ Allowances are based on the needs for the middle year in each age group (5, 8, 11, 14, 18) and are for moderate activity and for average weight at the middle year of the age group.

Table 12. HOW DAILY ALLOWANCES OF SPECIFIC NUTRIENTS CAN BE MET

Daily food needs of school-age children	Principal contributions made by these foods
Milk, ¾ to 1 quart (one generous serving of hard cheese is about equal to 1 cup of milk in food value)	An excellent source of protein, calcium, and riboflavin
Potatoes, one or more servings	A good source of vitamin C and an economical source of calories; sweet potatoes are a good source of carotene (the provitamin from which the body makes vitamin A)
Other vegetables, at least two servings, with emphasis on green and yellow vegetables and salad greens	From dark-green, thin-leaved vegetables, carotene (vitamin A) and iron; other green vegetables and deep yellow ones are valuable chiefly for carotene (vitamin A); raw green-leaf vegetables are valuable for vitamin C
Fruits and tomatoes, two servings (one of which should be citrus fruit or tomatoes)	An excellent source of vitamin C (of which citrus fruits are the best source); yellow-fleshed fruits are valuable also for carotene (vitamin A); dried fruits are good sources of iron; most fruits and vegetables are excellent sources of roughage for good elimination
Meat, fish, or poultry (at least one serving); eggs, one (at least three or four during week)	Excellent sources of protein, iron, thiamine, and niacin; eggs and liver are good sources of vitamin A; salt-water fish and shellfish supply iodine
Whole-grain or enriched bread and cereals, one or both at every meal	Calories and protein; good sources of B-complex vitamins, iron, and roughage
Butter and other fats, 1 to 3 tablespoonfuls	Calories; butter and enriched margarine are good sources of vitamin A
Fish-liver oil (in amounts prescribed by physician)	Fish-liver oils are the only excellent food sources of vitamin D, and they also are excellent sources of vitamin A
Sugar, sirups, and preserves, in moderate amounts for flavorings and desserts	Calories; food value of desserts, other than calories, depends upon the ingredients used
Water, 4 to 6 glasses	To aid in balancing daily loss of water through the processes of removing waste products and excess heat

allowances of specific nutrients for men and women according to degree of activity and for children according to age. That part of the table which applies to boys and girls of school age is reproduced as Table 11.

For many years, enough has been known about the composition of foods to group them according to their most important contributions to the food needs of the body. This has been done in Table 12. By meeting the daily food needs of school-age children shown in this table, the allowances of specific nutrients recommended by the Food and Nutrition Board (Table 11), as well as minerals and vitamins for which the requirements are less well known, will be provided.

Observing the Nutritional Status of School Children

Nutritionally needy children may be suffering from all-round undernourishment (Table 13) or from some specific deficiency caused by an

Table 13. PHYSICAL SIGNS RELATED TO GENERAL NUTRITIONAL STATUS

Point of observation	Good nutrition	Poor nutrition	Possible nutritional deficiency
Growth record	Progressive gains in weight and height at the established rate of gain for the individual child, taking into consideration periods of decelerated and accelerated growth (see Stages and Rates of Growth under Physical Growth and Development, in Chap. 2)	Failure to show measurable gains in weight and height over several months; any sudden change in the rate of growth	Slow intake of protein or calories, or an all-round poor or unbalanced diet *
General appearance and behavior	General impression of physical fitness, vigor, and enjoyment of life; alert, happy facial expression; good skeletal and muscular development; good functional posture; moderate amount of well-distributed fat (curves rather than angles); good appetite, good digestion, good elimination, restful sleep	Fatigue posture, round shoulders, winged shoulder blades, protruding abdomen; small or flabby muscles; excessively thin (angles rather than curves), excessively fat, or poor distribution of fat; strained, worried look; listless and inactive or high-strung and overactive; easily fatigued and possibly irritable and difficult to manage	Same as above

* While a diet supplying all essential nutrients in the right amounts is necessary for good nutrition, other causes may be responsible for poor nutrition; for example, acute or chronic illness, or an endocrine imbalance, or prolonged worry or other emotional disturbance, which may interfere with the consumption, assimilation, or utilization of essential food elements.

insufficient intake of one or more of the essential food elements. If any one of these elements is lacking or supplied inadequately in the diet, the organs or tissues needing it in the greatest amounts will suffer most.

It is seldom nowadays that school children show signs and symptoms of severe nutritional deficiency except in regions where the customary diet is completely lacking, or is seriously deficient, in one or more essential food elements. In mild form, however, nutritional deficiencies are not infrequent, and some severe cases still occur.

The chief food sources of the most important food elements and what may happen when a person does not get enough of each one are given in Table 14. Teachers may use this table as a guide in observing children. However, it must be remembered that the signs of nutritional deficiencies may be present in many other conditions. Also, nutritional biochemists are now learning through animal experimentation that the requirements for specific nutrients can be changed with alterations in the amount consumed of other nutrients. It may be possible, for example, to show the signs indicating a particular vitamin or mineral deficiency not because one is not getting enough of that vitamin or mineral, but because one is getting too much or not enough of some other food element.

Another important thing to remember is that the screening out of nutritionally needy children is a highly technical procedure. Teachers and nurses can do no more than to call attention to the obvious warning signals that are commonly associated with malnutrition and specific nutritional deficiencies. In referring a child for suspected malnutrition, it will be helpful to the physician to know what the teacher and nurse can tell him about the child's living habits in general, and more particularly about his dietary habits. This information provides a valuable supplement to tests made to measure nutritional status and may be used in planning the reclamation of children whose vitality has been allowed to burn low because of poor nutrition.

Nutrition Education

Convincing children of the importance of good nutrition and helping them to learn how to attain it requires teachers who are well grounded in the subject. Although everyone knows that one must eat to live, no one knows intuitively what and how much one must eat to be as healthy as possible. That knowledge must be acquired. Many authorities believe that all teachers should receive adequate training in nutrition as part of their preparation for the teaching profession and also should be provided with consultation services in this field.

But no matter how skillfully nutrition is taught, school and home must

Table 14. GOOD FOOD SOURCES OF SPECIFIC NUTRIENTS AND CONSEQUENCES
OF INSUFFICIENT INTAKE

Food elements	Good food sources	What may happen if children do not get enough
Starches.....	Grain foods: breakfast cereals, rice, tapioca, and all foods made of flour or meal (breads, macaroni, spaghetti, noodles, crackers, pancakes, etc.) Vegetables: potatoes, root vegetables (carrots, turnips, beets, etc.), legumes (peas, beans)	Underweight Listlessness Fatigue Hunger Lack of interest in work and play
Sugars......	Sugar in practically pure form: table sugar, sirups, honey, molasses, jams, jellies, candy Fruits: most kinds, dried or fresh Sweet desserts	Lessened ability to utilize vitamins (resulting in certain vitamin deficiencies) and minerals
Fats........	Animal products: bacon, other fat meat, lard, cream, butter, cheese made from whole milk or cream, egg yolk Plant products: salad and cooking oils, mayonnaise, margarine, nuts, chocolate	
Proteins.....	Animal products: milk (all kinds), eggs, all cheeses (except those made from cream only), meat, fish, poultry Plant products: dried peas and beans, bread and cereals, nuts and peanut butter	Stunted growth Muscular weakness Decreased vitality Mental and physical fatigue Lowered resistance to infection
Calcium.....	Animal products: milk and dishes made with milk, cheese Plant products: all green leafy vegetables (except spinach, beet greens, and Swiss chard)	Abnormalities in bone growth (for example, bowlegs and chest malformations) Possibly poor teeth Stunted growth
Iron........	Animal products: lean meat, liver, heart, kidneys, oysters, egg yolk	Nutritional anemia Pallor Easy fatigability

Table 14 (Cont.). GOOD FOOD SOURCES OF SPECIFIC NUTRIENTS AND CONSEQUENCES
OF INSUFFICIENT INTAKE

Food elements	Good food sources	What may happen if children do not get enough
Iron (cont.)....	Plant products: green leafy vegetables, whole-grain and enriched bread and cereals, dried beans and peas, potatoes, dried fruits	Nutritional anemia Pallor Easy fatigability
Iodine.......	Sea food, iodized salt	Simple goiter Swelling in neck below Adam's apple
Vitamin A....	Animal products (in form of active vitamin A): liver, fish-liver oils, egg yolk, butter, cream, whole milk, cheese made with cream or whole milk	Rough scaly skin Papular eruption (like goose flesh) on skin
	Plant products (in form of carotene): yellow and green vegetables and fruits, such as sweet potatoes, yellow corn, pumpkin, bananas, cantaloupe, apricots, yellow peaches, spinach, watercress, string beans, peas, and green peppers	Dry, coarse, brittle, lusterless hair Inflammation of eyelid margins (blepharitis) Night blindness and glare blindness
	Margarine fortified with vitamin A	Retarded growth
Thiamine (B_1).	Animal products: liver, heart, kidneys, lean meats (especially pork and ham), oysters, milk, eggs	Nervous irritability Headaches
	Plant products: whole-grain and enriched bread and cereals; wheat germ, peanuts, green or dried beans (especially soy beans), and peas	Fatigue Limited ability to concentrate Listlessness Loss of appetite Faulty digestion Constipation due to poor intestinal muscle tone
Riboflavin (B_2)	Animal products: liver, heart, kidneys, fish, milk, cheese, egg yolk	Redness at angles of lips with scaling and fissuring (cheilosis)
	Plant products: whole-grain and enriched bread and cereals, green leafy vegetables, peanut butter	Sore, beefy red or magenta tongue (glossitis)

Table 14 (Cont.). GOOD FOOD SOURCES OF SPECIFIC NUTRIENTS AND CONSEQUENCES OF INSUFFICIENT INTAKE

Food elements	Good food sources	What may happen if children do not get enough
		Tiny red lines (engorged capillaries) extending around or across cornea and inward toward pupil (keratitis)
		Inflammation of eyelid margins (blepharitis)
		Eye fatigue and sensitivity to light
		Lowered resistance and vitality
Niacin......	Animal products: heart, liver (especially pork liver), kidneys, lean meats, poultry, fish	Dermatitis (pellagra)
	Plant products: whole-grain and enriched bread and cereals; beans (especially soy beans), peas, peanuts, almonds, bananas	Gastrointestinal disturbances (diarrhea, for example)
		Mental depression
Ascorbic acid (vitamin C)	Plant products: canned, frozen, or fresh citrus fruit (oranges, grapefruit, lemons, and limes), raw apples, strawberries, cantaloupe, papayas, tomatoes (canned or fresh), raw cabbage, raw green peppers and other raw vegetables, potatoes (baked or boiled in skins)	Tender, swollen, bleeding or spongy gums (subclinical scurvy) Easily bruised skin Sore joints
Vitamin D....	Animal products: the oils of many different bony fishes (cod, halibut, etc.), irradiated (vitamin-D) milk (Egg yolk, butter, and cream contain vitamin D in very small amounts. These amounts are increased when hens and cows are exposed to summer sunlight or are fed irradiated substances.)	Rickets Malformation of bones and teeth

work together if children are to get the full benefits of nutrition education. Guiding children in food selection requires an intimate knowledge of their food habits. Also what the children learn can be put into practice only when nutrition education is carried into the home and the cooperation of the parents obtained. Essential contact with the home may be made by encouraging parents to visit the school to observe the school lunch in operation or to talk over their children's eating problems, and by having a teacher or school nurse or school nutritionist visit homes for the purpose of giving guidance and help in the solution of family food problems.

THE KIDNEYS AND THEIR WORK

The parts of food that cannot be digested and hence cannot be absorbed into the blood and lymph streams are simply pushed out of the body by way of the colon and rectum. Metabolic wastes, on the other hand, are the end products of the various processes involved in the use of food elements by the body cells. These end products would be harmful if they were allowed to accumulate. They consist chiefly of the carbonic acid (carbon dioxide dissolved in water) and excess heat produced in energy metabolism, and the nitrogenous wastes produced in protein metabolism.

As we have seen, the lungs excrete the carbon dioxide and the skin excretes the excess heat produced in the oxidation of glucose and fatty acids. We are now to consider the body's remarkable provisions for getting rid of the metabolic wastes produced through the breakdown of amino acids.

Urine and Its Excretion

The water-soluble wastes produced in protein metabolism are excreted by the kidneys in urine. The kidneys are brownish bean-shaped organs, each of which is about as big as a fist. They hang loosely on the back wall of the abdomen, one on each side of the lower portion of the spine (lumbar region). The kidneys clear the blood of several end products of protein metabolism literally by filtering blood plasma.

The Nephron. The nephron is the functional unit of the kidney. In each human kidney there are about a million nephrons. Each nephron consists of a twisted skein of capillary loops called the glomerulus, and a tube leading from it called the renal tubule (Fig. 56). The glomerulus is thrust like a clenched fist into the closed cuplike upper end of the tubule. This upper blind end is called Bowman's capsule after its discoverer, Sir William Bowman, an English physician (1816–1892).

Beyond Bowman's capsule the renal tubule pursues a tortuous course, including two series of snakelike convolutions and an abrupt hairpin turn, before it emerges to join a branch of the treelike system of urine-collecting conduits. The length of a single nephron, when strung out in a straight line, is between $1\frac{1}{2}$ and 2 inches. The estimated total length of the nephrons of both kidneys is some 45 miles.

Under ordinary circumstances large numbers of the million nephrons in each kidney are not working. This luxurious surplus of labor is an indication of the importance to the body of urine excretion. One kidney can be removed if the other is uninjured, and the amount and composition of the urine remain practically unaltered. Indeed, two-thirds of the kidney substance can be put out of commission before there is serious impairment of kidney function.

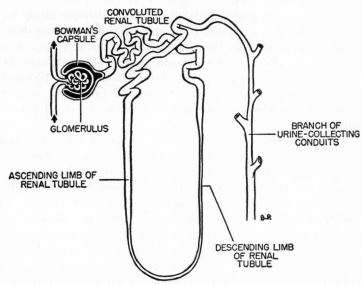

FIG. 56. A nephron, one of the two million filtering units of the kidneys.

How Urine Is Produced. Fluid containing everything in blood plasma *except the plasma proteins* passes from the glomerulus into Bowman's capsule and on through the capsular membrane into the renal tubule. About 170 liters of this filtrate is formed in 24 hours. This is more than fifty times the total volume of blood plasma. As the filtrate drains through the tubules, 99 per cent of this huge quantity of fluid is actively reabsorbed, leaving between 1½ and 2 liters of fluid to be excreted as urine. This means that every 24 hours 168½ liters of water is salvaged, together with about 33⅓ ounces of salt (NaCl), about 5½ ounces of sugar, and small quantities of other dissolved substances of value to the body.

The substances absorbed with water as the filtrate passes through the tubules are either absent from the urine or present in extremely small amounts. However, they appear in the urine in greater amounts if their concentration in the blood plasma is too high. The sugar found in the urine in diabetes is one example. Another is the more than usually large amount of salt present in urine when excess amounts are eaten. By removing surpluses of this kind the kidneys help to offset harmful changes in the composition of the blood and body fluids.

The substances that are reabsorbed in very small quantities, or not at all, are the ones that are highly concentrated in the urine. As we should expect, they consist mostly of the metabolic wastes that it is the duty of the kidneys to excrete. Of these, urea is present in the urine in by far the largest amount. Urea is made from the basic nitrogen group which is split off in the form of ammonia from an amino acid during deaminization (see How the Body Uses Proteins, earlier in this chapter). Ammonia has a highly toxic effect on the nervous system. It must have its teeth pulled, so to speak, before it can be allowed to enter the blood stream. This is done chiefly in the liver. There the poisonous ammonia is changed into urea, which is one of the least toxic of all nitrogenous compounds.

How Urine Is Removed from the Body. Drops of urine drip from the renal tubules into a system of collecting conduits, arranged like the spokes of a wheel, which convey the urine to the kidney pelvis. From this basinlike sac the urine enters a slender tube (ureter) which opens into the urinary bladder. The ureters (one for each kidney) contract rhythmically in peristaltic waves which squirt the urine into the bladder. The latter is a balloonlike muscular organ lined with mucous membrane. Sensory nerves of the autonomic nervous system end in the bladder wall in delicate little bulbs.

Distention of the bladder is responsible for the desire to urinate. Normally this stimulus acts on the sensory nerve endings in the muscular bladder wall when about half a pint of urine more or less (250 to 300 cubic centimeters) has collected.

Urination is essentially a reflex act, but after infancy and early childhood it is normally controlled by the will. That is, it can be voluntarily started, stopped, or interrupted. Ordinarily, the healthy child or adult can wait to empty the bladder until there is opportunity to do so. If the wait is too long, however, a feeling of fullness and discomfort culminating in pain results.

When the voluntary restraint on urination is lifted, the reflex operates automatically. The sphincter that guards the orifice leading into the urethra (the canal leading from the bladder to the outside) relaxes, and the urine is expelled with considerable force.

Normal Variations in Urine Excretion. The volume of urine excreted in 24 hours depends upon many different factors. Among them are diet, the quantity of fluid drunk, environmental temperature and humidity, posture, exercise, mental excitement, weight, age, and sex. The healthy adult usually excretes about 1½ liters of urine in 24 hours. Young children excrete three to four times more urine for their weight than adults. A diet high in protein results in a greater output of urine. The caffeine in coffee acts as a powerful diuretic, that is, a promoter of urine excretion. Drinking large quantities of water causes the urine output to increase manyfold. Copious sweating on warm days and exercise reduce the urine output. More urine collects when a person is lying down than when he is standing up. Also exposure to cold and various psychic influences may make the bladder more sensitive to tension.

Abnormal Variations in Urine Excretion

There are several abnormal conditions that have an effect on the quantity of urine excreted. For example, the amount may be reduced below normal in fever and in acute nephritis (see further on). It is almost always increased in diabetes (see Diabetes, in Chap. 3) and often in nervous states.

Frequency of urination, regardless of the amount excreted, also may have significance. In diabetes and in some nervous disorders frequency of urination is increased. In pyelitis (inflammation of the kidney pelvis) the bladder is very irritable. A child with this condition may not be able to get to the toilet between the time he feels the need to urinate and the time he is forced to let go.

Unwise toilet training in early childhood may prolong involuntary urination beyond the time it usually stops (between the ages of two and one-half and three years). In most cases this occurs at night (nocturnal enuresis, or bed wetting). Some children may "wet their pants" to get attention or to express resentment.

Observing Deviations from Normal in Kidney Function. The most valuable observations regarding kidney function which teachers can make are those which indicate a *persistent* change in a child's toilet habits. Requests to leave the room to go to the toilet which *persistently* occur more often or less often than usual should be reported to the nurse or physician serving the school. Frequently repeated complaints of excessive thirst or mention of the need to urinate more often than usual also should be reported.

Acute Kidney Inflammation

Acute inflammation of the kidneys goes by the general name of nephritis, that is, inflammation of the nephrons. When the glomeruli are primarily affected, the inflammation is called glomerular nephritis. When the tubules are involved the condition is called tubular nephritis, or nephrosis.

Acute glomerular nephritis is usually preceded by a streptococcal infection, such as scarlet fever, streptococcal sore throat, or a streptococcal skin infection. The streptococcal toxin causes inflammatory changes in the glomeruli which produce the signs and symptoms of this form of nephritis. These changes permit serum albumin and red blood cells to escape from the blood into the kidney tubules. Hence the most reliable signs of acute glomerular nephritis are albumin and red blood cells in the urine. They can be detected only through urinalysis (see further on).

The onset of acute glomerular nephritis may be so slow that it is detected only through a routine urinalysis. Or the child may suddenly show signs of severe illness and have to be treated as an emergency case until arrangements can be made to have him taken home or to a hospital for medical diagnosis and treatment.

Edema and reduction of the urine output are characteristic of acute glomerular nephritis. The edema is caused by the loss of serum albumin from the blood plasma. This loss lowers the osmotic pressure of the blood (see Circulation Survey, in Chap. 4), with the result that large amounts of fluid escape from the capillaries into the tissues. The decrease in urinary output is caused by the inflammatory changes which put large numbers of the kidney filtering units out of commission.

If so many nephrons are incapacitated that kidney function is seriously impaired, urea may pile up in the blood and cause urea poisoning, or uremia. This unhappy event occurs very seldom in children. With proper treatment acute glomerular nephritis usually results in complete recovery. However, there may be relapses in some cases, and in others the acute form of the disease may progress to chronic glomerular nephritis (chronic Bright's disease). The chronic form, however, is rare in children. It is mostly a disease of middle and old age.

Nephrosis, or tubular nephritis, is usually not preceded by an infection. It may be the second stage of a transient glomerular nephritis so mild that it was not detected. Nephrosis is marked by degenerative changes in the mucous-membrane covering (epithelium) of the renal tubules. The manifestations of nephrosis vary widely. Usually they include edema and albumin in the urine, but the urine output is not reduced. Many cases of nephrosis are very mild and clear up by themselves. However, there may be many recurrences marked by edema over a period of years.

Urinalysis. Because of the efficiency with which the nephrons in healthy kidneys act as selective filters, it is easy to see why a urinalysis is a valuable tool in diagnosis. For example, if serum albumin—which makes up about 50 per cent of the plasma proteins—is found in the urine in appreciable amounts, kidney damage is suspected because normally no plasma proteins are allowed to pass through the kidney filtering units. Other things looked for besides albumin and sugar (which may indicate diabetes) include the specific gravity of the urine (which indicates the quantity of solid substances contained in it), acid-alkali reactions, fragmented or whole red blood cells, white cells (pus), and bile pigment.

Children with a history of acute nephritis should have their urine examined periodically for red blood cells. This requires a microscopic examination of the sediment.

The physicians of an earlier day placed very great stress upon the appearance, odor, and volume of the urine. Sometimes they ventured to predict the outcome of a sickness (prognosis) simply by looking at and smelling the patient's urine. A flask of urine held aloft was the sign manual of the medieval physician, as the stethoscope around the neck is that of the modern physician.

Even now the physician can learn a great deal about the functioning of the kidneys by noting the amount, clearness or turbidity, and color of the urine.

DO YOU KNOW?

1. Suppose you were correcting the papers of high school students who had been given a "supply the missing words" test on the digestive system and you found the following mistakes. Make the corrections.

   a. The contraction and relaxation of __peristalsis__ regulates the passage of food through the alimentary canal.

   b. The wavelike motions of __sphincters__ are responsible for pushing food along the digestive tract away from the mouth toward the anal canal.

   c. Large food molecules are chemically taken apart during digestion by hormones.

   d. The __pepsin__ in saliva starts the digestion of starch.

   e. The enzymes in __pancreatic__ __juice__ begin the splitting up of protein molecules into __grape__ __sugar__ .

   f. Chemical digestion is completed in the __large__ intestine .

   g. Pressure on the walls of the __duodenum__ gives the stimulus for defecation.

2. Select the correct ending for each of the following incomplete sentences:

   a. Peristaltic waves operating in reverse from the upper end of the stomach cause (1) halitosis, (2) belching, (3) anorexia.

   b. Hunger is caused by (1) an empty stomach, (2) a good appetite,
      (3) smelling appetizing odors.
   c. Jaundice is caused by the presence in the blood of an excessive
      amount of (1) hemoglobin, (2) ptyalin, (3) bilirubin.
   d. Food infections are caused by bacilli belonging to the (1) *Shigella*
      group, (2) *Salmonella* group, (3) *Brucella* group.
   e. The most important factor in the spread of undulant fever in our
      country is (1) failure to wash the hands before eating, (2) drinking
      raw milk, (3) drinking polluted water.
   f. The most effective method of preventing hookworm infection is
      (1) to keep intestinal discharges off the ground, (2) to wash the
      hands after toilet, (3) to drink only pasteurized milk.
   g. Water-soluble protein wastes pass into the kidney tubules from the
      (1) ureters, (2) glomeruli, (3) urinary bladder.

3. Match each word or term in Group A with the word or group of
   words in Group B you associate with it:

Group A	*Group B*
Cheilosis	Gum inflammation
Herpes simplex	Salivary-gland infection
Mumps	Periodontal-membrane infection
Dental caries	Cold sores
Sodium fluoride	Production of enamel-dissolving acids
Lactobacilli	A substance used in preventive dentistry
Malocclusion	Failure of upper and lower teeth to meet properly
Gingivitis	Riboflavin deficiency
Pyorrhea	Tooth decay

4. What deficiency or deficiencies in the diet would you suspect if a
   doctor told you that a poor or unbalanced diet was responsible for
   underweight and listlessness in a child? lowered resistance to infection?
   rickets? nutritional anemia? simple goiter? blepharitis? constipation
   due to poor intestinal muscle tone? cheilosis? pellagra? spongy, bleeding gums?

SUGGESTED ACTIVITIES

1. Review your own eating habits as objectively as possible. Leading
   questions to ask yourself are: Do I take time to eat a good breakfast?
   Do I allow enough time to eat lunch unhurriedly? Do I unfailingly
   wash my hands with soap and warm water before eating? Do I brush

my teeth, or at least rinse my mouth, after eating whenever possible? Do I rest before eating when I am very tired? Do I avoid eating when I am emotionally upset? Do I endeavor to make mealtimes cheerful pleasant times for my table companions? Do I avoid indulging in sweets too often between meals? Do I take time to relax for a little while after meals whenever possible? Have a panel discussion on the incentives which do, or might, move you to practice what you are supposed to teach about eating habits. Then plan a unit for an elementary or high school class with the object of motivating children to practice good habits of eating.

2. Keep a careful record of everything you eat for one day. How does your record compare with the table of daily allowances for specific nutrients recommended for school children (Table 12)? Using Tables 11 and 12 and any book in which food values are given (for example, Taylor's "Food Values in Shares and Weights," listed as a reference), plan well-balanced meals for yourself for one day. How do these meals compare with those you ordinarily eat? Do you need to give more attention to your daily selection of food?

3. If your laboratory or practice school (or the school in which you teach) has a cafeteria, make a note of the kinds and quantities of foods selected for lunch by three or four children. Ask each child observed to tell what he or she had for breakfast. The next day, ask each one what he or she had for dinner or supper the night before. Decide whether or not the specific nutrients in the foods selected for lunch on the day of observation adequately supplemented the nutrients supplied by the other two meals. If not, how would you help the children to make better choices of food for lunch?

4. If some children bring lunches from home, observe what they have in their lunch boxes on one day. Then carry out the other activities suggested in project 3.

5. Have a member, or committee, of the class report on the history of the school-lunch movement in America. Then make a plan for gaining the interest of the parents in providing a hot school lunch for school children in a community that does not have this service.

6. If possible, arrange a visit to a dental clinic in the school or community, to observe the dental examination of school children, prophylactic cleansing of teeth, the topical application of sodium fluoride solution, and the instruction given on toothbrushing methods. If this is not possible, invite a dentist to visit the class and demonstrate the dental examination of a school child. Also invite a dental hygienist

serving a school to give a talk on the ways in which she can cooperate with teachers in the dental health education of children.

7. Have class discussions on ways of helping a child who is known to have:
   a. Constipation due to irregular toilet habits
   b. Tartar at the necks of the teeth due to neglect of toothbrushing
   c. Spongy, bleeding gums due to a vitamin-C deficiency
   d. Rampant dental caries aggravated by excessive indulgence in sweets
   e. Lack of appetite at meals due to the habit of eating between meals
   f. Loss of appetite due to overconcern on the part of his parents

SELECTED REFERENCES

AMERICAN DENTAL ASSOCIATION, COUNCIL ON DENTAL HEALTH: *Fluoridation in the Prevention of Dental Caries,* Chicago, 1951.

AMERICAN MEDICAL ASSOCIATION: *Wonder Stories of the Human Machine: The Fuel System (Digestion),* Chicago, 1948. (Pamphlet 6 in a series explaining how the principal organs of the body work.)

AMERICAN MEDICAL ASSOCIATION: *Wonder Stories of the Human Machine: The Exhaust (Waste Removal),* Chicago, 1948. (Pamphlet 7 in the series.)

BOGERT, L. JEAN: *Nutrition and Physical Fitness,* 6th ed. Philadelphia, W. B. Saunders Company, 1954.

CANNON, WALTER B.: *Digestion and Health,* New York, W. W. Norton & Company, Inc., 1936. (A classic on digestion by a distinguished physiologist.)

COOPER, L. F., E. M. BARBER, H. S. MITCHELL, and H. J. RYNBERGEN: *Nutrition in Health and Disease,* 12th ed. Philadelphia, J. B. Lippincott Company, 1953. (Application of basic theoretical principles of human nutrition to specific conditions.)

KOHN, LOUIS W.: *Your Digestive System,* New York, Blakiston Division, McGraw-Hill Book Company, Inc., 1945. (Information on the organs of digestion and their activities and the parasites that produce digestive disturbances.)

MARTIN, ETHEL AUSTIN: *Roberts' Nutrition Work with Children,* Chicago, University of Chicago Press, 1954.

NATIONAL RESEARCH COUNCIL, COMMITTEE ON DENTAL HEALTH: *Problem of Providing Optimum Fluoride Intake for Prevention of Dental*

Caries; a report of the Committee on Dental Health of the Food and Nutrition Board prepared by subcommittee on optimum fluoride levels, Washington, D.C., 1953.

TAYLOR, CLARA MAE: *Food Values in Shares and Weights,* New York, The Macmillan Company, reissue, 1954. (Contains tables giving the nutritive values of about five hundred foods.)

TAYLOR, CLARA MAE, and GRACE MACLEOD: *Rose's Laboratory Handbook for Dietetics,* 5th ed. New York, The Macmillan Company, 1949. (Food values and requirements.)

TODHUNTER, E. NEIGE: *Everyday Nutrition for School Children,* University, Alabama, University of Alabama, 1945.

U.S. DEPARTMENT OF AGRICULTURE: *Composition of Foods: Raw, Processed, Prepared,* Agriculture Handbook No. 8, Washington, D.C., 1950.

YAHRAES, HERBERT: *Your Teeth—How To Save Them,* Public Affairs Pamphlet No. 147, rev. ed. New York, Public Affairs Committee, 1949.

Organizations

American Dental Association
American Home Economics Association
Food and Nutrition Board of the National Research Council
U.S. Bureau of Human Nutrition and Home Economics

Chapter 7   THE BODY'S ENVELOPE

---

*Topography and Functions of the Skin, Hair,
    and Nails*
Observing Cutaneous Deviations from Normal
*Observing Deviations from Normal Mirrored by
    the Skin*
Skin Infections
Skin Infestations
Skin Injuries

TOPOGRAPHY AND FUNCTIONS OF THE SKIN, HAIR, AND NAILS

Normally the skin presents a relatively smooth, dry surface to the naked human eye. But an account of the travels of a mythical, ultramicroscopic pygmy wandering over the skin would include descriptions of mighty mountain ranges and deep valleys filled with pitfalls, of vast forests, of a wet, slippery terrain subject to sudden floods and quick unpredictable changes of climate, and of a highly varied fauna and flora. Some knowledge regarding the structure and functions of healthy skin will help teachers to understand what they see in observing various deviations from normal.

The skin has three major jobs. First of all, it forms a tight-fitting elastic protective envelope for the body. When unbroken and healthy, it serves to keep blood and other essential body fluids in and foreign substances, including bacteria, out. The second job is the regulation of body temperature. The skin forms an essential part of the mechanism by which wanted heat is kept inside the body and excess heat is permitted to escape. The third job is to act as a receiving set for the stimuli that evoke the sensations of touch, pressure, stretch, pain, heat, and cold.

"Upon the Skin"

The part of the skin we see is the extremely thin top sheet of the epidermis. Strictly speaking, the epidermis has no proper name of its own, since its name means simply "upon the skin." From the top downward, the epidermis is built up of a horny layer and a layer of living epithelial cells sometimes called the germinative layer.

312

The horny layer consists of sheet upon sheet of flat, dry, inert scales closely packed together and overlapping like the shingles of a roof. As the existing top sheet is rubbed or scrubbed off, the one next below takes its place and so on while life lasts.

The horny layer never wears out because it is continually being renewed from its underside with new sheets formed of cells pushed up

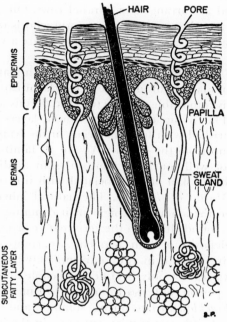

FIG. 57. Cross section of skin showing its three layers.

from the germinative layer. The deepest row of cells in this living layer is attached to the dermis or true skin underneath. The cells of the germinative layer are perpetually dividing. In this process the daughter cells are crowded upward. During their upward journey the strong, living nucleated cells become less and less virile as they get further away from their source of nourishment. Finally they undergo a process of hornification which changes their protoplasm into keratin, the substance of which the sheets of the horny layer are composed.

True Skin

The dermis, or true skin, contains blood vessels, nerves, muscles, connective tissue, in short, all the structures that go to make up what we call "flesh." The surface of contact between the epidermis and the dermis is undulating rather than flat and smooth. Miniature conical peaks called papillae project upward from the upper face of the dermis and fit into corresponding hollows in the underface of the epidermis. This arrangement locks the two surfaces together so that the epidermis cannot easily be rubbed off.

Fingerprints. Minute ridges that are seen on the palms and the soles owe their existence to the fact that the papillae are most prominent in these locations and are arranged in parallel rows. On the undersurfaces of the fingers and toes the papillary ridges form whorls which are peculiar for each individual. That is why the fingerprints are a valuable means of identification.

How the Skin Is Fed. The skin is nourished with materials brought to it by the blood circulating through the networks of capillaries enmeshed in the dermis. It is impossible to puncture the dermis anywhere without drawing blood. The living cells in the lower layers of the bloodless epidermis are nourished with food materials in the lymph or tissue fluid, which percolates up from the dermis. We are all familiar with the dewiness and bloom of well-nourished youthful skin as distinguished from the thin, dry, splotchy skin often associated with illness or aging.

The Coloring Matter of the Skin. The natural inherited color of the skin depends upon the amount of pigment it contains. This pigment, or coloring matter, is found chiefly in the germinative layer of the epidermis. In brunets the deposits of skin pigment are comparatively large; in blonds, comparatively small; in albinos, completely lacking. The amount of skin pigment varies not only in different people and in different skin areas of the same person, but also from time to time.

Sun Tan and Freckles. In late spring, summer, and early fall the children who have had a chance to play outdoors in the sun and wind will have coats of tan or crops of freckles. Exposure to the ultraviolet rays in sunlight increases the deposits of pigment in the epidermis. These deposits act as a screen to protect the more delicate structures underneath from further action of the ultraviolet rays. In fair children, especially redheads, the pigment in the skin is unevenly distributed. These children usually freckle instead of tan. They are much more susceptible to sunburn than are children whose skins tan evenly. The redness of sunburn is caused by the dilation of the blood vessels of the skin by histamine which is released under the influence of ultraviolet irradiation.

Flesh Color. In the white-skinned races the epidermis is translucent like a very thin sheet of horn or a pane of ground glass. The red color of the blood in the blood-vessel networks in the dermis shining through the epidermis produces the "flesh color" or tone, beloved of artists, which reflects the luster, tint, and vitality of healthy human skin. In places where the epidermis is thinnest and the network of minute blood vessels in the dermis very abundant, as in the center of the cheeks, the red tints are most pronounced.

Normally, there is a wide variation in skin color. There is a tendency amounting almost to an obsession in some of us to think of rosy cheeks as denoting good health and of pale cheeks as indicating poor health. Yet many healthy children in whom the epidermis is comparatively thick or heavily pigmented may have a naturally creamy, sallow, or olive complexion with little or no pink in the cheeks.

Mucous Membrane. In the soft, moist skin that lines the eyelids, the lips and mouth, and all body tubes and cavities, the dermis is thinner and more loosely built than elsewhere, and the epidermis has no horny surface layer. Hence the red color from the underlying blood vessels shows through more clearly. This modified skin is called mucous membrane.

The Fatty Layer of the Skin

The subcutaneous, or fatty, layer of the skin serves as the connecting link between the dermis above the muscles and other tissues below. It acts as a shock absorber against possible injury caused by falls or blows and as an insulating material. It furnishes rotundity to body contours, which is considered advantageous or disadvantageous depending upon its quantity and its distribution.

The tone of the skin—its firmness and texture—depends partly on the cushion of fat below the dermis and partly on the elastic fibers in the skin itself. The elasticity of the skin can easily be observed by pinching up the skin between thumb and finger and then releasing it. This elasticity is not so great, however, that it can accommodate itself to considerable variations in tension. If a plump person loses a great deal of weight, for example, his skin does not retract, or shrink, and become as smooth and tense as it was before. Hence, it tends to look baggy or wrinkled.

The wrinkled, thin, overstretched skin in old age is usually due both to the depletion of subcutaneous fat and to loss of elasticity from the skin. In healthy well-nourished children the skin looks smooth and firm, and the body is delightfully rounded, with curves rather than sharp angles.

The Skin's Secretory Apparatus

Readers of "Gulliver's Travels" will remember that Gulliver in discussing the complexions of the natives of Lilliput was told by one of these diminutive people that his own face upon close inspection was at first a very shocking sight. He said

> "he could discover great holes in my skin;
> that the stumps of my beard were ten times
> stronger than the bristles of a boar, and my
> complexion made up of several colours alto-
> gether disagreeable. . . ."

We know that the "great holes" so distressing to the Lilliputians, to which we give the name pores, are the openings of deep-rooted sweat and oil glands.

The Sweat Glands. The total number of sweat glands is about two million. From each one a long duct, which is spirally twisted like a cork-screw as it passes through the epidermis, leads to the surface of the skin. Although the secretion of sweat is continuous, it is seldom noticed because it evaporates faster than it is produced (insensible perspiration). Either increased heat production within the body or a rise in environmental temperature calls for increased sweating as a means of stepping up the amount of body heat lost through evaporation (see Reactions to Internal Temperature Changes, in Chap. 3). When sweat does not evaporate as fast as it is secreted, it becomes visible in the form of drops standing on, or running off, the oily surface of the skin (sensible perspiration).

The Sebaceous Glands. The oily coating of the skin comes from sebaceous (fat) glands lodged in the dermis, or true skin. Occasionally their ducts open directly upon the surface of the skin. More frequently they open into the hair follicles, and their secretion passes out to the skin surface along the hairs. The fat glands connected with the hair follicles are called pilosebaceous glands ("pilo-," meaning "hair," plus "sebaceous," meaning "fatty"). Sebum, as the secretion of the fat glands is called, is squeezed slowly out of the glands by pressure exerted across them by minute strands of the "hair-raising" muscles, much as tooth-paste is squeezed out of a tube by the pressure of the fingers on the tube. The function of sebum is to keep the skin and hair soft, pliable, and waterproof. In smooth velvety skins the amount of sebum, or oil, secreted is just about right—not too little, not too much. But many individuals have skin that is either too dry or too oily. Fair, "thin-skinned" children are the ones who are most likely to have dry skin. Also dryness of the skin is sometimes associated with a nutritional deficiency.

The Hair and Nails

Hair and nails are appendages of the skin. Hair is found in all regions of the skin except that of the palms, the soles, the lips, and the backs of the finger tips and toe tips. There are three kinds of hair: (*a*) the short, soft, downy hairs usually seen on the face, trunk, and limbs; (*b*) short, strong or bristly hairs such as those of the eyebrows and eyelashes; (*c*) and the long hairs of the scalp, beard, and armpits.

How Hair Grows. The follicles, or sockets, out of which hair grows are formed by a dipping down of the epidermis into the dermis. The part of the hair showing above the surface of the skin is the hair shaft and the part contained within the follicle is the hair root. The lower end

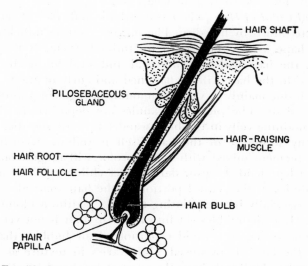

HAIR SHAFT

PILOSEBACEOUS GLAND

HAIR - RAISING MUSCLE

HAIR ROOT

HAIR FOLLICLE

HAIR BULB

HAIR PAPILLA

FIG. 58. One hair and the structures that oil and move it.

of the root, which is thicker than the upper part, is the hair bulb. The bottom end of the hair bulb fits like a snug cap over a tiny mound containing blood vessels which is called the hair papilla. For a short distance above the hair papilla the hair is a mass of succulent living cells similar to that of the surrounding dermis. The cells in dividing and multiplying push upward. As they move farther and farther away from the papillae from which they get their nourishment, they become horny like the upper layer of the epidermis.

Goose Flesh. A tiny muscle is attached to each slanting hair follicle. As we have seen, the pressure of strands of the muscle upon the sebaceous glands draining into the hair follicle distributes sebum over the hair shaft. When stimulated by cold or fear, the muscle pulls the slanting hair follicle erect. The result is the puckering of the skin known as goose flesh.

Goose flesh is a survival from a time when human beings had more body hair than they do now and could increase their protection from cold by erecting it. Many mammals and birds can do this. For example, the sight of sparrows perched with their feathers ruffled is a familiar one in city parks on a cold day. The sensation of the hair lifting on the scalp at moments of extreme fright gave rise to the expression, "his hair stood on end," in describing terror-stricken behavior. Goose flesh is a common accompaniment of the shivering and chattering of the teeth which occur when the body is chilled as a result of very cold atmospheric temperature or in a disturbance of the body's heat-control mechanism at the onset of an infectious fever (see Fever, in Chap. 3).

Shape and Color of Hair. The natural shape and color of each person's hair are determined by heredity. The narrow slanting follicles mold the hair into shape as the roots push up through them. If the follicle is cylindrical, the hair will be cylindrical and straight; if the follicle is oval or flattish, the hair will be flattened and curly or wavy. The color of the hair is due mainly to varying amounts of pigment granules present in the hair shaft. The pigment granules are deposited in the hair as pigment-containing cells in the bulb wander upward and die. The color of the horny substance of the hair itself is yellow. According to the amount of pigment mixed with it, hair color will range from blond to black. Light hair tends to grow darker after childhood. The presence of tiny air bubbles in the central portion of the hair shaft also may affect hair color, especially in contributing toward "platinum blond," gray, or white hair. How air bubbles get into the hair shaft is not yet known. It is presumably owing to a rapid evolution of air bubbles that "sudden graying of the hair" is produced. Hair varies in texture as well as in shape and color. Redheads have the coarsest hair, and blonds the finest.

The Life Span of Hair. The hair of the scalp grows about four or five inches a year. There is a very wide variation in the length of life of individual hairs—from 6 months to 4 years. When a hair reaches the end of its life span it becomes detached from the papilla and falls out, to be replaced by a new one growing from the same papilla.

Fingernails and Toenails. Nails protect the tips of the fingers and toes, and fingernails help in the picking up of things. The growth of fingernails and toenails is much like that of hair. At the base of the nail the epidermis folds under to form a slot which corresponds to the hair follicle. Out of this slot the nail grows from a collection of living cells called the matrix. The half-moon at the base of the nails represents the upper limit of the matrix. The cells of the matrix are continually being pushed outward by new cells forming behind them. Gradually their food supply is cut off, with the result that they are changed to horny plates. Beyond the matrix the nail rests on the nail bed, over which it is pushed as the cells in the matrix divide and multiply.

OBSERVING CUTANEOUS DEVIATIONS FROM NORMAL

The skin, at least of the face and hands, and its appendages, hair and fingernails, are practically always open for observation. What can be learned from the skin and its appendages depends upon observing them from several different points of view. This section is devoted to various conditions and defects more or less closely associated with their structure or function.

Skin Troubles

"Threadbare" Skin. In some individuals the process of hornification of the epidermis (see earlier in this chapter) runs into trouble. Rows upon rows of cells, as they push upward from the germinative layer, do not lose their nuclei; rather they form sheaths or scales that break away readily. These scales are shed in appreciable quantities, and the outer skin mantle becomes "threadbare" in spots. This state of affairs is due in most instances to a skin disease of many varieties, which is labeled psoriasis because it is characterized by the formation of bright red patches covered with silvery scales (*psōriasis,* in Greek, means "a scabby disease of the skin").

Psoriasis may attack any or all parts of the body, including the scalp. Although it is fairly common, it is fortunately rare in children. Usually it first appears after adolescence. Its cause is unknown. In some families there may be a tendency to develop it, but it cannot be stated with certainty that it is a hereditary disease. It is definitely *not contagious.* The chief distress caused by it is its unsightliness. Although there is as yet no sure cure, the recently developed drugs cortisone and ACTH may be useful in its treatment.

Wheals. The small blood vessels of the skin are extremely sensitive to stimulation by mechanical and other agencies. If a blunt-pointed instrument is drawn lightly over the skin of the forearm, a white line will quickly appear along the path taken by the instrument. This "white reaction," as it is called, is caused by the contraction of the capillary walls. If the instrument is drawn more firmly over the skin a red line instead of a white line appears. This "red reaction" is caused by the dilation of the capillaries. An unusually strong stimulus, like a slap, calls nervous mechanisms into play and the arterioles dilate, with the result that there is a spreading flush or flare surrounding the path of the stroke.

A still more intense stimulus, like severe whipping, raises wheals on the skin. Wheals are white elevated patches which follow the red reaction in two or three minutes and are surrounded by the red flare. They are

due to increased permeability of the capillary walls which permits fluid
from the blood to seep into the tissues. Hence wheals are a localized
edema. They disappear as the fluid disappears into wider areas of the
skin. The stimulus of an allergen from within may raise wheals similar
to those caused by a strong mechanical stimulus from without (see Hives,
Table 15).

Blisters. Sometimes the fluid in a wheal collects between the horny
top layer of the skin and the layer underneath. When this occurs, the
one is lifted away from the other. This is called a "blister." Blisters
frequently develop as a result of burns or mechanical rubbing or pinching. If the blister is filled with clear fluid, the injury is confined to the
epidermis. If it contains bloody fluid—a blood blister—we may be sure
that the dermis also is involved, because there are no blood vessels
whatever in the epidermis.

Vesicles and Pimples. Small blisters, not larger than a split pea, are
called vesicles. Usually the skin around a vesicle is red, in which case
it may look like a small dewdrop on a rose petal, but occasionally the
red area is lacking. The formation of vesicles is associated with many
different conditions—for example, small burns, sunburn, chickenpox, and
ivy or oak poisoning or other forms of dermatitis.

Pimples are small, solid elevations of the skin, sometimes called papules.
Pimples usually begin as a result of irritation and pressure from the waxy
plugs obstructing the flow of sebum from the fat glands. These plugs have
much the same effect as any foreign body in the skin, a splinter, for
example. It is easy for germs to get in under the plugs of sebum and
start an infection. When infected pimples or vesicles become filled with
yellowish pus, they are called pustules.

Blackheads and Whiteheads. Blackheads, or comedones, are simply
hard plugs of sebum and other debris protruding from blocked fat-gland
ducts. Their blackness is caused by oxidation of that portion of the plug
which is exposed to air and not by negligence in face washing as is popularly supposed. A whitehead, or milium, is white because the gland
involved has no excreting duct and so the tip of the waxy plug is not
exposed to oxidation.

Warts. Warts are very common in children. They are located most
frequently on the hands and fingers, less frequently on the face and
scalp. A wart is an overgrowth of epidermal cells which does not break
through the thin dividing line between the epidermis and the underlying true skin. It is roughened, like a cauliflower, and grayish or blackish
in color.

There is evidence that a virus may be involved in the production of warts. It is common knowledge that warts often appear in crops. Also, one or two warts may be followed by others through self-inoculation. For example, a row of warts sometimes develops along a scratch on the hand on which other warts are present. Also warts on the soles sometimes occur among school children almost in epidemics. Warts in this location are very painful because of the pressure exerted on them in walking. The peculiar thing about some warts is the suddenness with which they appear and disappear. This has led to innumerable superstitions regarding their treatment. Any hocus-pocus may seem to succeed in a condition that naturally disappears as if by magic.

Warts are not dangerous except in the rarest instances. If they are uncomfortable or unsightly, medical treatment will give relief.

Moles. Moles belong to a class of skin blemishes called nevi (singular, nevus). Actually they are small birthmarks consisting of collections of densely packed skin cells which are brown or black in color because they contain more pigment than ordinary skin cells. Almost everyone has one or more moles. In the great majority of cases they are not dangerous or disfiguring—indeed, they were once called "beauty marks." The custom of wearing tiny black patches to accentuate some alluring facial line or dimple may have had its origin in observations of the pleasing effect of fortunately placed moles.

There are, however, many kinds of moles, and some of them may constitute cosmetic blemishes that will worry youngsters as they grow up, or may develop later into malignant growths. Any mole, but more particularly the black or blue-black variety, is potentially dangerous if it is located in a place where it is subject to frequent irritation. Young people should learn to leave moles alone—not to pick at them or try to remove them with caustics. If they wish to get rid of a mole or birthmark because of its unsightliness, they should be advised to consult a physician —preferably a dermatologist—not a beauty specialist. When a mole, either spontaneously or as a result of friction or other injury, shows signs of irritation, or change of color, or further growth, competent medical advice and care should be sought at once.

Chapping. In dry-skinned children, especially, chapping in cold weather is often troublesome. Chapping is a familiar form of inflammation of the skin, or dermatitis, to give it its technical name. It does not ordinarily occur in warm weather because at that time the sebaceous and sweat glands are most active and keep the skin thoroughly oiled.

In chapping, the skin first gets red and tender with some scaling, and then develops painful cracks and fissures. Like leather, skin cannot stand up when dry under conditions that it easily endures when properly oiled.

Failure to dry the skin thoroughly after washing and before going outdoors favors chapping, because the rapid evaporation of the water by
the dry cold air of winter causes sudden dryness of the skin.

To prevent or relieve chapping, children susceptible to it should learn
to dry their hands and faces thoroughly and then to rub in cold cream,
petroleum jelly, or any bland oil such as olive oil or mineral oil. The
use of superfatted toilet soap instead of ordinary toilet soap or strong
laundry soap may be suggested.

The squirming and twisting of dry-skinned children during the winter
months may be caused by the uncomfortable itchy feeling of extremely
dry skin, aggravated in some cases by winter underwear. Such children
may relieve their itchiness by rubbing the entire body once or twice a
week with a cloth moistened with oil.

Chilblains. Exposure to cold damp weather also may produce chilblains on the fingers, toes, heels, or ears of some children. Chilblains are
painful red spots which itch intensely, especially in a warm room. The
redness is due to congestion of the skin capillaries. Chilblains sometimes
develop when the frozen area of the skin is thawed out too quickly in
frostbite (see Frostbite under Skin Injuries, in this chapter).

Oily Skin. In oily skins the texture of the skin is usually coarse, the
pores large, and the face and hair greasy. Hence, an oily skin is a handicap because it detracts from personal appearance and predisposes the
skin to many troublesome conditions such as acne and boils.

Young people who have excessively oily skins should learn that they
cannot change the texture of their skins, but they can do a great deal to
improve their appearance by proper care of the face. Following the
directions for cleaning the face given below in the section on adolescent
acne will be helpful for young people troubled with an oily skin.

Acne. During adolescence, hormonal influences arising in the sex
glands activate the pilosebaceous glands (see p. 316) of the face, chest,
and back which are relatively inactive during infancy and childhood.
While this is going on, the excreting ducts or the external outlets of the
pilosebaceous apparatus may not enlarge fast enough to take care of
the increased production of sebum. Or the hair-raising muscles may be
too weak to squeeze out the sebum fast enough. Or an alteration in the
viscosity of the sebum itself may contribute to its stagnation within the
glands or their ducts. The result may be the development of acne, an
unsightly skin condition which is of great concern to adolescent boys
and girls.

The signs of acne—blackheads, whiteheads, oily skin, distended pores,
pimples, and scars of healed pimples—singly or all together make up

what is called a bad complexion. No wonder that boys or girls troubled with acne may be left with worse scars on the psyche than on the face!

Unfortunately acne disfigures the complexion at the very time when an attractive appearance counts the most. Young people afflicted with it worry inordinately about their bumpy, pimple-studded faces and are likely to pick at or squeeze blackheads and pimples in an attempt to get rid of them. Understanding teachers can do a great deal to help these troubled young people by giving them the facts about acne.

In the first place, acne is a temporary condition in the great majority of cases. Just as soon as the fat-gland ducts and their outlets grow large enough to take care of the increased secretion of sebum, the acne will clear up. But it is not necessary to wait for that happy event. A young person should know that his regular doctor or a skin specialist can do much to improve his present appearance and spirits and to prevent permanent scars. Also there are many things he can do to help himself.

One of the most important helps is to keep the hands away from the face at all times except when washing it. In persons with acne who sit with the face resting on the hand, it has been observed that the acne is most pronounced where the hand touches the skin, because the heat of the hand increases sebaceous secretion. Also contact of the fingers with the face leads to picking at or squeezing pimples until they break. This practice serves to spread the infective matter with which they are filled. Wherever this material is "planted"—on the skin near the original pimple or on some other part touched with soiled fingers—another pimple may grow. Also squeezing fingers may serve to spread infective material into the surrounding tissues. When this happens the pimple may become larger and harder to get rid of and eventually leave an ugly scar. As a means of breaking the habit of picking at the face, physicians often tell their young patients to avoid looking into a mirror until the face has improved.

Another great help is to keep the skin as healthy as possible by getting enough of all the known essential food elements in the daily diet. No special vitamins will cure acne; all are important for the health of the skin. Rich greasy food seems to encourage acne. The greatest offender is chocolate. This means chocolate in any form—in ice cream, cake, candy, and beverages (chocolate "malteds," hot chocolate, chocolate ice cream sodas, and cola drinks). A young person troubled with acne should be encouraged to "swear off" chocolate for a trial period anyway. Other prime offenders are nuts and heavily fried foods. It seems logical to assume that, if more oil than usual is being formed by the fat glands of the skin, it is wise to decrease the amount of fat in the food eaten.

Also face creams and ointments with an oily base simply add more grease to already grease-clogged pores and should be avoided.

Skin cleanliness is the third great help in controlling acne. It stands to reason that keeping the pores and hair-follicle openings cleared of debris will promote better drainage of sebum. Washing the face morning and evening with a thick lather of soap and hot water is enough to clear up many cases of simple acne. Two latherings with a hot rinse between and a cold rinse afterward is the procedure recommended. A soft cloth should be used to apply the lather. In stubborn cases, the physician may prescribe a medicinal preparation for use after the cold rinse.

General measures that will put the body as a whole in better fighting trim to overcome acne are adequate sleep, vigorous daily exercise, fresh air, and direct sunshine.

Hair and Fingernails

Normal variations in hair are legion. Natural hair color ranges from platinum blond to coal black. Natural hair shape ranges from stick-straight to tightly curled. Hair texture may be "as coarse as a horse's mane" or "as fine as silk." In addition to noting that a child has naturally straight, yellow, fine hair or naturally curly, black, coarse hair as an inheritance, we see also the effects of variations in grooming and in style of hairdo on appearance.

But whatever may be the normal variations on the theme of hair, all healthy well-cared-for hair has something in common. It is clean and glossy; it has a shine; it looks alive. Many departures from good health may be first evidenced by changes in the texture and amount of hair because the nutrition of the hair, like that of the skin, depends upon the adequate functioning of other organs of the body.

Falling Hair. The normal cycle of hair growth (see above) may be interrupted by sickness or complications resulting from neglect or abuse. Excessive falling out of a child's hair should always be brought to the physician's attention. However, a moderate amount of hair shedding is to be expected. Normally, one may lose as many as 50 to 100 hairs a day.

Dry Hair and Oily Hair. Dry lusterless hair is due to a lack or shortage of oil deliveries from the pilosebaceous glands of the scalp. This condition may be natural in dry-skinned children. But it is important to observe and report changes from customary sleekness or glossiness to a condition of dryness, coarseness, brittleness, and lack of luster. Vitamin-A deficiency and an acute or chronic illness are among the factors that may be responsible for producing these changes.

Flat greasy hair is due to an overproduction of natural hair oil. This condition is often seen during adolescence as an accompaniment of acne. Frequent shampoos are necessary to remove the excess oil.

Simple Dandruff. Both in excessive dryness and in excessive oiliness of the scalp, dandruff may be especially bothersome. Simple dandruff is the constant scaling off of the topmost horny layer of the epidermis of the scalp. It is the same sort of scaling as that which goes on less noticeably from other areas of the skin. Almost everyone at one time or another has been annoyed by the showers of untidy little dandruff flakes that are so noticeable on the collars and shoulders of dark-colored coats and dresses. If the scalp is very oily the flakes are usually moist and sticky and hence difficult to brush off. Aside from appearance, there is nothing to worry about in simple dandruff of the dry or sticky variety. Usually it can be controlled by keeping the hair clean and well brushed. However, a persistently greasy, scaly scalp which itches constantly calls for medical investigation.

Fingernail Defects. The white spots that sometimes appear in the fingernails are usually formed by bubbles of air between the cell layers. They may have no significance or may be caused by injury to the nail or by a nutritional deficiency. Severe injury to the matrix may cause loss of the nail, but if the lower layers of living cells are not destroyed, a new nail will be formed.

Any abnormal brownish or whitish discoloration or grooving or pitting of the fingernails, or nails that curve over the ends of the fingers, should be called to the attention of the nurse or physician.

Hangnails. The thick skin around the nail is called the cuticle. It is imperfectly oiled and for this reason cracks easily. The urge to pick at or bite a cracked or rough cuticle is hard to resist, and that is why hangnails are such common afflictions.

Children should learn how to care for their nails, both for the sake of appearance and to prevent the formation of hangnails. A little cold cream or oil rubbed into the cuticle from time to time helps to keep it soft and smooth. It is also helpful to keep the cuticle pushed back from the nail. This may be done easily with the blunt end of an orange stick when the cuticle is soft after a bath. If hangnails form they should be removed with sharp clean manicure scissors, taking care to cause no bleeding.

Nail Biting. It has been found that nail biting, far from being just a bad habit, is often used unconsciously by a child as an outlet for some suppressed emotion—aggression, for example. Also, nail biting has frequently been observed in irritable, restless children whose trouble is a nutritional deficiency. Children who persistently bite their nails need thorough medical study.

OBSERVING DEVIATIONS FROM NORMAL MIRRORED BY THE SKIN

Since the skin is an organ and shares with the other organs in whatever affects the whole body for good or ill, it often reflects good health or poor health as clearly as the skin itself is reflected by a mirror.

Changes in Skin Color

Observation teaches us that the color of the skin in any individual is not a static thing. It registers the play of emotions and of physical ups

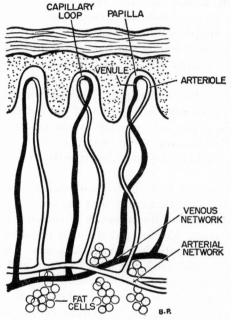

FIG. 59. The arrangement of blood vessels in the dermis.

and downs as the color of water registers the effects of sunshine or shadow or the ruffling wind.

Changes in skin color depend largely upon changes in the circulation of blood in the skin. The skin's blood supply is influenced by the number and arrangement of the blood vessels in the dermis, the amount of blood in the blood vessels, and the character of the blood itself.

As the arterioles approach the bases of the papillae in the topmost layer of the dermis, they shed their muscle coats and form capillary loops. The arterial branch of each capillary loop ascends into a papilla, makes a hairpin turn, and descends as the venous branch. Upon reaching the base of the papilla the venous branch joins with the venous branches of other capillary loops in the neighborhood to form a venule. The venules unite with one another to form a rich network which runs horizontally beneath the bases of the papillae. The venous networks drain into deeper veins.

When the blood vessels of the skin are dilated or widened, they can hold far more blood than when they are constricted or tightened up. Hence the intensity of the skin color will be deeper when the blood vessels are dilated, lighter when they are constricted.

The red color of the blood is intensified when the hemoglobin in its red cells is rich in oxygen. After the hemoglobin has given up part of its oxygen in the tissues, the blood takes on a bluish shade—becomes duskier. When the flow of blood through the blood vessels near the surface of the skin is rapid, there is not so much chance for the hemoglobin to give up its oxygen. Then the hue of the skin will be reddish. When the flow is slow, the amount of oxygen given up will be increased considerably. Then the hue will be slightly bluish. Hence the hue or tint of the skin at any time will depend upon the rapidity with which the blood is coursing through the cutaneous blood vessels.

Normal Temporary Changes in Skin Color. Almost everyone has had the experience of temporarily "changing color"—flushing with embarrassment or getting red from exercise, or white with rage or fear, or blue with cold. These temporary changes in skin color take place, as we have seen, when the blood vessels in the dermis dilate or contract in response to temperature changes, increased physical activity, or strong emotions.

Observant teachers will notice that there are wide temperamental variations in the rapidity with which different children change color in response to emotional stimuli. Some children normally change color very little or not at all. At the other extreme is the occasional child who changes color rapidly. He blushes at the slightest compliment or criticism, or turns pale when only mildly annoyed or frightened. Such a child may have "nervous blood vessels." He is likely to suffer from temperature changes and have frequent colds.

Abnormal Changes in Skin Color. The observant teacher quickly becomes familiar with normal skin color and tone in her children. Reference has already been made to several common changes in color, such as unnatural pallor, blueness, and a yellow hue which are associated with illness. Abnormal color is rarely the only sign of trouble. Almost always it is accompanied by other signs and symptoms, such as lassitude or drowsiness, complaints of feeling ill (malaise), circles under the eyes, sore throat, excessive underweight or overweight, and fatigue posture. The skin of a child returning to school after an illness is quite likely to look pale or sallow and flabby or doughy, both from the effects of the illness and from the confinement indoors (Plate 2).

Feverish Flushing. Besides the healthy flushing of the skin on a hot day or during vigorous exercise or as the result of embarrassment, the skin is usually flushed when any form of fever is present. In a number of acute infectious diseases—scarlet fever and measles, for example—the skin becomes red in patches. Such patchy flushing is called a rash. Rashes typical of different acute infections (see Table 7*A*) rarely appear at the onset of the disease. The teacher is much more likely to be alerted to the need for medical attention by earlier signs and symptoms than to be presented with a rash as the first warning that something is wrong.

Changes Due to Nutritional Deficiencies

The skin pictures the nutritional status of the child much better than any other organ. The skin itself is nourished by food brought to it by the blood, and it is easy to tell whether it looks healthy and well nourished. We can tell, for example, whether there is enough fat in the lowest layer of the skin to fill out the upper layers so that the skin looks smooth and the body nicely rounded with curves rather than sharp angles. Observation teaches us that the aging process is reflected in wrinkled, thin, overstretched, dry skin as opposed to the dewiness and bloom of youthful skin. Hence, the appearance in children of any of the skin conditions that are unnatural in youth—bagginess or flabbiness, wrinkles, cracks, extreme dryness, yellowish spots, for example—should make us suspect that all is not well.

The complexion is influenced by the skin's blood supply as well as the amount and distribution of pigment in the skin. A good supply of healthy blood depends upon good nutrition. One outward sign of a good blood supply is the pinkish color of the mucous-membrane lining of the mouth and eyelids, of the ears as seen against light, and of the fingernails. Whatever may be the natural color of the skin, the cheeks of healthy children will have a ruddy tinge after play outdoors.

In several nutritional deficiencies the skin or mucous membrane is involved (Table 14 and discussion in Chap. 6). When a physician suspects that a nutritional deficiency is to blame for a certain skin condition, he studies the child and his habits carefully before making his diagnosis. However, some children needing such careful study may not get to a physician unless teachers are quick to notice suspicious skin changes. A case in point is that of Anne (Plate 8). The teacher noticed a persistent cracking and slight redness at the corner of Anne's mouth. Also, Anne's general appearance and posture indicated chronic fatigue. The teacher referred Anne to the school physician for a medical examination. The physician discovered that Anne was suffering from inadequate nutrition, and more particularly from a vitamin-B deficiency.

Changes Due to Allergic Reactions

The shock tissue (see Defense Reactions of Physical Origin, in Chap. 3) in many forms of allergy is the skin or the walls of the skin capillaries (see Table 15). Any child who is subject to skin inflammations, puzzling rashes, hives, and so on, which suggest sensitivity to one or more substances, needs careful study by a physician to determine the cause or causes. Besides taking the child's history and giving a complete and thorough physical examination, the physician will perform a series of skin tests for the purpose of determining sensitivity to various suspected substances.

SKIN INFECTIONS

The outermost horny layer of the skin of every human being at any one time is covered by a vast flora and fauna in the form of microorganisms, or germs, of various families. Some are transients picked up on things touched with the bare hands or other exposed areas of the skin; others are more or less permanent residents. Some families are harmful; others are not. Some are harmful only when they are present in unusually large numbers, or when one group gangs up with another group, or when the previously established balance of one group with other groups is upset. Some germs are able to do harm only when the biologic defenses of the skin falter, or when the epidermis is broken, as in a cut or raw blister, or when its impenetrability is weakened.

The acidity of the skin is disagreeable to many bacteria and fungi which do not thrive in an acid medium. Sebum, which gives the skin its oily coat, and perspiration, which gives it its moist one, are responsible for the fact that the surface of the skin has an acid reaction. Perspiration is in itself slightly acid, and the decomposition of sebum, which is continually going on, yields acids.

Skin-dwelling microorganisms lead a precarious existence. They barely get established when the terrain that they occupy lifts, separates from the new horny layer next below, and is shed. With the constant scaling off of the epidermis, myriads of germs are removed from the skin. This process is expedited considerably whenever the skin is washed with soap and water. The rubbing and scrubbing mechanically loosens the dirty worn top sheet of the epidermis, and the warm soapy water breaks up its oily coating into tiny oil droplets and keeps them from coalescing again. The latter process is called emulsification. The oil droplets con-

Table 15. COMMON ALLERGIC SKIN REACTIONS

Type	Causative agents (allergens)	Shock tissue	Manifestations	Method of diagnosis
Contact dermatitis	1. Plant oils, such as those of poison ivy and ragweed. 2. Chemicals, dyes, and other materials found in manufactured articles or used in industrial processes. Examples are cosmetics, toilet preparations, matches, newsprint, shoe polish, insecticides, materials used in cleaning or dyeing furs, and materials used in the stuffing of mattresses, pillows, and upholstered furniture.	The epidermis. The cells of the epidermis swell and fluid forms between them when the allergen comes in contact with the skin.	Redness, vesicle formation, and itching. "Weeping" occurs as the vesicles break. Itching leads to scratching and further skin injury.	Identification of the specific offending substance, or substances, is made from the history and by means of patch tests.
Eczema (familial, or allergic dermatitis). The term "eczema" comes from a Greek	1. Usually a protein food, such as eggs, milk, cereals, etc. 2. Less commonly an inhalant, such as	The walls of the skin capillaries. The allergen is brought to the skin by the blood. Fluid seeps	Redness, papule formation, itching, and a watery discharge which tends to dry into scales and crusts. (The signs of eczema	Identification of the offending substance, or substances, is made from the history and by means

word meaning "boiling out."	pollen, animal danders, house dust, etc. Many other factors, besides specific allergens, may be involved both in predisposing a person to eczema and in perpetuating it. That is why eczema may persist even when an offending substance (or substances) has been discovered and removed.	into the tissues through the capillary walls.	are so much like those of many other skin diseases that actually no form of dermatitis is called eczema unless similar conditions have been ruled out by painstaking examinations.)	of scratch and intradermal tests.
Hives (urticaria). The term "urticaria" is derived from the Latin word for "nettle," probably because grasping a stinging nettle results in the raising on the skin of lumps or wheals similar to urticaria.	1. Usually a food, such as shellfish, pork, cheese, butter, eggs, strawberries, mushrooms, and tomatoes. 2. Certain drugs, especially opium, morphine, and penicillin. 3. Serum injections, if the person has been sensitized to the animal serum used. 4. Less frequently, an inhalant.	The walls of the skin capillaries. The allergen is brought to the skin by the blood. Fluid seeps into the skin tissues through the capillary walls.	The sudden development of wheals ranging in size from a dot to a dime or larger. The wheals may run together forming huge irregular welts. They are usually whiter than the surrounding skin, but may be pink in color, and itch, sting, or burn intensely. They usually last for only a short time—from several minutes to a few hours—and disappear as rapidly as they appeared.	Identification of the offending substance, or substances, is made from the history and by means of scratch or intradermal tests.

taining tatters of skin and the particles of dirt and germs adhering to them are held in the lather or suds and can be easily flushed off.

Although soap in itself may kill several different kinds of harmful germs, everyone seems to agree that the principal way in which soap and

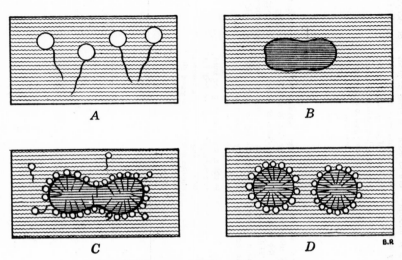

FIG. 60. The emulsifying action of soap.

A. A soap molecule. Its head dissolves in water but not in oil. Its tail dissolves in oil but not in water.
B. A drop of oil surrounded by water.
C. The tails of the soap molecules dissolve in the oil and split it into droplets.
D. The heads remain on the outside of the droplets and keep them from coalescing.

water help to fight them is by the ability of this combat team to reduce their numbers simply by loosening and rinsing away the top sheet of the epidermis upon which they have established themselves.

Staphylococcus and Streptococcus Skin Infections

Of all the germ families that pick quarrels with the skin, the staphylococci and the streptococci (see The Causative Agents of Respiratory Infections, in Chap. 5) are the most frequent offenders. Staphylococci (Greek *staphyle*, meaning "bunch of grapes," plus *coccos*, meaning "berry") are round bacteria which group themselves in clusters.

More than any other bacteria, streptococci have a tendency to act as accomplices of other pathogenic (disease-causing) microorganisms, that is, they often help, or are helped by, some other family of bacteria or viruses in setting up infection. On the skin the favorite allies of the streptococci are the staphylococci. There they live in such close harmony that whenever one is caught in the act of doing mischief, the other is almost sure to be found also. Injury to, or lowered resistance of, the skin greatly favors the development of infections caused by this infamous team.

Successful invasion and effective occupation of the skin at various levels by streptococcal-staphylococcal troops result in a great variety of skin infections. The two that are most commonly found in children of school age are impetigo contagiosa and furunculosis.

Impetigo Contagiosa. The name impetigo comes from the Latin verb meaning to "attack," and contagiosa is added to signify that impetigo is highly contagious, or "catching." Although impetigo may affect persons of any age, children seem to be most susceptible to it.

The lesions, or sores, of impetigo appear mostly on the face (especially at the corners of the mouth, nose, and ears) and on the hands. Occasionally they are widely scattered over the body. Any break in the continuity of the skin, including a scratch or an area from which adhesive tape has been removed, may become infected.

The lesions arise on highly inflamed skin areas from which a thick, sticky yellow or brown liquid oozes (Plate 11). Scabs or crusts are built up as this purulent liquid dries on the sore and on the surrounding skin. As the lesions cause intense itching, the crusts may contain blood drawn in the act of scratching to relieve the itch. The dried blood gives the crusts a black or dark brown discoloration. Eventually the epidermis of the affected areas is lifted completely off its base, as in blistering, and the crusts are shed. The naked dermis thus exposed looks painfully red and "weepy."

It is important for teachers to know that impetigo is spread not only by direct contact with the lesions but also indirectly by handling anything which the infected child has handled. "Anything" includes pencils, paper, schoolbooks, doorknobs, desk or table tops, towels, and many other objects touched or handled in the course of the school day. Whether the child evidently has a skin infection or not, he should learn to be careful about keeping exclusively for his own use all articles that he personally owns. If he has impetigo or some other infectious skin disease, he should know that it is necessary to keep his fingers away from the lesions both to prevent spread of the infection to other regions of his own body and to protect others.

In some school systems children are excluded from school until the sores have healed. Usually healing occurs after only a few days of vigorous treatment. Red spots may remain on the skin for some time after the sores have healed and the danger of infection is past. Such spots disappear gradually as the epidermis returns to its normal thickness.

A child with impetigo should be under the care of a physician. Neither the parents, the school nurse, the teacher, nor any other lay person should attempt to treat this disease without medical advice. There are several reasons for this:

1. Other more serious skin infections or serious systemic diseases may be accompanied by lesions similar to those of impetigo. The sooner such conditions are recognized by the physician, the better are the chances of successful treatment.
2. Long-lasting impetigo may sensitize the child to streptococci and staphylococci. Since these bacteria are very prevalent, heightened susceptibility to them may have serious consequences.
3. The physician is best able to teach the child and his parents what they must do to lessen the danger of spreading the infection.

In this connection it is worth saying that impetigo is a medical problem and not a socioeconomic one. No one in any status of life is immune from it, and no child who has it should be made to feel that it is disgraceful.

There are very effective ointments for the treatment of impetigo to be applied after the crusts or scabs have been cleared away. The choice of ointment and the method of removing the crusts should be left to the physician in each case. For cases that appear to be alike, directly opposing measures may be indicated.

Furuncles. Practically everyone at one time or another has had a boil. The scientific name for boil is furuncle (from the Latin *furunculus,* meaning "petty thief"). Properly speaking, every localized staphylococcal infection that starts within the tiny openings of the sweat gland ducts or sebaceous gland ducts is a furuncle. Names vary, however, according to the size or locality of the furuncle. A boil on the eyelid margins, for example, is called a sty (see Sties, in Chap. 8); a very small furuncle is usually called a pimple; a large and extensive one, including several hair follicles, is called a carbuncle (from the Latin *carbunculus,* meaning "little coal"). Since the ducts of most sebaceous glands drain into the hair follicles, boils occur most commonly on hairy areas of the skin.

A furuncle, be it lowly pimple or arrogant carbuncle, is an excellent example of one of the body's most important and interesting defense mechanisms. As soon as boil-producing staphylococci (frequently accompanied by streptococci) establish a beachhead in a pore or hair follicle opening or in a practically invisible break in the skin, two things happen almost simultaneously. Cells in the neighborhood start multiplying to wall off the theater of operations from the rest of the body, and shock troops consisting of great numbers of white blood cells, or phagocytes, are rushed into the area by the blood.

The redness and tenderness of the spot in the skin where a boil is forming is explained by the rush of blood to that spot and by the pressure of the white cells, the extra blood, and the rapidly multiplying bacteria against the delicate nerve endings in the dermis. The pus which forms as the boil "comes to a head" is made up of phagocytes that have "mopped up" the bacteria by engulfing them and have thereby lost their lives on the field of battle. The liquefaction of the dead phagocytes softens up the area of operations and the overlying layer of skin. Eventually the skin breaks and lets out the pus. As soon as this occurs, pain is relieved by the removal of pressure. Eventually the core of the boil, consisting of the protective wall and the closely packed white cells and bacteria not yet dissolved, is discharged or slowly absorbed.

The drama of phagocytosis, if successfully confined to one small walled-off theater in the skin, saves the body as a whole from bacterial invasion. But if the protective wall is broken down and the bacteria escape into neighboring tissues, or into the lymph and blood streams, a very serious infection—even septicemia, or blood poisoning—may be the outcome. Squeezing or pinching a boil to evacuate the pus, or amateur attempts to open it, may very well break down the wall. That is why children should learn that "hands off" is the only safe policy in dealing with any boil, small or large.

Some individuals seem to be especially susceptible to boils. Why this should be so is not always clear. In some cases the skin may harbor a particularly tough family of staphylococci; in others, the chemical reaction of the skin itself may favor the multiplication of the bacteria responsible. Also several different systemic diseases may be accompanied by outcroppings of boils.

Any child who has one boil after another or crops of boils should certainly have a complete medical check-up. The treatment of the boil itself should be carried out by a physician. The use of the sulfas and penicillin or other antibiotics has largely displaced the slow, painful, and sometimes hazardous treatments of the past. However, the drug must be given properly—that is, in the proper doses, by the proper method, and at the proper times. Otherwise, the patient may have a serious reaction, or the bacteria may build up resistance against the drug.

Infectious Dandruff. There is one form of dandruff that is infectious, although this form is not so common as advertisers of antiseptic hair lotions would have us believe. It is caused by an infection of the sebaceous glands of the scalp. The discharge from the infected glands collects in yellowish, greasy, thick scales which adhere rather closely to the scalp.

When the scales become loosened and fall off, the skin beneath looks red and sore. Usually there is considerable itching. This form of dandruff, if allowed to continue, results in gradual thinning of the hair and possibly even in baldness. It is spread by hats, combs and brushes, and unsterilized barbershop or beauty-parlor instruments.

Ringworm Infections

Ringworm is a widespread communicable disease of the skin caused by microscopic plant parasites called fungi. There are several different types of these fungi, some of which usually affect only human beings (the human types) whereas others affect both human beings and animals (the animal types). Ringworm caused by any one of the animal types usually gives little trouble, as it responds very well to local treatment with the proper ointment. Human-type infections are not so easy to control.

Different types of ringworm fungus prefer to live on different areas of the skin. The diseases they produce are named according to the skin areas on which they usually grow, for example, ringworm of the general surface of the body, ringworm of the scalp, and ringworm of the feet (athlete's foot).

Many skin conditions resemble ringworm and are confused with it. For that reason a teacher should not state that a child has ringworm even though she strongly suspects it. The diagnosis in each case should be left to the physician. Prompt referral to a physician of children who have skin sores of any description will help greatly in checking the spread of ringworm as well as other skin infections.

Ringworm of the General Body Surface. The infection begins as a rounded, sharply limited, slightly elevated, red patch on the skin. It creeps out from its center in concentric circles. As the patch tends to heal in the center, its circumference has the appearance of a reddish ring, thus giving the disease its name.

The fungus causing the infection is spread from one person to another by direct skin-to-skin contact and indirectly by clothing and by any surface on which scales from the lesions, or sores, have been shed. Sometimes children catch animal-type ringworm from infected cats or other pets.

Ringworm of the Feet. Cases of fungus infection of the feet are not likely to be observed directly by the teacher. However, a child may tell the teacher of symptoms suggestive of this infection before medical attention has been obtained. Also, the health education of all children should include precautions to be taken in preventing it and the importance of medical care in its treatment.

Because of popular advertising, it is taken for granted by the average American that any red, irritated, itching, skin lesions on the feet, especially if they are between the toes, are "athlete's foot." However, many skin conditions popularly regarded as athlete's foot are not caused by a fungus, but are actually due to any one of a variety of other causes. Medicines advertised, or recommended by friends, as effective in the treatment of so-called "athlete's foot" may irritate the skin of some individuals and prolong the condition rather than cure it. Hence, any abnormal condition of the skin of the feet should be seen by a physician for diagnosis and treatment.

True ringworm of the feet is easy to acquire and difficult to get rid of, because the type of fungus causing it is present everywhere and starts growing whenever conditions are favorable. It grows best when it is supplied with darkness, moisture, warmth, and food. Shoes that completely cover the foot provide the first three conditions, and the macerated dead skin between the toes and the moist leather of leather shoes provide the food. It has been noted that athlete's foot is relatively uncommon among girls and women who wear open-toed shoes.

Keeping the feet clean and dry helps to eliminate some of the conditions which favor fungus growth between the toes. The skin between the toes should always be dried *thoroughly* after bathing and after getting the feet wet in any other way. Talcum powder sprinkled between the toes helps to dry these areas and to keep them dry. Changing into clean socks or stockings every morning and giving shoes a good airing after each wearing will also help.

Walking barefoot on wet or damp floors or pavements, where it is customary for many persons to go barefoot, is a wide-open invitation to infection. For that reason children should learn to protect their feet with bathing slippers or sandals immediately after taking off their ordinary footwear in the locker rooms or dressing rooms of bathing pools, gymnasium showers, and the like.

Conditions of the skin between the toes of which a person with an early ringworm infection of the feet may complain are itching and slight redness, slight scaling, and perhaps some cracking. More severe cases are characterized by intense itching, deep fissures or cracks, and blisters that weep or ooze moisture when broken. Raw red places are left as the blisters dry up and scale off. Any child who reports troubles of this kind should be referred to the physician. If the diagnosis is ringworm of the feet, the teacher should be given any information that will help her to supervise the child properly and to guard others from the infection.

Ringworm of the Scalp. Most epidemics of ringworm of the scalp among school children are caused by a human-type fungus (*Microsporum audouini*). This type of infection is rare after puberty. The theory has been advanced that the increased activity of the sebaceous glands associated with adolescence has some power to kill the fungus responsible. All children up to fifteen years of age are susceptible to human-type infection. There is no immunity after cure; hence reinfection is common.

Adults as well as children are susceptible to the animal-type fungus (*Microsporum lanosum*), which is spread by contact with the lesions, or hairs from the lesions, of cats and dogs. Ringworm of the scalp caused by animal-type fungi responds much more readily to treatment than do infections caused by the human type.

The fungus of human-type ringworm of the scalp invades the hair and the hair follicle, multiplies, and travels down the walls of the follicle and the hair root to the point where the hair bulb begins. The hair breaks off at its weakest point, which is just above the surface of the scalp. As long as the bottom end of the infected hair remains in its follicle the infection goes on. However, the hair papilla, which is responsible for the reproduction of new hair, does not become involved.

A typical fully developed patch of ringworm of the scalp in the majority of cases is rounded, grayish, somewhat scaly, and slightly but often imperceptibly elevated (see Plate 12). It is covered with the stubs of broken-off hairs. In some cases the patch may have a puffed or goose-flesh or plucked-fowl appearance.

The treatment usually recommended for human-type infections consists in getting the infected hairs completely out en masse, either by plucking them out by the roots (manual epilation) or by treating them with x-rays so that they fall out by the roots (x-ray epilation), followed by applications of a fungus-killing medicine (fungicide) to the scalp over a period of weeks. In a certain proportion of cases the use of a fungicide alone may work a cure.

X-ray epilation makes the child's hair fall out entirely. He will be bald temporarily, but new hair will begin to grow back in about a month if the treatment is given properly. Because of the great danger that the reproductive portion of the hair may be destroyed by inexpert treatment, x-ray epilation, when advised, must be done only by, or under the supervision of, an experienced dermatologist.

The spread of ringworm infection to other parts of the scalp is easily brought about. Thousands of fungi and their spores are present on even the smallest piece of hair that breaks off. Broken-off hairs falling on new regions of the scalp or skin start other areas of infection. The fungi and their spores are readily transmitted from one child to another by direct contact during play; by the interchange of caps, mufflers, combs, and brushes; by unsterilized barbershop instruments; and by the backs of seats in movie theaters, public conveyances, classrooms, and so on, which have been previously used by infected youngsters.

The presence of ringworm of the scalp can seldom be detected in its early stages without the use of a special type of lamp called "Wood's light." The light from this lamp, which was invented by Robert William Wood, an American physicist, is obtained by passing ultraviolet light rays through a special glass filter. The infected hairs of a child with ringworm of the scalp fluoresce, or glow, in a characteristic manner when the scalp is exposed to the filtered ultraviolet light in a darkened room.

When human-type ringworm appears in a community it almost always spreads rapidly and is extremely difficult to check. Specific methods of control usually recommended are as follows:

1. *Detection of cases.* Authorities agree that it is very important for teachers, school nurses, and parents to be familiar with the appearance of ringworm of the scalp, so that the first case, or cases, can be spotted in time to put into operation the drastic measures required to prevent its spread. Upon the discovery of a case of ringworm of the scalp, home, school, and other contacts of the infected child should be inspected and, in addition, examined under a Wood's light at regular intervals until 1 month after the last case is detected. If the condition is found to exist in two or more classrooms in a school or in more than 2 per cent of the children in a single classroom, the entire population of the school under fifteen years of age should be screened periodically by means of suitably filtered ultraviolet light. A Wood's light may be acquired by the school authorities or by the health department. The school nurse may be trained in the technique of using it to examine the scalp.

2. *Preventive measures.* The exclusion of infected children from school is not considered to be practical, as recovery in many cases may require months. Such children should be under medical treatment, however, with periodic visits to a physician or clinic. The schools in some epidemic areas provide separate isolated classrooms for infected children. Young children in epidemic areas should be surveyed by a Wood's light before entering school. Special measures during epidemic outbreaks include the education of parents and children and the enlistment of the services of doctors and nurses for diagnosis.[1]

3. *Supervision of children.* Each infected child should wear at all times a cotton stocking cap, or other type of tight-fitting head covering, which must be sterilized by boiling after each wearing. The public health authorities may advise the wearing of such caps by

[1] "Control of Communicable Diseases in Man," American Public Health Association, 8th ed., pp. 152–153, New York, 1955.

all children under fifteen (infected and noninfected alike) when playing with others, and while at school, in the movies, on public conveyances, in children's clinics, and so on.

The nurses serving the school and, when appropriate, the teachers should help to educate the parents regarding the ways in which this highly communicable disease is spread and the measures for its control. Cleanliness of the scalp and hair is very important. Clippers should not be used on the hair in barbershops, because these instruments are difficult to sterilize.

Parents of infected children should know that the treatment takes a long time and must not be discontinued until the child is pronounced cured. After cure, precautions must still be taken to prevent reinfection.

SKIN INFESTATIONS

Infestation means an invasion of the surface of the body with animal parasites which are not microscopically small and which produce mechanical effects. It differs from the term infection, which is reserved for an invasion of microscopically small plant or animal parasites (germs, microbes, or microorganisms) which produce chemical and toxic effects within the body. Itch mites and head lice are responsible for the skin infestations most often found in American school children.

Mites

Long before medical scientists made the acquaintance of microscopic skin-dwellers, practically everyone was familiar with a family of living skin irritants which affected high and low alike until modern facilities for cleanliness and modern methods of treatment became generally available. These barely visible, less than pinhead-sized parasites are the itch mites which cause scabies (Latin for "itch").

Mites are the smallest members of one of the great divisions of the animal kingdom, the Arthropoda. They belong specifically to the order *Acarina* which includes both ticks and mites. The itch mite has an important place in medical history. It was first discovered by Avenzoar, a great Jewish physician of the twelfth century; rediscovered in 1687 by Cosimo Bonomo, an Italian physician; and finally and permanently connected with the itch in the first half of the nineteenth century.

Scabies. Infestation with the itch mite occurs during a period of close bodily contact with already infested persons or with their clothing or bedding. The female itch mite burrows molelike in the skin, producing a minute, slightly elevated, black trail. These burrows are located most commonly on the inner sides and webs of the fingers, the wrists and back of the hands, the armpits, the abdomen, and the inner sides of the thighs. Scratching inflames the infested areas and may produce signs mistaken for those of eczema, poison ivy, "stomach rash," or almost any other form of dermatitis.

The female mite burrows in the horny layer of the epidermis, immediately starts laying her eggs there, and dies after 6 or 7 weeks. Baby mites hatch out of the eggs in 3 to 5 days and excavate their way into the sides or floor of the burrow. When grown up they crawl over the skin, and the females make other small burrows. Itching is caused by the irritation of stout spines or bristles on each of the eight legs of these parasites, and in addition, by a highly irritating fluid released from their skin.

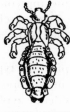   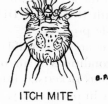

HEAD LOUSE   ITCH MITE

FIG. 61. The two chief offenders in skin infestations (highly magnified).

The itching when it starts is so intense as to be almost unbearable, especially at night. Scratching, scratch marks, or raw red patches in the areas where the burrows are most commonly located should suggest the possibility of scabies. Casual diagnosis of scabies, however, is impossible because there are probably a thousand odd causes of itching and certainly the itch mite is not always the culprit. In dealing with children found by a physician to be infested with the itch mite, the safest procedure is to exclude them from school until disinfested. Several satisfactory medicines for external application make the cure of scabies relatively easy when carried out faithfully under medical supervision.

Harvest-mite Infestations. Close relatives of the itch mite are the harvest mites. Probably the best known harvest mite is the chigger (chigo, chigre, jigger), which is found in the Southern United States. Other common types are the harvest bug and the red bug. Harvest mites burrow into the skin and cause itching as itch mites do, but their reproductive cycle is not so efficient and they tend to die out rather promptly. Their disappearance is hastened by medical treatment. A history of being in harvest fields or in underbrush during the season in which harvest mites are prevalent in a locality will help the physician to make a diagnosis of harvest-mite infestation in children suffering from it.

Lice

The Latin name for louse is *pediculus*. Hence, the medical term for infestation with lice is pediculosis. There are three kinds of lice for which man is the natural host—body lice, head lice, and pubic lice (crabs). Of the three, head lice are by far the most common in American school children.

Body Lice. Body lice really should be called clothing lice, because they live and lay their eggs in the seams of clothing and come out on the skin only when they want a meal of blood. Like other skin parasites, they cause intense itching and scratching which often lead to a dermatitis, or skin inflammation, of one kind or another. The possibility of body lice infestation is another good reason for never ignoring complaints of itching and the act of scratching in school children. Fortunately, treating clothing with 10 per cent DDT powder now makes delousing a comparatively simple procedure.

Body lice are responsible for the spread of epidemic typhus fever wherever conditions favor outbreaks of the virulent European type of this dangerous rickettsial infection. Fortunately, epidemic typhus is now nonexistent in our country.

Head Lice. Head lice are rarely involved in the spread of communicable disease from one person to another. However, they are exceedingly unpleasant, if not dangerous, guests and by their bites may cause considerable irritation of the scalp. Also, as a result of scratching the head the germs responsible for folliculitis of the long hairs (a form of impetigo) and carbuncles may gain a foothold.

Head lice usually stay on the head, but they may wander all over the body, infecting other hairy parts. The nits, or lice eggs, are seen as tiny glistening lumps connected rather firmly to the hair a short distance from the scalp. The nits hatch in about ten days.

One child harboring head lice may be responsible for the infestation of large numbers of his schoolmates unless he is discovered and speedily disinfested. Children literally "put their heads together" so often in school and at play; so freely borrow and lend their combs, brushes, caps or hats, mufflers, coats or sweaters; and so frequently hang their outdoor clothing cheek by jowl in cloakrooms, that there is little wonder that head lice have always been one of the most vexatious school health problems.

One of the chief objectives of formal morning inspections was, and in some schools still is, the discovery of children with head lice. However, an effective search involves the use of a fine-tooth comb and, if this seems advisable, should be done by the school nurse or teacher in privacy, or at home by the parents, to avoid embarrassment for the child. Persistent scratching of the head should be a signal for this thorough inspection. In boys, especially, the nits may sometimes be seen on the hair behind the ears.

The insecticide DDT makes it much easier than formerly to get rid of lice. The preparation usually recommended by physicians is 10 per cent DDT dusting powder. This powder is perfectly safe when dusted into hair, garments, or on the skin. It may be applied with an ordinary shaker-type container. After the hair has been dusted, the head should be kept covered for several hours with a towel or cap. The hair should then be combed with a fine-tooth comb. After a week has passed, without washing the hair, the dusting should be repeated to destroy lice which have hatched from nits in the meantime. The parents of a child who has lice should be given instructions for applying DDT powder.

Like impetigo and scabies, pediculosis has often been looked upon as a disgrace. Actually it is a small part of the bitter that goes with the sweet of communal living.

SKIN INJURIES

"Youth," as Robert Louis Stevenson remarked, "is wholly experimental." And as youngsters, especially boys, are more venturesome as well as less experienced than their elders, their skins get harder usage and more frequent exposure to many different forms of abuse—cuts, bruises, scratches, burns, bumps, abrasions, blisters, and so on.

In schools where a nurse is available, it is usually her duty to care for all minor skin injuries. For major wounds such as wounds with severe bleeding, puncture wounds, and severe or extensive burns, a physician should, of course, be consulted immediately.

In schools where a nurse is not at hand to deal with minor mishaps to the skin, the teacher should be prepared to do the simple things necessary to bring relief and prevent infection. As surgeons found out long before the era of asepsis, any break in the skin, even as small as a pinprick, quite literally may be a "door open to death."

First-aid Supplies

Practically everyone associated with children will have to deal, at one time or another, with skinned knees, little cuts and scratches, blisters, and so on. Supplies to have on hand for these injuries are

Sterile gauze in sealed packages
A roll of ½-inch adhesive tape

A number of 1-inch gauze compresses on adhesive tape in individual
  packages
A mild skin antiseptic (for example, 2 per cent iodine in individual
  ampules)
A small package of sterile cotton
A tube of petrolatum
A box of baking soda
A pair of scissors
Soap

Abrasions, Cuts, and Scratches

First wash your own hands with soap and water. Using pieces of sterile
gauze or cotton, cleanse the surrounding skin with soap and water. Swab
away from the edges of the wound so as not to wash more dirt into it.
Use a fresh piece of gauze or cotton for each swabbing. If loose dirt is
in an abrasion, it may be flushed out under a running water tap. Next,
paint the wound with a mild skin antiseptic. When it is dry, cover it
with a sterile gauze compress and fasten with adhesive. In case of a deep
or lacerated cut or an abrasion in which dirt or gravel is ground into the
flesh, the child should see a physician for the thorough cleansing of the
wound and other measures required to prevent infection.

Tetanus. Any deep wound with a narrow or sealed opening or any
deep lacerated wound in which chips of glass, wood splinters, or grains
of dirt have become embedded carries with it the danger of tetanus, or
lockjaw. This disease is caused by a toxin produced by bacilli which
multiply rapidly in the absence of oxygen. Favorable conditions for the
growth of tetanus bacilli occur when these organisms are driven into the
tissues where they are sealed away from the air.

Tetanus bacilli are present in the feces of some of the domestic animals. They are common inhabitants of the superficial layers of the soil
in many localities, especially in the earth of cultivated and manured
fields and gardens. They exist in the soil as spores developed by the
bacilli as a protection from deleterious influences. Tetanus spores may
remain alive and virulent for many years.

Tetanus toxin, produced by the bacilli living and growing within the
tissues, has an affinity for the central nervous system. Having reached
there, it exerts an action that produces spasmodic (tetanic) contractions
of the muscles. In the acute form of tetanus, the incubation period
elapsing between the time of infection and the development of the first
symptoms may be only 3 to 4 days or may be 10 to 14 days; most commonly it is about 7 days. In the so-called chronic form the incubation
period may be more than a month.

To counteract, or neutralize, the toxin, the body develops antitoxin. Tetanus antitoxin produced by immunizing horses (or cows) is used in treatment to supplement the antitoxin already being produced in the body of a person sick with tetanus. It is also used in the passive immunization (see Immunization, in Chap. 3) of persons with wounds carrying the danger of tetanus. The most effective safeguard, however, is the active immunization of individuals most likely to be exposed to infection with tetanus bacilli. As children in the rough-and-tumble stage are in this category, it is considered advisable to begin the active immunization of all children with tetanus toxoid in babyhood (see Table 4, Immunization Timetable, in Chap. 3).

Animal Bites

A child bitten by a dog or some other warm-blooded animal should have medical attention promptly because of the possibility that the biting animal has rabies.

Rabies is primarily a disease of warm-blooded carnivorous animals (chiefly dogs, but also cats, foxes, coyotes, and similar animals). It is caused by a virus that is found in the saliva, salivary glands, and central nervous system of the infected animal. When a person is bitten by a rabid animal, virus-bearing saliva enters the body through the break in the skin. The virus appears to take the same route as tetanus toxin along the nerve trunks to the spinal cord and brain. Bites on surfaces covered by clothing are the least dangerous, and bites on the head, arms, and hands are the most dangerous.

The incubation period is variable, depending upon the severity of the bite and its location; it usually ranges from 2 to 6 weeks, but may be prolonged to 6 months or more. The development of rabies *after* exposure through a break in the skin to the saliva of a rabid dog, or other rabid animal, or any animal suspected of being rabid, may be prevented by the prompt institution of prophylactic antirabic vaccination. Louis Pasteur was the first to prepare and use antirabic vaccine successfully to protect both dogs and human beings (1885) from rabies after exposure.

First-aid treatment of animal bite consists in cleansing the wound thoroughly with soap under running water to remove the animal's saliva. Medical aid must then be sought promptly so that the required further treatment of the wound may be given and an investigation made to determine whether antirabic vaccination should be given. This preventive treatment should be started in every doubtful case. It may be discontinued if the biting dog is well at the end of the prescribed period of observation, usually 10 days.

Blisters and Small Burns

Unless there is danger that a blister may be accidentally ruptured, it is best to leave it alone until it dries. The intact horny layer of epidermis is the best protection from infection while a new horny layer is being manufactured to take its place.

If a blister caused by pinching or friction is located where it is extremely likely to break (on the heel, for example), gently cleanse the area around it with soap and water, apply a small amount of mild skin antiseptic, and cover the blister with a sterile gauze compress fastened with adhesive. This will lessen the danger of infection if the blister should rupture.

For small minor burns characterized by reddened unbroken skin or surface blisters, apply a paste of baking soda and water or sterile petrolatum and cover the area with a sterile gauze dressing. This will relieve pain and lessen the danger of infection if the blisters should rupture. For severe burns—deep burns and all extensive burns—get medical aid as quickly as possible. Emergency treatment should be given by someone trained in first-aid procedures.

Bruises

A bruise is caused by a fall or blow which ruptures the capillaries in the dermis without breaking the epidermis. The bruised area first looks red and swollen because the blood has oozed into the tissues. It becomes discolored—"black and blue" and later "green and yellow"—as the blood clots and is eventually absorbed. To relieve the pain and swelling of a bruise, apply cloths wrung out in cold water. If the blow or fall that caused the bruise was severe, a physician should examine the child.

Frostbite

The color of the flesh in a frostbitten area is a peculiar waxy white because blood cannot circulate in the frozen blood vessels. The skin is numb and feels cold to the touch. The frozen part must be handled gently in order to prevent further injury. It should be warmed as rapidly as possible by placing it in lukewarm but *not hot* water or by wrapping it in warm blankets. Do not expose the frozen part to heat from a stove, hot-water bottle, or heat lamp. Do not rub it, as frozen tissues are easily bruised or torn, with the result that gangrene may develop. After thawing occurs in frozen fingers or toes, the child should be encouraged to exercise them.

Insect Bites and Stings

The bites of most insects are not dangerous as a rule, but often cause swelling and pain or itching. To relieve the discomfort of bee, hornet, wasp, yellow-jacket, and mosquito bites, cover the bite with a thick paste of baking soda and water.

DO YOU KNOW?

1. If you were exploring the skin from the top downward, in which layer should you expect to find keratin? papillae? sweat glands? hair bulbs? sebaceous glands? the topmost layer of living cells? fat cells? blood vessels and nerves? pigment? pores?
2. What would you say to a child who asked you

   a. Where do freckles come from?
   b. Why can't I have curly hair like Jane's?
   c. What makes me break out in goose pimples when I'm cold?
   d. Why do I get red and sweaty after playing hard?
   e. What makes my hands get rough in cold weather?

3. From the three structures named after each of the words given in the list below choose the one you associate with it.

   a. Wheals: sweat glands, capillaries, arterioles
   b. Blackheads: pores, papillae, fat-gland ducts
   c. Acne: pilosebaceous glands, hair bulbs, venules
   d. Dandruff: hair follicles, horny layer of epidermis, germinative layer of epidermis

4. In each of the following groupings of diseases or conditions there is one that does not belong with the group. Select the one that is out of place and tell why.

   a. Warts, psoriasis, athlete's foot
   b. Impetigo, ringworm of scalp, furunculosis
   c. Scabies, acne, pediculosis
   d. Epidemic typhus, rabies, tetanus
   e. Eczema, hives, comedones

5. Tell the difference between

   a. Infection and infestation
   b. Dermis and epidermis
   c. Cutaneous and subcutaneous
   d. Dermatologist and beauty specialist

SUGGESTED ACTIVITIES

1. Measure the amount of space that is devoted in one month's issue of several popular magazines to advertisements of products (soaps, cold creams, lotions, cosmetics, dentifrices, etc.) sold for the care of skin, hair, nails, and teeth. Discuss in class the motivating value of the emphasis placed on an attractive personal appearance in helping young people to cultivate cleanliness and good grooming.

2. Plan demonstrations of hand washing, shampooing, and manicuring which would be suitable as a class activity for children in an elementary grade. If possible, have the children in your class in laboratory or practice school put on these demonstrations.

3. Ask the nurse serving the practice or laboratory school to stage nurse-teacher and nurse-parent interviews before the class on a child with impetigo, a child with pediculosis, and a child with ringworm of the scalp. Students may play the part of teacher and parents.

4. Discuss ways in which you would help a child who

   a. Has adolescent acne
   b. Has chapped hands in cold weather
   c. Has excessively oily skin and hair
   d. Complains of itching all over in winter
   e. Is being taunted for having head lice
   f. Has B.O.
   g. Is worried about a noticeable skin blemish

5. Discuss the scientific reasons (as opposed to social reasons) for the admonition: "Always wash your hands with soap and warm water before eating or preparing food and after using the toilet."

SELECTED REFERENCES

AMERICAN MEDICAL ASSOCIATION: *Wonder Stories of the Human Machine: The Body Finish (Skin)*, Chicago, 1948. (Pamphlet 9 in a series explaining how the principal organs of the body work.)

BEHRMAN, HOWARD T., and OSCAR L. LEVIN: *Your Skin and Its Care*, New York, Emerson Books, Inc., 1948.

LEVIN, OSCAR L., and HOWARD T. BEHRMAN: *Your Hair and Its Care*, New York, Emerson Books, Inc., 1945.

Chapter 8 STOP! LOOK AND LISTEN

What "Meets the Eye" in Observing Eyes
Seeing Right and Seeing Wrong
Vision Testing
Observations about the Ears
Hearing Right and Hearing Wrong
Hearing Testing

WHAT "MEETS THE EYE" IN OBSERVING EYES

Looking at her own eyes in a mirror will give the teacher a good idea of what she can observe in looking at the eyes of children. All that can be seen of the eye itself is the front curve of the eyeball. The normal eyeball is a small globe about an inch in diameter and slightly longer from front to back than from side to side, which fits snugly into a depression of the skull called the orbit, or eye socket. The size of a person's eyes—large, small, or medium—depends not upon the size of the eyeballs, which is about the same in everyone, but rather upon the length of the slit between the edges of the eyelids.

The eye is well protected in its bony socket. The cheekbone and forehead guard it against blows, and through reflex action the eyelids snap shut involuntarily when anything comes toward the eye. The eyelashes filter dust and foreign bodies from the air, and the eyebrows keep perspiration from running into the eyes from the forehead.

The Eyelids and the Skin below the Eyes

The eyelids are two movable folds of skin from the margins of which the eyelashes spring. Both the eyelashes and the margins of the eyelids are kept oiled with secretions from fat glands.

Eyelids cover the eyes in sleep and during the daytime protect them from external injury, foreign bodies, undue exposure, and bright lights. They also serve to spread over the surface of the eyeball the tears and other lubricating secretions that keep it moist and clean.

The Sandman. Waking up with tiny, gritty particles in the corners of the eyes is such a common experience for practically all children that it gave rise to the legend of the sandman who sprinkles children's eyes

with sand to put them to sleep. What really happens is that during
sleep some of the fluid normally present in the eyes dries on the eyelid
margins at the inner corners of the eyes. This dried secretion has the
appearance of yellow or greenish specks. Its presence in a child's eyes
in school usually means that the child either has not washed his face
that morning or has been careless about washing it.

Inflammation of the Eyelid Margins. Some children may have persistent redness and swelling of the eyelid margins, accompanied by the
appearance of scaly yellow crusts around the eyelashes. This may become
a chronic condition, especially in children suffering from a nutritional
deficiency (Table 14, in Chap. 6) or living in insanitary surroundings.

Children with inflammation of the eyelid margins (blepharitis marginalis) will probably say that their lids are stuck together when they
wake up in the morning. They may also say that their eyes itch or burn
or feel sore, that the light hurts their eyes, and that their eyes feel tired
after a period of reading or other close eye work. The teacher may
notice that such children frequently rub their eyes during the day.

If the condition is allowed to continue, it may result in loss of eyelashes or in drooping eyelids caused by thickening of the eyelid margins.
Hence early medical attention is important both for preventing dis-
figurement and for determining and removing the underlying cause or
causes of the condition.

Sties. A sty is an infection of one or more of the glands connected with
the roots of the eyelashes. The sign of a beginning sty is a red swelling
at the margin of the lid accompanied by pain and tenderness. Soon pus
gathers to form a yellow spot at the summit of the red swelling. Shortly
after the sty has come to a head, it breaks and the pus runs out. The
application of hot compresses hastens the gathering and evacuation of
the pus. Amateur attempts to prick open a sty with an instrument or to
squeeze it may result in a dangerous infection.

The recurrence of one sty after another at frequent intervals means
that medical attention is needed. Sties often appear in crops in children
whose general health is poor or who are suffering from eye fatigue (see
further on). A child with any eye difficulty is likely to rub his eyes
frequently and may thus infect the eyelid margins with germs from his
fingers.

Black Eye. The eyelids are easily bruised by blows on account of the
looseness of their subcutaneous connective tissue. The common name
for bruised eyelids is "black eye." The characteristic discoloration, which
is due to the escape of blood into the tissues from ruptured capillaries,
may not appear for several days after the injury. Usually it is of no

importance and clears up in one or two weeks. However, a certain number of black eyes are associated with damage to the skull or eyeball. To be on the safe side all black eyes should be examined by a physician. Cold compresses applied immediately after the injury will help to lessen the subcutaneous bleeding.

Circles under the Eyes. Of themselves, circles under the eyes have no significance. In some children, however, fatigue may produce changes in the skin below the eyes which result in the formation of shadows. These shadows may be most noticeable in children with fair complexion. Loss of skin tension in this region may be the cause in some cases; in others an actual change in skin color occurs. This change may be due to congestion in the small blood vessels close to the surface of the skin.

Shadowy circles under the eyes are most likely to be observed at the end of the day. When seen occasionally they are of no particular significance other than to suggest temporary fatigue. Children who have persistent circles under the eyes combined with evidences of chronic fatigue should have medical attention. Among the possible causes of fatigue are increased nervous tension at home or in school, loss of sleep, poor nutrition, or a beginning illness.

Puffy Lids. This condition may be seen in some children, especially in the morning, when it is usually due to congestion in the nose. It may have no particular significance if seen occasionally. But if this sign appears in a child who has never shown it before, together with other signs, such as pallor, sudden increase in weight, and a tendency to tire easily, he should be referred to the nurse or physician.

The Conjunctiva and Tear Glands

The inner surface of the eyelids is covered with a delicate membrane called the conjunctiva. At the upper edge of each upper eyelid and at the lower edge of each lower eyelid the membrane folds over to pass from the inner surfaces of the lids onto the front of the eyeball, which it completely covers. When the lids move up and down, the two surfaces of the membrane slide over each other. The surfaces are kept lubricated by a small amount of tear fluid.

Tears. It is not necessary to weep to observe that the eyes are always kept comfortably moist by tears. Tears consist of a slightly salty fluid which is manufactured and secreted by small almond-shaped glands (lacrimal glands) located in the outer angle of each eye socket. The tears are piped from these glands to the eyeballs, across which they are conveyed by winking into the minute openings of ducts, or tubes, that drain into the nose. If it were not for the constant washing of the surfaces of the conjunctiva by the tears, this delicate covering membrane would soon become dry and inflamed and the eye would eventually be destroyed (see Vitamin A, in Chap. 6).

"Running" Eyes. Emotions that arouse the impulse to weep and irritations of the eyes cause a flood of tears which the drains are too small to handle. Hence the tears overflow their banks and roll down the cheeks. "Watery," "weepy" eyes are a common occurrence in inflammations of the eyes due to mechanical irritations such as wind, smoke, bright sunlight, or foreign bodies in the eye.

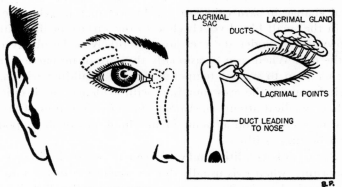

FIG. 62. Where tears come from.

Redness of the eyes and puffiness of the eyelids, accompanied by watering of the eyes and sneezing, are usually associated with the onset of communicable diseases affecting the upper respiratory tract, especially measles and the common cold (see Plate 7). The communication between the nose and the eyes by means of the tear ducts explains the frequent occurrences of eye symptoms and disturbances as a result of infections that involve the upper respiratory tract.

Bloodshot Eyes. In weeping or in irritations of the eyes, the normally colorless whites of the eyes become streaked with red wavy lines and the normally pale pink lining of the eyelids becomes red and swollen. The eyes are then said to be "bloodshot" or inflamed. This bloodshot appearance is caused by a temporary increase in the blood supply of the conjunctiva.

Sometimes after whooping cough or after bouts of violent sneezing one or two red spots may appear in the white of the eye. Such a spot is caused by the rupture of a small blood vessel in the conjunctiva as a result of the strain of coughing or sneezing. It is usually of no importance and will clear up gradually in a week or 10 days.

Exposure to wind, strong sunlight, smoke, dirt, and so on may make the eyes look bloodshot, but this effect usually clears up within 24 hours. In eye fatigue the conjunctiva, as well as the eyelid margins, may look inflamed, largely because the child is likely to irritate the conjunctiva by constant rubbing.

Conjunctivitis. Conjunctivitis, or inflammation of the conjunctiva, may have any one of a number of causes including mechanical irritation, an infection, a nutritional deficiency, or an allergic reaction.

Acute conjunctivits caused by the infection of the eyes themselves with one or more of a variety of germs is popularly called "pinkeye." It may affect only one eye, but usually both are involved. In pinkeye the conjunctiva is red, swollen, and watery, and later there is a copious discharge of pus. As the eyes itch and smart in pinkeye, it is difficult for the child to keep from rubbing them. Pinkeye is very contagious and may occur in epidemic form in school, especially during the spring and fall. It is caught by touching the eyes with fingers, towels, washcloths, handkerchiefs, in short, with anything soiled with discharges from the eyes of persons suffering from the infection.

It is important for a doctor to see all children who show signs of persistent or acute inflammations of the conjunctiva. Only a physician can select the right cause from several possible ones and prescribe the proper treatment or, if necessary, refer the child to a specialist in the care of the eyes.

The Wall of the Eyeball

The wall of the eyeball is built up of three layers or coats—an outer coat, a middle coat, and an inner coat.

The White of the Eye. The tough outer coat of the eyeball is called the sclera or "white" of the eye. The sclera is tough, opaque, and supplied with very few blood vessels. Its functions are to keep the eyeball in shape and to protect the delicate structures within. The sclera is comparatively thin in childhood. Hence the "whites" of a child's eyes are often bluish white in color, owing to the showing through of the dark pigment of the middle coat of the eyeball. A yellowish tinge is not normal, however, and should be called to the attention of the physician or nurse.

The Window of the Eye. Looking closely at the eyes, the observer sees a slightly bulging, clear, colorless disk covering the colored disk in the center of the white of each eye as a watch crystal covers the dial of a watch. This is the cornea, or "window" of the eye. It is the transparent part of the sclerotic, or outer coat, and its function is the same as that of a window in a house, that is, to let in light. There are no blood vessels in the cornea, but it is richly supplied with nerves, as anyone knows who has ever had it hit by a speck of dirt. Any cloudiness or opaque spots in the cornea calls for immediate attention. If the surface of the cornea is injured in any way a scar will form which, if large and in the line of vision, will cause blindness.

Among the possible causes of keratitis, or inflammation of the cornea, are nutritional deficiency (Table 14, in Chap. 6), infection, and allergy.

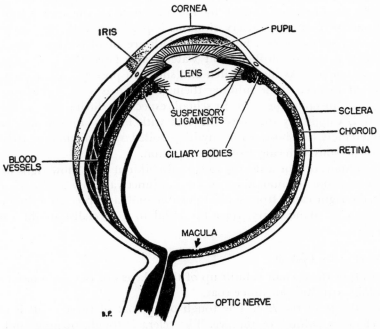

Fig. 63. Cross section of the eyeball with coats peeled at left to show the structure of the eye and its focusing apparatus. The macula is the point of clearest vision at the center of the retina.

The cause in a particular case can be detected only by ophthalmic examination. Some forms of keratitis are accompanied by pain (as if there were "something in the eye") and blurring of vision. Such symptoms are associated with several other forms of eye trouble. Needless to say, any child who complains of them should have immediate medical attention.

The Middle Coat of the Eyeball. The middle layer, or choroid coat, of the eyeball carries the largest number of blood vessels with which the eye is supplied. These very fine arteries and veins weave in and out to make a dark red tapestry which completely covers the eyeball except for a small peephole in front. This peephole is familiar to us all as the pupil of the eye.

The Shutter of the Eye. The circular band of the choroid coat which surrounds the pupil is also familiar to everyone because it gives the eyes their distinctive color. This colored disk is the iris of the eye. Its color is determined by heredity. Its function is similar to that of a window shade or a camera shutter, that is, it regulates the amount of light entering the interior of the eyes through the pupils. The pupil looks black because the inside of the organ which gives us the power to see is in itself dark. We cannot see the interior of the eyes through the pupils for the same reason that we cannot see the interior of a dark room by looking in through the windows. However, the structures inside the eye can be seen and examined by throwing light into each eye through the pupil by means of an instrument called an ophthalmoscope, much as the interior of a dark room may be seen and examined by throwing light through a window from a flashlight.

It is possible by close observation to see the motions of the iris in regulating the amount of light entering the eye through the pupil. These motions are carried out by means of tiny muscles in the iris which draw it in close to, or away from, the center opening, according to the amount of light striking the eyes. The visible effect is a shrinking or enlarging of the size of the pupil.

Changes in the size of the pupils, according to the amount of light striking the eyes, can readily be demonstrated. One way to do this is to place a child in a darker part of the classroom and cover his eyes with a card. After a minute or so remove the card, turn the child directly toward the light, and observe the shrinking of the pupils. Notice also how small the pupils are when a child is outdoors in the sunlight.

Excitement or fear will cause the pupils to dilate because the tiny muscles moving the iris curtain are controlled by the autonomic nervous system, which responds automatically to emotional stimuli. Also the healthy iris is extremely sensitive to variations in intensity of light. Sluggishness of action as shown by slowness of the pupils to change in size with changes in light intensity, or inequality in the size of the two pupils should immediately be reported to the nurse or physician.

The iris of the eye is normally clear and of its characteristic color— blue, brown, gray, hazel, and so on—and the pupil is normally coal black, regular in outline, and equal in size to its fellow. Dullness or discoloration of the iris, or redness around the iris, or contraction or grayness of the pupil, or sensitivity to light should be called to the attention of the nurse or physician.

The Inner Coat of the Eyeball. The layer of tissue that lines the interior of the eyeball is the retina. It is a highly sensitive film designed to convert the energy of light waves into the nerve impulses that are transmitted to the seeing center of the brain by way of a compact rounded bundle of nerve fibers called the optic nerve. Actually the retina is a nervous structure originating from the brain.

"Something in the Eye"

Pain and an increased flow of tears follow quickly after a particle of dust or other foreign body has lodged in the eye. First aid is confined to removing particles on the conjunctiva of the eyelids. Removing a speck on the eyeball should be done only by a physician.

It is best to send a child who complains of "something in the eye" to the nurse serving the school. But if professional help is not immediately available, instruct the child not to rub the eye and then proceed as follows to locate the speck.

First, inspect the conjunctiva of the lower lid by placing the thumb a little below the eye and pressing gently downward while the child looks up. If the speck can be seen, remove it with the corner of a clean handkerchief or a twist of sterile cotton moistened with water.

Inspection of the conjunctiva of the upper lid should not be attempted unless you have had training in first aid and are authorized to practice it in school. The first thing to do if a speck is located on the conjunctiva of the upper eyelid is to grasp the lashes of the upper eyelid gently while the child looks upward and pull the eyelid forward and downward over the lower lid. This may dislodge the particle so that the tears can wash it out. If this does not work and the necessary supplies are on hand, flush the eye from the inner corner to the outer corner with sterile water or baking soda solution (1 level teaspoonful of baking soda to 1 cupful of cool boiled water) from a sterile eye dropper. A little sterile olive oil, mineral oil, or castor oil dropped into the eye after a speck has been removed is soothing.

In removing a foreign body from the eye gentleness is absolutely necessary. If the child is nervous and resists inspection, or if the speck cannot be located or removed by the simple procedures described, arrangements should be made to have him taken to a physician. It is important that foreign bodies be removed promptly to prevent serious inflammation of the eyeball.

SEEING RIGHT AND SEEING WRONG

Light, eyes, and brain—all three—give us the gift of sight. Light waves reflected, or bounced back, from the objects through which they cannot pass enter the eye through the pupil and are focused upon the retina— the light-sensitive membrane, or film, that forms the inner coat of the eyeball. The retina is the terminal in the eye for millions of tiny nerve fibers which run via the optic nerve to a terminal in the brain. Over these one-way nerve tracks the impulses provoked by light speed from the retina to the seeing center of the brain, where they produce the sensation of sight.

Two-eyed Vision

In looking at the eyes one of the first things to catch the attention of the observer is the almost continuous motion of the eyeballs. They can

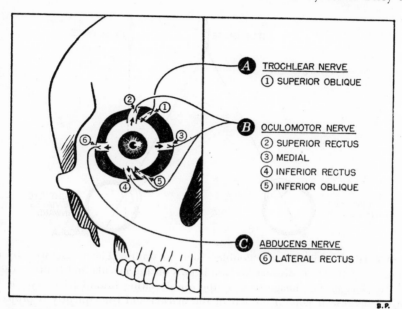

A TROCHLEAR NERVE
① SUPERIOR OBLIQUE

B OCULOMOTOR NERVE
② SUPERIOR RECTUS
③ MEDIAL
④ INFERIOR RECTUS
⑤ INFERIOR OBLIQUE

C ABDUCENS NERVE
⑥ LATERAL RECTUS

B.P.

FIG. 64. Diagrammatic representation of the muscles that move the eyeball and their controlling nerves.

be turned at will in many directions—right, left, up, down, up and right, up and left, down and right, down and left.

The motions of the eyeball are made possible by voluntary muscles attached at one end to the bones of the orbit and at the other end to the eyeball. These muscles work in antagonistic pairs. One muscle of a pair helps to turn the eyeball to the right, for example, and its fellow helps to turn it to the left. While one "fellow" works, the other relaxes.

Normally the action of the muscles of both eyes is synchronized so that they turn together to focus on the same spot. Even if one eye is covered it turns automatically to look in the same direction as the uncovered eye. That is why both eyes must be bandaged if it is necessary to keep one eye comparatively still.

Binocular or two-eyed vision enables us to see things in proper perspective. With one eye we have photographic vision (perception of length and breadth); with two eyes, stereoscopic vision (perception of depth or thickness as well as length and breadth).

Strabismus or Squint

When the external eye muscles do not function correctly to focus both eyes simultaneously on the same object, strabismus or squint is the result.

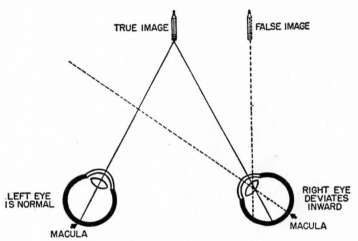

FIG. 65. Diagram illustrating double vision in squint. The image seen by the fixing eye (left eye) is distinct because it falls on the macula and hence is called the true image. The image seen by the eye deviating inward (right eye) is less distinct because it falls to the left of the macula and consequently is projected to the right as the false image.

The eye that is directed toward the object looked at is called the fixing eye; the other, the squinting eye. A true image is seen with the fixing eye and a false image with the squinting eye. Hence a person with a squint may have double vision. However, a child with uncorrected squint usually does not see double by the time he is ready to enter school because he has unconsciously learned to suppress the image from the squinting eye. If the condition is left uncorrected the vision in the squinting eye may become impaired, because progressive loss of function is the penalty nature exacts for disuse of function.

The Detection of Squint. Squint may be *manifest,* that is, readily observable, or *latent,* that is, not readily observable. In the most common forms of manifest squint, the teacher will observe that one of the child's eyes deviates inward toward the nose (convergent squint) or outward away from the nose (divergent squint) while the other eye is fixed on the object being looked at. Sometimes the eyes may take turns in deviating. This is known as alternating strabismus. Convergent squint is the most common form of squint and usually develops between the ages of one and four. Divergent squint usually develops in youth or early adult life.

The squint may be present all the time, or present at some times and absent at others; if intermittent, it may be most noticeable when the child is tired or in poor health. It may be greater for near vision than for distant vision or vice versa. If vision has been suppressed in the squinting eye, the child may not be able to see with that eye any of the letters or symbols on the vision-testing chart (see Snellen Test Charts, further on). Suppressed vision does not necessarily mean permanent loss of vision, but it does mean that the squinting eye has become "rusty" through lack of use and that the child will have to practice using it under the supervision of an eye specialist until it has regained its lost function.

In latent squint, one eye may tend to turn in, out, up, or down because of muscular imbalance. A child with latent squint may be able to overcome this tendency by muscular effort because of his strong desire to maintain binocular vision. In the milder forms, there may be no noticeable signs of squint. In more pronounced forms, there may be some evidence produced by the strain imposed in overcoming the difficulty. Tilting of the head may indicate the child's effort to correct double vision.

It is difficult for the untrained observer to detect latent squint. However, since both eyes under normal conditions turn in the same direction, even when one is covered, a tendency to squint may be detected if an eye that has been covered makes a sudden jump to change its position when the cover is removed. Another simple test may be helpful. The observer holds a pencil or other object in front of the child and asks him to look at it. If the child has a tendency to squint, only the fixing eye will follow the object when it is moved in various directions.

In strabismus (tropia) or latent squint (phoria), careful attention should be given to any difference in the visual acuity of the two eyes. If such difference exists, correctly prescribed and correctly fitted glasses may compensate for it and thus relieve unnecessary muscular effort. It is evident that the sooner any manifest or latent squint is brought to the attention of an eye specialist the greater is the possibility not only of correcting the difficulty, but also of preventing psychological reactions that may influence the child's adjustment to life.

Eye exercises under the supervision of a specialist in orthoptics are often helpful. It may also be necessary to cover the good eye so that the squinting eye will be forced to work. A child who is obliged to wear a patch or a "blacked-out" eyeglass lens over one eye should be watched to make sure that he keeps it on. A simple explanation of why Johnny or Jane must wear an eye covering may help to prevent teasing by the other children. In some cases, a surgical operation may be required to correct a squint.

The Focusing Apparatus of the Eyes

The focusing apparatus of the eyes, like that of the camera, is designed to take advantage of the fact that light rays are bent when they pass from one transparent medium, such as air, into another transparent medium of different density, such as glass or water. This bending is called refraction.

In the course of their progress from the air through the window of the eyeball to its back wall, light rays reflected from objects in the outside world pass through several refracting media: (a) the cornea, (b) the watery liquid between the cornea and crystalline lens, (c) the crystalline lens, and (d) the soft jellylike substance between the lens and the retina. The most important refracting device is the crystalline lens. The crystalline lens is a clear elastic body thicker in the middle than at the edges. Thus its shape is double convex, like that of an ordinary magnifying glass. The first person to describe the shape of the crystalline lens was the great Arab scientist Alhazen (962–1038), who said that it looked like a lentil seed. The English word "lens" comes from the Latin word for "lentil."

The center of the front surface of the crystalline lens coincides with the center of the pupil. The margin of the pupil is in contact with this surface. The lens is enclosed in a highly elastic capsule. Attached to the lens capsule is the suspensory ligament by which the lens is slung like a hammock from one side to the other of a circular zone of tissue extending from the choroid coat of the eyeball. This zone of tissue is called the ciliary body. It is made up chiefly of the ciliary processes and the ciliary muscle. The ciliary processes project outward like tiny fringes toward the lens, which they completely encircle.

Accommodation

Light rays coming from objects 20 feet or more away are nearly parallel when they reach the eye, and the curvature of the crystalline lens in the normal eye at rest is just right for focusing these parallel rays on the retina. But light rays coming from objects nearer than 20 feet are spread apart, or divergent, when they reach the eye, and in the normal eye at rest are focused *behind* the retina. How then can we see nearby objects distinctly? This is what happens: The ciliary muscle contracts and in doing so draws the choroid forward. This permits the ciliary processes to move forward and inward, thus reducing the diameter of the ring which they form around the lens. The pressure of the suspensory ligament and lens capsule upon the lens is thus relieved. Consequently, the elastic lens becomes thicker—more convex or spherical—just as the surface of a small rubber ball held tightly between fingers and thumb would round up when the pressure upon it was reduced. The more curved or bulging shape of the crystalline lens increases its focusing power.

The process by which the eye accommodates itself to near vision is called accommodation. It happens so smoothly and instantaneously that a person with normal vision is not aware of any change whatever taking place in his eyes when he turns from looking off into the distance to the reading of a book or other close eye work and vice versa.

Errors of Refraction

To see nearby and distant objects clearly and distinctly, the light rays reflected from those objects must be focused directly upon the retina of the eye. If the rays come to a focus in front of, or behind, the retina instead of exactly upon it, blurred vision is the result. Mistakes in vision caused by defects in the structure of the eye are called errors in refraction. Such errors can usually be corrected by placing glass lenses of the required type and strength in front of the eyes so as to bring the focal point just enough backward or sufficiently forward to land it squarely on the retina.

Table 16. PREVALENCE OF VISUAL HANDICAPS AMONG SCHOOL CHILDREN

Condition	Number of children
Blindness	7,000
Partial-sightedness (special educational facilities required)	67,000 *
Less serious visual defects (observation or treatment by an eye specialist required)	8,400,000

Source: Estimates furnished by the National Society for the Prevention of Blindness, New York, for preparation of "Impairments of Young People," in *Statistical Bulletin*, Metropolitan Life Insurance Company, Vol. 36, No. 8 (August), 1955. See also "The Nation's Handicapped Children," by Arthur J. Lesser and Eleanor P. Hunt, in *Am. J. Pub. Health*, Vol. 44, No. 2 (February), 1954.

* Special facilities were available to 8,000 in the public school system.

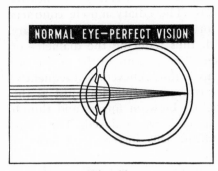

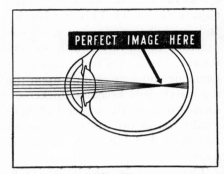

Fig. 66.   Fig. 67.

FIG. 66. Normal eye. The image is focused correctly on the retina. (*Figs. 66–70 from "Methods of Testing and Protecting Eyesight in Industry," Metropolitan Life Insurance Company.*)

FIG. 67. Nearsighted eye—blurred vision. In nearsightedness the eyeball is too long from front to back, and light rays entering the eye focus the image in *front* of the retina instead of exactly upon it. Nearsighted people can see objects close at hand, but distant objects appear blurred.

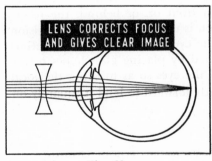

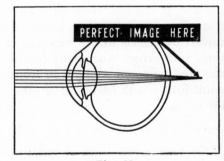

Fig. 68.   Fig. 69.

FIG. 68. Nearsighted eyes that have been fitted with concave lenses of suitable power will be able to see distant objects clearly.

FIG. 69. Farsighted eye—blurred vision. In farsightedness the eyeball is too short from front to back, and light rays entering the eye focus the image *back* of the retina. Farsighted eyes cannot see objects near at hand without giving considerable extra work to the muscles of accommodation. This often results in eye fatigue.

Farsightedness. The most common cause of farsightedness is the possession of an eyeball that is too short from front to back. Consequently, light rays come to a focus behind the retina even when the muscles of accommodation try to be accommodating.

Children are usually farsighted at birth because their eyeballs have not yet reached their full size. As they grow older they may become less farsighted, normal-sighted, or nearsighted. In some children, the eyeball may reach its full development at about the age of nine or ten, but it is not uncommon to find hyperopia, or farsightedness, in older children, even in high school students.

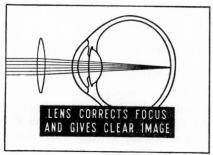

LENS CORRECTS FOCUS AND GIVES CLEAR IMAGE

Even to see distant objects distinctly, a farsighted person whose error is uncorrected by glasses requires some accommodation, that is, some alteration in the focus of his eyes. To see nearby objects, he must not only make the alteration required of a person with normal vision, but also an additional adjustment to compensate for his error. The unaided eyes of a farsighted person are *never* at rest as

FIG. 70. Farsighted eyes that have been fitted with convex lenses of suitable power can see nearby objects clearly without overworking the muscles of accommodation. Eye fatigue from the defect of farsightedness is thus avoided.

long as he can see clearly, because to see clearly his eyes must work constantly. No wonder he has eye fatigue!

Very often the testing of a farsighted child's vision does not indicate that anything is wrong with his refracting apparatus. By making an extra effort he may be able to pass the test successfully. Screwing up the eyes when looking at distant objects, holding the book far away when reading, and signs and symptoms of eye fatigue observed by the teacher may be the only indications of trouble of this kind.

Nearsightedness (Myopia). A person to whom distant objects appear blurred and nearby objects more or less clear and distinct is said to be nearsighted. In nearsightedness the eyeball is too long from front to back so that light rays come to a focus in front of the retina. A child is rarely born with nearsightedness. However, it usually begins at an early age and nearly always gets worse (see Table 17). Nearsightedness is found in more than 10 per cent of children in the primary grades and increases to 20 per cent or more between the ages of ten and twenty.

Many children who are nearsighted may be able to do close work comfortably and show no symptoms except indistinct vision for distance.

Table 17. CHANGES IN PROPORTION OF CHILDREN HAVING SPECIFIED REFRACTIVE ERRORS
UPON REEXAMINATION 2½ YEARS LATER (AVERAGE) *

1,481 white school children of Washington, D.C.

| | Per cent |
Refractive error	change
Simple hyperopia.........................	−18.7
Simple myopia	+70.4
Hyperopic astigmatism.....................	+39.7
Myopic astigmatism.......................	+63.6

Source: "The School Child: Health Progress and Needs," Metropolitan Life Insurance Company
(after Ciocco).
* Based upon examination of the right eye after administration of a cycloplegic.

Such children can see to read at their desks without difficulty, for example, but may not be able to see clearly what is written on the chalkboard or the details of wall maps or charts. Others may have to hold their books closer to their eyes than the usual 14 inches (Plate 13), look as if they were writing with their noses, and say that their eyes feel tired after doing close work for only a short time.

The pupils of a nearsighted child are likely to be larger than the pupils of a child with normal vision or farsightedness. Hence more light gets into his eyes, and he may complain that strong light or glare hurts them. Also, he may tend to squeeze his eyelids together in an effort to shut out some of the light and so obtain clearer vision. This "squinting" of the eyes in order to see more distinctly is a common sign of nearsightedness.

Whereas farsighted eyes may improve their near vision by making an extra effort to accommodate, or alter their focus, nearsighted eyes cannot improve their focus for distance without the help of lenses of the correct type and strength. In other words, nearsighted eyes are permanently focused for near objects. Hence, eye testing with the Snellen chart at 20 feet will nearly always detect nearsighted children.

Astigmatism. Astigmatism is usually caused by some irregularity in the curvature of the cornea or the lens of the eye. As a result some light rays are bent more sharply than others, so that all the rays are not brought to a sharp focus anywhere on the retina. The astigmatism may be hyperopic, myopic, or mixed.

To persons with astigmatism, details appear blurred and the outlines of objects look hazy as in a photograph out of focus. The image conveyed to the brain resembles that of an object seen through a windowpane which is uneven or wrinkled. The decrease in acuteness of vision caused by astigmatism is present both for distant vision and near vision. Hence, children with astigmatism are subject to constant fatigue, both in using their eyes for close work and in looking at distant objects. A nearsighted child or a farsighted child who is also astigmatic may have all the troubles associated both with farsightedness and nearsightedness.

Efforts to reduce or neutralize the effect of astigmatism are likely to give rise to the symptoms of severe continuous eye fatigue and extreme nervousness or irritability in children. A small amount of astigmatism may cause greater eye fatigue than a large amount because the child with severe astigmatism gives up the struggle to see clearly, whereas the child with mild astigmatism continues his straining effort to see clearly.

Eye Fatigue

The constant and excessive fatigue to which the eyes are subjected in trying to overcome errors of refraction or a tendency to squint may affect not only their own well-being but also that of the whole body. Among the signs and symptoms of eye fatigue are frequent headaches; dizziness; watering eyes; continual blinking; a scowling expression; tired, droopy eyelids; a blurring of near vision; sensitivity to light; and sties and inflammations of the conjunctiva and margins of the eyelids usually caused by constant rubbing—as if by rubbing one might clear away the fog before one's eyes.

Reading Difficulties

The child's behavior when reading or during lessons involving the use of the chalkboard, wall charts, or maps also may indicate a visual disturbance. Significant signs other than those already mentioned (continual blinking when reading, squinting at the page, holding the book too far from or too close to the face) include moving the book backward or forward, stopping the effort to read after a brief period, shutting one eye or covering it with the hand, frequently losing the place on the page, and confusing the following letters in reading or spelling: o's and a's; e's and c's; n's and m's; h's, n's, and r's; f's and t's.

A visual disturbance, however, is not the only possible cause of a child's failure to read as easily or as well as the average of his class. Many poor readers of normal or superior intelligence have normal or nearly normal vision. In some cases the disability is associated with left-handedness, especially if an attempt has been made to change left-handedness to right-handedness (see Handedness under The Brain in Speech, in Chap. 5). The child may confuse one consonant with another, as b with d and p with q; or see syllables, words, or entire sentences in reverse (as in mirror writing); or completely fail to recognize a word.

The condition is aggravated by the criticism of the child's teacher or parents, with the result that various emotional problems may develop.

The cause of reading difficulties, in the absence of visual disturbances, subnormal intelligence, or organic brain damage, is not clearly understood. It is believed that emotional factors, such as fear, anxiety, jealousy, feelings of inferiority, or hostility for teachers or parents, play an important role in creating them. Endocrine imbalances and dietetic errors also may be involved.

Some ophthalmological authorities are of the opinion that the substitution of the so-called "flash" method of teaching reading for the phonetic method is an important contributory factor.[1] In one study, three times as many cases of reading difficulty were found among children taught by the "flash" method as among those taught by the phonetic method. The "flash" method strains the child's powers of attention and concentration to the limit, and minor difficulties of vision, such as slight farsightedness or latent squint, assume greater significance than under the older methods. With the great emphasis on speed in the "flash" method, the children who for one reason or another cannot keep up may develop a subconscious feeling of defeat which leads to failure in further efforts.

An appraisal of the advantages and disadvantages of various methods of teaching reading, as related to the development of reading difficulties, presents a problem for the ophthalmologists and the educators to solve. Children who actually have difficulty in learning to read for no readily detectable reason are best treated by specialists familiar with all aspects of the problem. Special tutoring by the teacher or parents seldom does much good because of the psychological complications usually involved.

Wearing Glasses

It would be a very unusual class in which no children wore eyeglasses or needed to wear them. Information regarding eyeglasses—what they are for and what they mean to the wearer in terms of comfort and clearness of vision—is an important part of the health education of all children. The wearers, to whom glasses may not seem to be an unmixed blessing, should be helped to develop a sense of responsibility for wearing their glasses under the circumstances prescribed by the eye specialist and for taking care of their glasses properly. Proper care means keeping the glasses clean and protecting them from bending of the frames and scratching or breaking of the lenses. When not in use glasses should be

---

[1] "Reading Disabilities in Children," *J.A.M.A.*, Vol. 142, No. 15 (Apr. 15), 1950, p. 1218.

kept in their case, and when taken off temporarily they should be placed in a safe position on the frames.

The nonwearers of glasses will not be so likely to tease the wearers if they realize how fortunate they are to have good vision and how wonderful it is that glasses make it possible for others with poor vision to see as well as *they* do.

The teacher should have the information that will help her supervise children for whom glasses have been prescribed. She should know, for example, whether a child wearing glasses is supposed to wear them all the time or only when he is reading or doing other close work. She can then cooperate with the eye specialist and the parents in seeing that the child gets the full benefit of his seeing aid.

VISION TESTING

Long after spectacles first came into use (about 1300) each individual did his own vision testing. The peddler's pack or hawker's tray was not complete without an array of spectacles, and from it the sufferer picked out the pair that suited him best. The optical errors to which the living eye is subject were not accurately described until the time of the great Dutch ophthalmologist Franz Cornelius Donders (1818–1889). Donders instituted the system of prescribing and fitting eyeglasses which is now in use. Hermann Snellen, an ingenious clinician and clever surgeon, who became Donders' "right-hand man" and later his successor to the chair of ophthalmology in the University of Utrecht, invented the test types that are still in use for testing acuteness of vision.

The method used for estimating the refraction of the eye with trial lenses and test types is known as the subjective method. The patient must cooperate with the examiner in determining the nature of his optical error, or errors, and say which lens or combination of lenses aids his vision most. Anyone who has had an eye examination knows how difficult it is sometimes to decide this question. For this reason great value is attached to instruments that help the examiner to determine objectively the kind and amount of errors of refraction and accommodation and other eye difficulties.

The Ophthalmoscope

The first instrument of this kind to be invented was the ophthalmoscope. It is based on the fact that under certain conditions light entering the eye through the pupil is reflected from the fundus, that is, the back part of the eye opposite the pupil, thus making it possible for an observer actually to see the interior of the eye. From earliest times the glowing appearance of the eyes of certain animals (notably the cat) when seen in a dim light had attracted notice. The glow was supposed to be due to the spontaneous development of light within the eye. The famous German scientist Hermann Helmholtz (1821–1894), in his lectures on physiology at the University of Königsberg, found it necessary to discuss the theory of the emission of light from the eye. The experimental study in which he demonstrated the falsity of this theory resulted in 1851 in the invention of the ophthalmoscope.

This instrument is a device consisting of a perforated mirror or reflector mounted on a handle. The mirror serves to reflect light into the interior of the eye, while the aperture allows a portion of this light, after returning from the patient's eye, to pass into the eye of the observer. A disk containing convex and concave lenses for use in scrutinizing the fundus is set behind the aperture. This disk can be rotated by means of a finger applied to its edge so that any lens on the disk can be placed behind the perforation in the mirror.

It is said that Helmholtz did not at first fully realize the epoch-making character of his invention. It was the brilliant German opthalmologist Albrecht Graefe (1828–1870) who first grasped this. According to a story told in 1886 by Donders, when Graefe, "the greatest of all eye surgeons," used an ophthalmoscope for the first time and saw the background of the eye with its nerve entrance and its blood vessels, his cheeks reddened, and he called out excitedly, "Helmholtz has unfolded to us a new world."

The ophthalmoscope has been greatly improved since its invention, and many other instruments have been devised for examining a patient's eyes objectively for evidence of optical errors or disease. The most accurate objective method for determining errors of refraction now in use is retinoscopy, sometimes called the "shadow test." The retinoscope consists of a perforated plane or concave mirror, which can be rotated. The mirror is used to throw light into the patient's eye through the pupil, with the result that the fundus is illuminated. By looking through the sight hole of the mirror, the observer sees the illuminated area and the shadow bounding it. The state of refraction of the patient's eye can be determined by observing the direction of movement of the illuminated area and the shadow when the mirror is rotated.

Before using the ophthalmoscope or retinoscope in examining the eye, the physician often uses a drug (called a cycloplegic) to paralyze the muscle of accommodation (ciliary muscle). While the effects of the drug last, the eye pupil remains dilated.

Eyesight Conservation

The most significant advances in eye care during the past generation have been along the lines of sight conservation. The eye in trying to overcome errors of refraction is subjected to constant fatigue which may affect not only its own well-being but also that of the body of which it is a part. For this reason the early detection of errors of refraction and the correction of such defects by glasses or other means, after a complete examination by an eye specialist, are of great importance.

The Teacher's Part in Vision Testing

Classroom teachers have proved that they can test children's vision with a reasonable degree of accuracy in discovering gross visual defects when these tests cannot be given by a physician or nurse. The records of such tests, with observations made in the classroom, should be reviewed by the physician serving the school in order to determine which children should be sent to an eye specialist. It should be remembered, however, that many abnormal eye conditions cannot or may not be detected in periodic tests of visual acuity. Many times the teacher's observations are of greater significance than the acuteness of vision as measured by the test. In addition to signs and symptoms of fatigue, the extent of the child's power to concentrate, to keep up with the class in reading ability, to work without tiring easily or acting irritable or inattentive, and to play games requiring both distant and near vision without noticeable awkwardness may also serve as criteria in judging the effectiveness of the child's visual apparatus.

Visual acuity tests may be depended on to screen out the nearsighted children, those with some forms of severe to moderate astigmatism, and a percentage of farsighted children. On the other hand, a slightly astigmatic or farsighted child who is able by straining his eyes to overcome an error of refraction may "pass" the test successfully.

Snellen Test Charts

The Snellen test for visual acuity at 20 feet is most commonly used to test the acuteness of vision of school children. Entire letters of the alphabet or a series of E's are reproduced on Snellen charts.

Snellen Letter Chart. Square-shaped letters are arranged upon a chart, the size of the letters diminishing from above downward. A small numeral at the side of, or above, each row of letters indicates the number of feet away from the chart at which the normal eye should be able to read letters of that size. In the charts ordinarily used in testing the vision of school children, the single top letter is of a size that can be read by

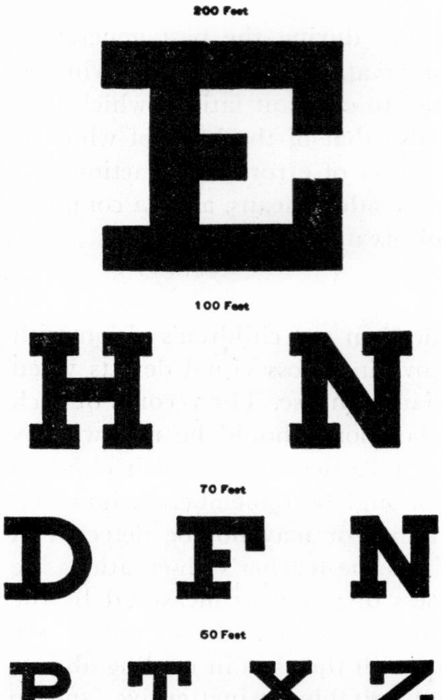

200 Feet

E

100 Feet

H N

70 Feet

D F N

60 Feet

P T X Z

40 Feet

F Z T D U

30 Feet

D F N P T H

20 Feet

P H N U T D Z

15 Feet

N P X T Z D F H

10 Feet

D Z H L N P T

FIG. 71. Letter chart, Snellen scale. (*Courtesy of National Society for the Prevention of Blindness.*)

the normal eye at a distance from the chart of 200 feet.[2] Then come rows of letters that can normally be read at 100, 70, 50, 40, 30, 15, and 10 feet, respectively (Fig. 71). The standard distance for testing acuteness of vision is 20 feet from the chart, because rays of light reflected from objects at that distance are nearly parallel when they reach the eye and a minimum amount of accommodation is needed to focus them on the retina.

Acuteness of vision is expressed by a fraction, the numerator of which corresponds to the number of feet separating the child from the chart. Hence, for testing vision at the standard distance of 20 feet, the numerator is 20. The denominator corresponds to the number indicating the line of smallest letters that the child can read without mistake at that distance. If he can read with one eye the row of letters numbered 20 (that is, letters of a size that the normal eye can read at 20 feet), his sight is normal in that eye and is expressed by the fraction 20/20. If he can read only as far down as the fourth row from the top with the other eye (that is, letters that the normal eye can see at 50 feet), the vision of that eye is 20/50. If he cannot read lower than the top letter, it is 20/200. If none of the letters can be read at 20 feet, the child should approach the card until he can read the largest letter at the top. The dis-

[2] In some schools the top letter of the chart used may be of a size that can be read by the normal eye at 100 feet.

stance at which he stands to read
that letter will serve as the numerator of the fraction, for example
10/200.

Snellen Symbol Chart. On this
second type of chart a series of E's
heading downward, upward, to the
right and to the left (Fig. 72) are
printed on numbered lines in sizes
corresponding to those of Snellen's
test letters. Acuteness of vision is
determined by the smallest symbols
of which the child, standing at the
standard distance of 20 feet from
the chart, can correctly tell the direction in which the symbols are
open. The Snellen symbol chart is
used to test the vision of young
children who cannot read and is
often preferred to the Snellen letter
chart in testing all children. The
reasons given for this preference
are that the judgment required is
simple; the E's of the same size do
not vary in visibility as do letters;
the symbols are not easy to memor-
ize; fatigue is not produced; and the
results can be interpreted by anyone.

In testing with the E chart the
child is asked either to tell in which
direction the shafts of the E point
(up, down, right, or left) or to show
with his hand which way the arms
of the E point. To make it easier for
the child to concentrate on one
symbol, "window cards"—that is,
cards with round holes of varying
diameters—should be used to expose
only one symbol at a time. The part
of the chart not in use should be

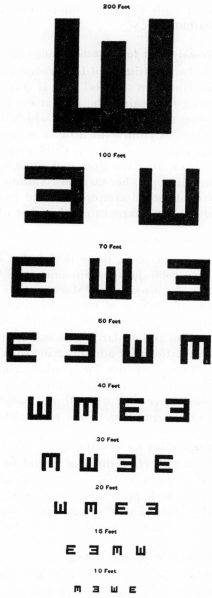

FIG. 72. Symbol chart, Snellen scale.
(*Courtesy of National Society for the
Prevention of Blindness.*)

covered with a cover card. Dull-finished white cover cards should be used with daylight illumination and soft gray with artificial illumination.

Wheel Chart for Detecting Astigmatism

A chart consisting of lines radiating from the center of a circle as spokes radiate from a wheel hub is used to detect astigmatism. The chart is hung flat against the wall at eye level under adequate light. The child being tested is asked to tell which lines across the chart look darker than others. A child with little or no astigmatism will notice little or no difference. Occasionally a child with a significant amount of astigmatism will say that the lines look alike to him. In that case the teacher must depend upon her own observations of the child's behavior or the child's complaints of symptoms of eye fatigue to determine whether the child should be referred to a physician who can apply more exact tests.

Other Testing Devices

In recent years, other devices for testing the vision of school children have come into use in some schools. The best known are the series of tests known as the "Massachusetts Vision Test" and a battery of tests that make use of the "telebinocular" (a machine developed from the stereograph) and a series of slides. Such tests are designed to detect astigmatism and ocular muscle balance (fusion) as well as errors of refraction. Instructions for administering such tests come with the apparatus.

The procedure for administering the Snellen test is described here both because it is the simplest to administer and because "it gives as good agreement with clinical judgment as any of the multiple-test procedures, and better than most, although its referral rate is lower." [3]

Preparation for Eye Testing

In health class, the eyes should be the subject for study and discussion in preparation for vision testing. The children should be told what is going to happen and why and be encouraged to ask questions. Also, a demonstration of vision testing may be given so that the children will know exactly what they are to do.

Procedure for Eye Testing

Place the eye-test chart on the wall. The intensity of illumination on the chart should be equal to 10 foot-candles evenly diffused without glare. The illumination of the surrounding areas should be as nearly equal as possible to the light on the chart and never less than one-fifth

[3] "Screening School Children for Visual Defects," report of a study conducted in St. Louis, Mo., 1948–1949, Children's Bureau Publication No. 345, United States Department of Health, Education and Welfare, 1954, p. 54.

as much. Too much light on the chart, or spot lighting of the chart, may compensate for some errors of refraction and keep them from being discovered. To avoid contrasts, no bright light should be within the child's field of vision. With daylight illumination the chart should be hung opposite a window and the child placed with his back to the window.

Using a tape measure or yardstick, measure a distance of 20 feet from the wall on which the chart is placed, and mark the 20-foot line on the floor with chalk or adhesive tape. Have each child being tested stand on the 20-foot line exactly in front of the chart or sit in a chair placed on the line. The eyes should be at about the level of the 20-foot row of letters or symbols. The chart may be raised or lowered with the varying heights of the children.

Test each eye separately. While one eye is being tested have the child or a helper hold a card or a folded clean sheet of paper (about 2½ by 3 inches when folded) over the eye that is not being tested. Each child should have his own card or paper to avoid the spreading of infection. Show the children how the eye cover should be held. It should be grasped at the edge and placed so that it rests obliquely across the nose. It should not be pressed against the eyeball. Tell the children to keep both eyes open during the test. When the cover is lifted, note whether the eye that has been hidden makes an abrupt movement in order to focus. If so, mention the fact in recording the results of the test.

Test the right eye first, then the left eye, then both eyes together. If the child wears glasses, have him take the test first with his glasses, and then without. This gives the child a chance to do his best on the first test. Have the child start at the top of the chart and read downward.[4] The number of the lowest line of letters on the Snellen letter chart which the child can read without difficulty will be the denominator of the fraction recording the acuity of vision for that eye.

If the symbol E chart is used, expose one vertical and one horizontal symbol on a line and move down to the next. In the lowest line read correctly, or in the 20-foot line, expose all four symbols, one at a time. Reading three out of four symbols correctly is considered to be satisfactory evidence that the child can see the symbols on that line.

Observe the child carefully while he is taking the test. If he shows signs of straining to see, do not allow him to continue. Record the lowest line correctly read with each eye and any evidences of straining to see. Signs to look for include thrusting the head forward or tilting it to one

---

[4] As young children find it hard to concentrate for long periods, the upper part of the chart may be covered down to the 50-foot line unless there is other evidence of an eye difficulty.

side, watering of the eyes, scowling or squinting, and rapid blinking of the eyes.

Record results of the test for each eye immediately in the form of a fraction such as, for example, "R. 20/20, L. 20/40." These figures should not be interpreted as representing a fraction of normal vision. They are simply a record of acuteness of vision at a given distance (20 feet). Vision of 20/40 in the left eye, for example, is not one-half of normal vision, but is merely a manner of recording the fact that the best the child can do is to see with his left eye at 20 feet letters or symbols that normally he should be able to see at 40 feet.

Also record all other findings, including any signs of eye fatigue or straining to see. For children wearing glasses, record the vision for each eye with and without glasses. It will be helpful also to state how long the child has worn glasses, when his glasses were last checked or changed, and whether he wears his glasses continuously or not. To get this information it may be necessary to consult the school nurse or the child's parents.

A summary of observations made in the classroom should be appended (later, if there is no time to do it during the test), as this will help the physician or nurse who reviews the record cards to determine which children should be sent to an eye specialist for a thorough professional examination.

OBSERVATIONS ABOUT THE EARS

The External Ear

The part of the ear we see and wash is an appendage of cartilage covered with skin and known as the pinna, or wing. Its function is to scoop up sound waves and direct them into the outer ear canal. This winding passageway extends inward and about 1 inch downward to the delicate membrane called the tympanum, or eardrum, which is stretched tightly across its inner end. The walls of the outer ear canal secrete a thick yellowish wax which acts like flypaper in catching and holding dust and insects that might otherwise injure the eardrum.

"Something in the Ear." The outer ear canal may be temporarily clogged by impacted wax, by water caught in it during swimming, by small objects which young children have been known to push into their ears, or by a pimple, boil, or other swelling.

If a child starts to rub or pull at an ear, or to shake the head as if to dislodge something in the ear, or to complain of fullness or stuffiness in the ear, something may be obstructing his outer ear canal. A child usually will confess the details of his ear-plugging experiment, if that is the trouble, when he begins to get a painful or uncomfortable reaction. A live insect usually advertises its presence in the ear canal by its buzzing. Sometimes it is possible to see an obstruction in the outer ear canal by gently pulling the upper part of the ear upward and backward and looking into the opening.

The removal of a foreign body or plug of wax from the outer ear canal can be done safely only by a physician. It is dangerous to poke into the canal with a hairpin, toothpick, match, or other pointed instrument in an effort to get it out. Not only may you push the object further in, but also you may scratch the lining of the ear canal and thereby prepare the ground for an infection.

The Middle Ear

The inner end of the outer ear canal is completely sealed by the eardrum. Beyond the eardrum lies the middle ear, a tiny chamber filled with air. The eardrum cannot vibrate properly under the impact of sound waves unless the pressure of air on each side of it is equal. Hence in evolving the architecture of the ear some method had to be devised to let air into the middle-ear chamber in order to equalize the pressure of air on the two sides of the drum. This was accomplished by connecting the middle ear with the nasopharynx (the meeting place of nose and throat) by a tube called the eustachian tube after its Italian discoverer, Bartolommeo Eustachio, a sixteenth-century anatomist. Before his day, the eustachian tube was unknown in human beings, although some acquaintance with it in animals may have led to the quaint theory that we breathe as well as hear with our ears. Physicians of ancient Egypt believed that "the breath of life enters by the right and that of death by the left ear."

The eustachian tube is about 1 to 1½ inches wide at its narrowest point. It is lined with mucous membrane which is a continuation of that which lines the nose and throat. It opens into the back of the throat and behind the soft palate. This opening, which flares outward like the mouth of a trumpet, is ordinarily kept closed. However, the mouth of the tube opens in swallowing, yawning, or when high pressure is created in the nasopharynx, as in blowing the nose forcibly or in exhaling forcibly with the mouth and nostrils closed. Practically everyone has had the experience of hearing his ears "pop" when going very far up or down from the place on the earth's surface to which he is accustomed. In going up, as in an elevator or an airplane, the air pressure on the outside of the eardrum decreases and the air in the middle ear drives the eardrum outward. Swallowing or yawning lets air of the same pressure as that on the outside of the drum enter the middle ear via the eustachian tube and the drum snaps or pops back into its original state of tautness. In going suddenly down from a high level to a low one, the pressure of air on the outside of the drum increases and the drum is

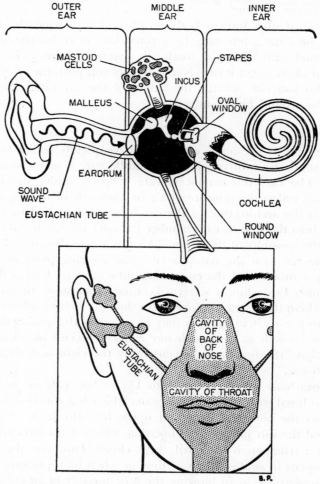

Fig. 73. Diagram showing divisions of the ear, with inset showing location with reference to nasopharynx.

driven inward until the air pressure on both sides of the drum is equalized by swallowing or yawning.

When the eustachian tube is closed temporarily by the swelling of its mucous-membrane lining, as often happens when one has a cold, the pressure of air in the middle ear is below that of atmospheric air. In that event air is gradually absorbed from the middle ear into the blood stream and the partial vacuum thus created causes the drum membrane to retract or push inward. This is the cause of the stuffy dull feeling in the ears and the dullness of hearing that so often accompany a head cold.

Middle-ear Infections

As we have seen, the eustachian tube is an ingenious device. Its only drawback is the opportunity it permits for the entrance of bacteria into the middle ear from the nose and throat. Infection of the middle ear is the chief cause of impairment of hearing.

An acute cold in the head, sinusitis, tonsillitis, grippe, scarlet fever, measles, and other acute infectious diseases involving the upper respiratory tract may lead to middle-ear infection.

Earache. Severe earache is usually caused by inflammation or abscess of the middle ear (acute otitis media). The pressure set up by pus in the middle ear causes the eardrum to bulge outward. If left to itself, the pressure of the pus perforates or ruptures the eardrum. The ear surgeon prevents this spontaneous rupture, if he sees the child in time, by making an incision near the edge of the drum to allow free drainage. A surgical incision usually heals soon, leaving no loss of hearing. Spontaneous rupture, on the other hand, may result in a large or jagged opening in the eardrum which may heal slowly and in some cases fail to close entirely. In the latter case the ear may discharge more or less continuously or whenever the child has a cold.

The ears also may ache or feel sore or stuffy during a head cold or at the onset of some other communicable disease affecting the upper respiratory tract. Other possible causes of earache are mumps, a decayed molar tooth, inflammation of the eustachian tube, inflammation or an abscess or boil in the outer ear canal, and inflammation of the mastoid bone back of the ear. Needless to say, medical attention is required for any child who complains of earache.

"Runny Ear." A child whose ear is "running" is quite likely to have a plug of cotton in the affected ear (see Plate 14). In chronic infections, however, the drainage may be indicated only by persistent slight moisture. The teacher should make sure that a child with a discharging ear (acute or chronic) is being looked after by a physician, as this condition may have serious consequences if neglected.

A child with a discharging ear who is free of pain and fever may be permitted by his physician to attend school. In supervising such a child the teacher may find the following information helpful. Usually a physician does not wish to have the ear canal tightly plugged with cotton, as free drainage is important. Cotton may be placed very loosely in the

outer portion of the ear canal to absorb the discharge and prevent dripping. The skin area exposed to a persistent discharge tends to become
red and raw. Petrolatum or some other bland ointment is often recommended as a help in protecting the skin from an irritating discharge.
It is also important to keep the area clean and to encourage the child
to keep his fingers away from it.

A severe head injury may result in a watery blood-tinged discharge
from the ears or nose. This is a serious sign, as it may indicate brain
damage (see Accidental Injuries Involving the Head and Back, in Chap.
9). A physician should be summoned at once for any child who has been
dazed, even momentarily, by an injury to the head.

Chronic Otitis Media. Far more insidious than acute middle-ear infection, which usually makes itself known in accents of severe pain, is
chronic inflammation of the middle ear. Sometimes this condition is
called chronic catarrh. Repeated or prolonged cold and other long-
continued irritations of the nose, the nasal sinuses, the throat, or the
passage to the ear may keep the membranes lining the middle ear in
a state of constant low-grade inflammation—a sort of mild resentment of
the constant nagging which is not provoking enough to cause a full-
blown flare-up, but which will result eventually in a thickening of the
membranes lining the middle ear and a stiffening of the joints of the
three miniature bones bridging it (see further on). The result will be progressive loss of hearing unless the condition is cleared up in time.

Mastoiditis. Nearly always some of the cells in the honeycomblike
mastoid bone which connects with the middle ear are involved in acute
middle-ear infection. The mastoid bone may be felt as a hard ridge
behind the external ear. Extensive inflammation of the mastoid process
results in mastoiditis. In children with a running ear or a recent history
of one, complaints of pain and tenderness back of the ear may be
symptoms of this infection. Acute or chronic mastoiditis is a serious condition which may now be prevented or treated successfully with sulfa
drugs or one of the antibiotics, such as penicillin, although a surgical
operation also may be necessary.

HEARING RIGHT AND HEARING WRONG

Hearing Right

The organ that makes possible the sensation of hearing is located in a
chamber about as big as a pea and shaped like a snail shell, which is
hollowed out of the bone of the skull. Its scientific name is the cochlea,
which means, literally, "snail shell."

The Organ of Hearing. The cochlea is a spiral canal which makes
two and three-quarters turns around a central pillar of bone. A ledge

of bone winding around this pillar, like the thread of a screw, divides the spiral canal incompletely throughout its entire length into an upper and a lower compartment or gallery, like this:

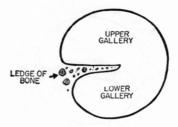

To complete the partition into two compartments, a membrane called the *basilar membrane* extends from the tip of the spiral bony ledge to the outer wall of the canal, like this:

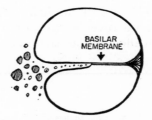

The basilar membrane is built up of a series of parallel fibers, called the auditory strings, of gradually decreasing length like the wires of a diminutive spiral piano. However, the standard grand piano has only 240 strings, whereas the human cochlea has 24,000!

A second membrane, called the vestibular membrane, stretches from the upper surface of the spiral ledge of bone to a point a short distance above the outer attachment of the basilar membrane.

So we see that the original bony canal is divided throughout its entire length into three spiral compartments or galleries. Giving them their proper names we now label the cross section like this:

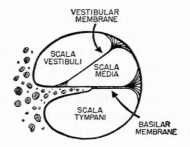

The organ of hearing (organ of Corti) lies on the floor (basilar membrane) of the scala media, or middle gallery of the canal, like this:

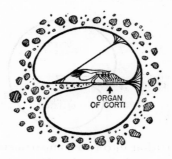

The organ of Corti consists essentially of rows of sensory sound receptors called hair cells because the surface of each one is equipped with fine hairlike processes. The tips of the hair cells are embedded in the under surface of a delicate covering (tectorial) membrane, and their bases are connected with the auditory strings of the basilar membrane, like this:

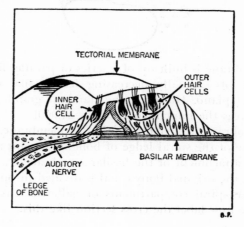

Both the upper gallery (scala vestibuli) and the lower gallery (scala tympani) are filled with lymph called perilymph ("peri-" means "around") to signify that this lymph lies around the middle chamber (scala media). The scala media also is filled with lymph called endolymph ("endo-" means "inside of").

The open end of the scala vestibuli is called the oval window, and the open end of the scala tympani is called the round window. Both the windows are covered tightly with curtains of membrane.

A diagrammatic longitudinal section of the cochlear canal as it would appear if straightened out may at this point help to make its structure clear:

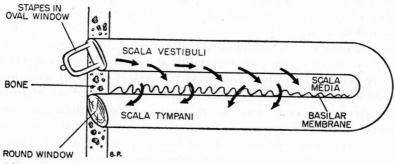

(After Best and Taylor, "The Human Body and Its Functions," p. 375.)

Ossicles of the Middle Ear. The membrane forming the eardrum and the membrane covering the oval window are connected by a bridge of three miniature interlocking bones, called ossicles, which are thrown across the gap of the air-filled middle ear (Fig. 73). The ossicle attached to the eardrum is the malleus, or hammer. Its club-shaped head articulates with the incus, or anvil, which in turn articulates with the head of the stapes, or stirrup. The base of the stapes is inserted into the oval window.

What Happens When We Hear. What happens when we hear is something like what happened in the nursery tale when, given the proper stimulus, the water began to quench the fire, the fire began to burn the stick, the stick began to beat the dog, and so on.

The eardrum vibrates when struck by sound waves set up in air by vibrating bodies just as a drumhead vibrates when struck with drumsticks. The vibrations of the eardrum are conducted over the bridge of interlocking ossicles spanning the middle ear to the membrane covering the oval window. The rocking of the stapes against this membrane sets up waves in the perilymph in the scala vestibuli. The impact of the miniature "water waves" against the delicate tectorial membrane roofing the organ of hearing sets up similar oscillations in the endolymph. These oscillations cause the basilar membrane, which forms the floor of the scala media, to move up and down. In this way the vibrations of the eardrum are reproduced in the basilar membrane. Thence they are transmitted through the perilymph of the scala tympani to the round window. The membrane of the round window, located between the scala tympani and the middle ear, acts as the shock absorber of the whole system, since it yields readily to pressure.

Each auditory string of the basilar membrane, like each piano string, is tuned to a sound (or note) of a particular wave length. Hence it vibrates in sympathy when a sound of the corresponding wave length makes the eardrum vibrate. The frequency of vibration, that is, the number of oscillations, or cycles, per second, determines the pitch of the sound we hear.

The auditory cells seated upon the vibrating auditory strings respond to tiny variations in pressure by sending impulses to the brain, via the auditory nerve, where the sound is recognized. A different sensation is received for every sound because the auditory cells seated on each string have their own separate nerve fibers. In the case of complicated sounds a number of auditory strings are thrown into vibration at the same time, the impression conveyed to the brain being the sum total of them all.

The longest and thickest auditory strings are at the top of the cochlea. They vibrate at the rate of about 16 oscillations (cycles) per second. The shortest and most delicate strings are at the base of the cochlea. They vibrate at from 20,000 to 30,000 c.p.s. (cycles per second). The ear is most sensitive to pitches ranging from 2,000 to 5,000 c.p.s., that is, for the upper two octaves of the piano.

When a sound is very loud it is felt as well as heard. Feeling is highest for sounds of low frequency, lowest for sounds of high frequency. Hence, a low rumbling sound is felt more than heard, while a high-pitched shrill note causes a very painful feeling in the ear.

The faculty of hearing sounds of high frequency is most highly developed in children and declines as persons grow older. A child with normal hearing can detect sounds of 20,000 c.p.s.; at thirty years of age the number is decreased to 15,000; and at fifty, to 13,000.

Hearing Wrong

Loss of hearing is a major handicap to learning and to normal child development. It is often the underlying cause of undesirable behavior or lack of progress in school. If loss of hearing is not recognized, a child may be scolded for seeming stupid, indifferent, or stubborn. As a result of feeling misunderstood at home and in school, he may become emotionally maladjusted—accept the idea of failure and seek compensation in undesirable ways.

Loss of hearing may result from a defect or disease in any part of the auditory mechanism. When the trouble is located in the outer ear canal, eardrum, or middle ear—the sound-conducting portions of the ear—the resulting loss of hearing is called transmission, or conduction, deafness. This is by far the most common form of hearing loss.

Loss of hearing due to a lesion of the auditory nerve is called nerve deafness. If the lesion is located along the auditory pathways leading to the auditory center in the brain, or in the auditory center itself, the resulting loss of hearing is called central deafness.

To distinguish one form of deafness from another, several tests have been devised which can be given and interpreted only by a physician. The teacher or nurse is concerned only with signs and symptoms that indicate loss of hearing whatever the type or cause.

Observations Leading to Detection of Loss of Hearing

As the teacher has no way of observing what is going on in the ears, it is easy to miss indications of loss of hearing. However, she has opportunities to make other observations that will serve as valuable leads when reported to the physician or nurse. Signs indicating chronic nose or throat trouble and early symptoms of chronic middle-ear inflammation should always be brought to the attention of a physician, since trouble of this kind so often leads to progressive loss of hearing.

Early symptoms of chronic middle-ear inflammation include a persistent feeling of heaviness, dullness, fullness, or stuffiness in the ear; and queer head noises such as buzzing, hissing, or ringing. However, these symptoms may develop so gradually that the child gets used to them before he realizes that he has good grounds for complaint. Hence other things to watch for are the characteristic behavior and appearance that usually accompany some loss of hearing. The teacher may suspect hearing difficulty when any one or more of the following signs are noted:

1. Asking to have words or phrases repeated; cocking an ear toward the speaker when addressed; answering questions incorrectly; seeming to be stupid in understanding instructions or making numerous mistakes in carrying them out; appearing to be inattentive to conversation going on about him
2. Failing to respond when called or failing to locate the source of a sound as shown by going in the wrong direction when responding to a call
3. Watching others before beginning to work or copying from other pupils
4. Bewildered facial expression showing that the child is not fully aware of what is going on about him; a look of "watchful waiting" (see Plate 14)
5. Faulty articulation out of proportion to age (a child who cannot hear words distinctly will not be able to pronounce them correctly); unnatural pitch of the voice—too high, too low, too loud, or monotonous

6. Retardation in school or poor progress in school (repetition of grades is on the average directly proportional to the hearing loss)

HEARING TESTING

The ordinary hearing tests that can be given in school do not show how much a child hears, but only the distance at which a sound can be heard. In several states a hearing test is required by law at or near the beginning of each school year. Probably most children with significant hearing loss will be discovered if all children are given a standardized audiometer test at least three times during their elementary school life, with special

Table 18. PREVALENCE OF HEARING DEFECTS

Hearing loss	Percentage
Nationwide survey of school children, 1944–1945 *	
Failure at 9 decibels...	4.4
Philadelphia fourth- and sixth-grade children, 1945–1946 *	
Hearing loss exceeding 10 per cent...	3.8
Survey of 12,360 school children in six counties of Tennessee, 1951–1952 †	
Minor defects (hearing loss without interference with perception of communication and without evidence of potentially progressive disease)............................	14.5
Major defects (hearing impaired below 15 decibels and/or history or evidence of chronic pathological condition)..	3.5

* "The School Child: Health Progress and Needs," Metropolitan Life Insurance Company.
† "Public Health Aspects of a Speech and Hearing Program," by Robert M. Foote, in J.A.M.A., Vol. 150, No. 14 (December 6), 1952.

tests between routine examinations for children who are suspected of hearing difficulty by the teacher or nurse or both.

Audiometric Testing

The audiometer is designed upon principles similar to those used in constructing radio sets. The test tones are generated electrically and conveyed by wires to the ear of the person being tested. The tone is varied in intensity or pitch by means of dials upon the front of the instrument.

Group Testing. The phonograph audiometer is used to test the hearing for speech of groups of children. Speech sounds from a phonograph record are led through the instrument and then to a receiver applied to the child's ear. From 30 to 40 children may be tested at one time.

In testing with the phonograph audiometer, the level of sounds at which speech sounds either are not heard or are heard incorrectly represents a child's degree of hearing sensitivity. Hearing loss is expressed in terms of sensation units. Children with normal hearing have no sensation-units loss.

Individual Testing. The pitch-tone, or pure-tone, audiometer is used for making individual tests. A series of pure tones, as in the tuning-fork test, are employed. It is a more reliable instrument for detecting hearing loss than the phonograph audiometer. Its frequency and intensity ranges are greater, and a given intensity can be maintained for repeated applications. It makes possible the detection of an ability to hear specific tones which range below and above the speech sounds heard in ordinary conversation. Early hearing loss frequently begins in the high-tone range. The hearing loss for each tone detected in a pitch-tone audiometer test is recorded on an audiogram.

The standard unit of measurement of sound intensity used in pitch-tone audiometer tests is the decibel, so named after Alexander Graham Bell, the inventor of the telephone. One decibel equals the least intensity or degree of loudness of any given tone at which that tone, or note, can be heard by the normal ear (normal threshold). The normal human ear has a range of auditory response of 120 decibels. In the pitch-tone audiometer, the intensity of tone is calibrated in intervals of 5 decibels.

The standard pitch-tone audiometer scale is logarithmic. Therefore, each step of 10 decibels represents ten times the previous step in decibel loss. If the loudness of a sound has to be stepped up to 10 decibels in order to make audible a sound that normally would be heard at 1 decibel (normal threshold), the amount of hearing loss is expressed as 10 decibels. A loss of 20 decibels means that the change in loudness required to hear the sound is 100 times that required at normal threshold; a loss of 30 decibels, 1,000 times; of 40 decibels, 10,000 times; and so on.

Preparation for Audiometric Testing. Many schools have their own audiometers [5] for testing the auditory acuity of children in groups and individually. In some states audiometers may be obtained on loan from the department of health or education, or representatives of the department of health or education may visit schools at stated times to conduct hearing tests.

For accuracy and efficiency it is necessary to have audiometric testing done by adequately trained persons. If the school is responsible for the testing, certain teachers or substitute teachers may be designated for special training in conducting the tests and in reading and recording the results.

In preparation for the testing of auditory acuity, the ears and their care should be the subject for study and discussion in health class. As

[5] Information concerning various types and models of audiometers can be obtained from the American Hearing Society and from its chapters and affiliates throughout the country.

in vision testing, the children should be told what is going to happen and why it is so important to find out how well they can hear.

The room selected for audiometric testing should be the quietest suitable room in the school building—usually a room on the top floor, or one with no room above, is best. The playgrounds should not be used, and there should be no marching or singing during the periods in which the tests are being given.

Results of Audiometric Testing. A child may show some hearing loss in one or both ears at the first or "sweep" test for any of the following reasons:

1. The child may actually have defective hearing.
2. Some extraneous noise may have distracted his attention.
3. He may have been unable to do his best because of nervousness. (Children unfamiliar with the use of a telephone are especially apt to be nervous.)
4. The receiver may have been improperly adjusted, or some condition, such as an acute cold, may have temporarily impaired his hearing.

Because of the many chances for error in a first test, all children who show hearing loss should be retested at least twice. One of these retests should be given on a later day, if the child has a cold at the time of the first test. Children who still show definite hearing loss are referred to their parents with the recommendation that medical advice be obtained. Usually children so referred after retesting with the phonograph audiometer are those with a hearing loss of 9 sensation units or more in the worse ear; with the pitch-tone audiometer, those with a hearing loss in the worse ear of 15 decibels for two or more of the tones of speech or a loss of 20 decibels or more for the higher tones.

Hearing Tests without the Use of an Audiometer

There are two types of rough-and-ready hearing tests that may be made by teachers in schools where it is impossible to obtain audiometric testing.

The Whisper Test. A whisper can usually be heard in a quiet room by a person with normal hearing at a distance of 20 to 30 feet, depending upon the loudness of the whisper. In making the whisper test, the residual whisper is employed. This is a whisper made with the air remaining in the lungs at the end of an ordinary expiration. It ensures the same degree of loudness of the whisper used in testing all individuals in a group.

In preparation for the whisper test, mark off a distance of 25 feet from the chair in which the child will be seated. At that distance and at intervals of 1 foot inward toward the chair, draw chalk lines parallel to one another. After the child is seated, blindfold him lightly or have him hold a card against the side of his face so that he cannot see your movements. Then instruct him to cover one ear tightly with his hand and to repeat after you each word or number that he can hear. Use either nouns of one syllable or numbers, but do not mix them. If nouns are used, tell the children in advance which ones you are going to whisper. Choose nouns that are familiar to the children. If numbers are used, the ones you are going to whisper should be recited in advance. Such numbers as 5, 19, 25, 26, 27, 33, 66, and 76 test hearing both for low tones and for sibilant sounds.

Be sure that the room is absolutely quiet. Then, standing at the line 1 foot away from the child and facing the ear being tested, whisper a few words or numbers. Enunciate clearly and breathe in and out after each whisper. If he repeats them correctly after you, move back a few feet and whisper different words or numbers. Continue moving back until the point is reached beyond which the child cannot hear. Record the greatest distance at which the child repeats the words or numbers correctly. Test both ears in this way.

The greatest distance at which about three-quarters of the class repeat the words or numbers correctly may be taken as the norm. It is not wise to use a standardized distance, such as 20 feet, as the norm because the "normal distance" will vary according to environmental noise and difference in the loudness of the whisper of the person giving the test.

Record the result for each child as a fraction of the norm. The numerator will be the greatest distance at which the sounds are audible to the child and the denominator the greatest distance at which they are heard by 75 per cent of the children under the same conditions. A hearing distance of even 3 feet less than the norm suggests some loss of hearing, and the child should be referred for medical examination.

The Watch-tick Test. A loud-ticking watch may be substituted for the residual whisper as a rough-and-ready hearing test. In quiet surroundings a loud watch is heard by the normal ear at a distance of about 3 feet. However, it is not safe to use this criterion, and the watch selected should be standardized by repeated trials on children with normal hearing. That is, if the majority of the children tested hear its tick at 3 feet, then 3 feet may be taken as the norm.

Seat the child to be tested, blindfold him, and have him cover one ear with his hand. Place the watch near the uncovered ear and ask him whether he can hear the tick. Move the watch away from his ear until the point is reached at which it ceases to be heard. From this point move the watch back toward the ear and measure and record the distance at which it is just heard. Test both ears in this way.

If a child's hearing distance is much less than the normal distance, the child should be referred for medical examination.

Referral for Otological Examination

If a hearing test given in school, together with the teacher's observations, indicates that a child's hearing apparatus should be checked by an ear specialist, it is considered unwise for the teacher or nurse to tell the parents or guardian the results of the test. The suggestion that an ear examination is advisable, without going into details, should be sufficient. It sometimes happens that findings which seem to indicate some loss of hearing, especially those of the whisper test or watch-tick test, are not confirmed by the specialist.

In making the referral for an otological examination it will be helpful to the physician making the examination to have the pooled observations of the teacher and school nurse. The record of such observations should include any history of frequent or prolonged upper respiratory tract infection, complaints made by the child of queer noises in the ears or head, and a description of behavior or appearance suggestive of hearing loss.

The Hard-of-hearing Child

In many cases of auditory loss, the hearing may be improved or progressive loss of hearing checked by early medical attention. Children whose hearing is irremediably impaired to the point at which the inability to hear constitutes a definite handicap may be helped by training in lip reading or by the wearing of a special hearing aid [6] recommended by the physician. In some school systems provision is made for lip-reading classes and for special instruction of hard-of-hearing children.

The teacher and school nurse should be informed of the otologist's recommendations in the case of any child whose hearing is impaired so that they can cooperate intelligently with the parents and physician in helping the child to make as good an adjustment as possible.

The child should know that he has hearing loss, but should not be pampered or made to feel self-conscious by too much attention. It is important for him to realize that defective hearing, like defective vision, is nothing to be ashamed of and that it is better to have others know

---

[6] The American Hearing Society gives information regarding the different hearing aids accepted by the American Medical Association. In some cities a person with impaired hearing may visit the offices of the local chapter or affiliate of this organization, try out hearing aids, and get advice. The Volta Speech Association for the Deaf provides inquirers with a list of approved hearing-aid clinics throughout the nation where audiometric testing is given and where hearing aids can be tried.

about it than to give a false impression of stupidity or stubbornness. His teacher and his schoolmates can be of great help by looking directly at him and speaking clearly when addressing him. His seat in the classroom should be assigned with a view to making it as easy as possible for him to see and hear the teacher.

Since loss of hearing imposes both a physical and a mental strain, a hard-of-hearing child should be watched carefully for signs of fatigue. Also the teacher should note on the child's health record any signs of change for the better or worse in his ability to hear and her observations as to his behavior and his success or failure in adjusting to the school situation.

DO YOU KNOW?

1. Match each structure of the eye or ear named in Group A with the condition in Group B which you associate with it.

Group A	*Group B*
Eyelid margins	Black eye
Middle ear	Pinkeye
Eyelash roots	Keratitis
Sound-conducting	Strabismus
apparatus of ear	Errors of refraction
Eyelids	Dullness of hearing during
Muscles of eyeball	head cold
Muscles of accommodation	Sties
Conjunctiva	Otitis media
Light-focusing apparatus of eye	Eye fatigue
Cornea	Blepharitis
Eustachian tube	Hearing loss (most common form)

2. Choose the correct ending for each of the following incomplete sentences:

   a. The only part of the eye that is sensitive to light is the (1) choroid coat, (2) cornea, (3) retina.
   b. The only part of the ear that is sensitive to sound is located in the (1) cochlea, (2) middle ear, (3) eustachian tube.
   c. Myopia results when (1) the eyeball is too short from front to back, (2) the curvature of the cornea is irregular, (3) the eyeball is too long from front to back.
   d. The most common cause of progressive loss of hearing is (1) acute otitis media, (2) chronic inflammation of the middle ear, (3) damage to the auditory nerve.

　　　e. A child with a hearing loss of 20 decibels should be referred for an (1) ophthalmological examination, (2) otological examination, (3) audiometric test.

　　　f. Vision of 20/40 in one eye means that the child (1) can see only half as well with that eye as he normally should, (2) must be twice as close to an object as he normally should be in order to see it clearly with that eye, (3) must be farsighted in that eye.

3. Which of the following statements are true and which are false? Rephrase each false statement so as to make it true.

　　　a. Progressive loss of hearing is always noticed by the child affected.

　　　b. A small amount of astigmatism may cause greater eye fatigue than a large amount.

　　　c. The teacher's observations are often of greater importance in detecting farsightedness than is vision testing.

　　　d. A child is likely to outgrow a tendency to squint.

　　　e. Myopia is nearly always a congenital defect.

　　　f. Children with hearing loss should be told that they cannot hear as well as other children can.

SUGGESTED ACTIVITIES

1. Obtain a vision-testing chart (letter chart on one side, symbol chart on the other) from the National Society for Prevention of Blindness. Using the vision-testing procedures outlined, take turns testing the vision of fellow students. Record the results in each case as described. If possible, arrange to test, under supervision, the vision of the children in your class in laboratory or practice school. Report in writing any observations of individual children which you think would furnish the nurse or physician serving the school with valuable supplementary information.

2. Have one student administer the watch-tick test of hearing and another the whisper test to the other students. Determine the norms for each method and record the results. Compare the two methods for consistency of findings. Then, if possible, arrange for the testing of the whole group with a phonograph audiometer. Compare the findings with those obtained from the watch-tick and whisper tests. Ask the trained person who administered the audiometric test to show the class how the instrument works and how findings are recorded. If possible, arrange also for a demonstration of the pitch-tone audiometer with a child as the subject.

3. Observe the children in your class in practice or laboratory school for the signs of possible hearing loss described in this chapter. Talk over with the nurse serving the school any children who, in your opinion, show indications of possible hearing loss.

4. As a class activity, plan ways in which you would prepare elementary school children for tests of vision and hearing.

5. Plan what you would do to help a child in your class who

   a. Was being teased by other children because he must wear a covering over one eye.
   b. Resented having to wear glasses.
   c. Did not take proper care of his glasses.
   d. Had "something in his eye."
   e. Had "something in his ear."
   f. Came in from recess with a black eye.
   g. Was hard of hearing.

6. Find out what facilities are available in your college town or your home town for providing eye examinations, otological examinations, needed eyeglasses, needed hearing aids, or instruction in lip reading for children who could not otherwise afford them. Are there special "sight-saving" classes in the local school system for children with vision defects of 20/70 or worse in the better eye after correction? If so, have a member, or committee of the class, visit one to observe and report the teaching materials and methods used.

7. Obtain from the Illuminating Engineering Society a copy of "American Standard Practice for School Lighting" (price 50 cents). Study the table giving standards of illumination in terms of foot-candles for various eye tasks in school. Then obtain a light meter from the superintendent of the local school system or from the local electric light company and measure the foot-candles of light supplied in your college or school for reading and other work at desks, tables, and other work areas in various classrooms, the library, laboratory, and workshops. Compare the findings with the standards of illumination recommended for the occupations carried on in the places surveyed. Discuss in class what teachers may do to help improve illumination in classrooms where it is inadequate.

SELECTED REFERENCES

DAVIS, HALLOWELL, ed.: *Hearing and Deafness: A Guide for Laymen*, New York, Murray Hill Books, Inc., 1947. (Anatomy and physiology of the ear, physics, and psychology of hearing, treatment of hearing loss, hearing tests, hearing aids, etc.)

Fox, SIDNEY A.: *Your Eyes,* New York, Alfred A. Knopf, Inc., 1944. (How the eye is constructed; how it focuses; how visual acuity is measured; common defects and diseases of the eye.)

HENDERSON, OLIVE G., and HUGH G. ROWELL: *Good Eyes for Life,* Tower Books edition, Cleveland, The World Publishing Company, 1943. (Methods of protecting vision in the school, home, office, and shop.)

NATIONAL EDUCATION ASSOCIATION (RESEARCH DIVISION): *Teaching about Light and Sight; a Handbook for Classroom Teachers in Elementary and Secondary Schools,* Washington, D.C., 1946.

OGG, ELIZABETH: *Save Your Sight,* Public Affairs Pamphlet No. 215, in cooperation with The National Society for the Prevention of Blindness, New York, Public Affairs Committee, 1954.

PHILLIPS, WENDELL C., and HUGH G. ROWELL: *Your Hearing—How To Preserve and Aid It,* Tower Books edition, Cleveland, The World Publishing Company, 1943. (An inexpensive edition of a well-known book by two authorities on the ears and their care.)

U.S. DEPARTMENT OF HEALTH, EDUCATION AND WELFARE: *Lighting School-rooms,* Office of Education Pamphlet No. 104, Washington, D.C., 1948.

U.S. DEPARTMENT OF HEALTH, EDUCATION AND WELFARE: *Services for the Child Who Is Hard of Hearing; a Guide for the Development of Programs,* Children's Bureau Publication No. 334, Washington, D.C., 1950.

U.S. DEPARTMENT OF HEALTH, EDUCATION AND WELFARE: *Screening School Children for Visual Defects,* Children's Bureau Publication No. 345, Washington, D.C., 1954.

Organizations

American Hearing Society. (This society publishes helpful and authoritative material on the ears and their care, audiometer testing, hearing aids, lip reading, etc. A list of the available books, pamphlets, and posters may be obtained from the society.)

National Society for the Prevention of Blindness. (This society publishes a set of selected publications on eye health of school children (mimeographed listing on request); inexpensive vision-testing equipment; and also a quarterly entitled *The Sight-Saving Review.*)

Chapter 9   ON GROWING STRAIGHT

> *Bones and Muscles*
> *Why Muscles Can Work Together in Moving and*
>   *Balancing the Body*
> *Posture and Its Appraisal*
> *Crippling Defects in School Children*
> *Common Bone, Joint, and Muscle Injuries*
> *Observing Children for Orthopedic Defects*

BONES AND MUSCLES

The strength and grace of healthy children are made possible by the working together of brain, bones, and muscles. Some acquaintance with this teamwork will help teachers to observe the deviations from normal that occur in children with orthopedic defects. Orthopedics comes from two Greek words meaning "straight" and "children." Orthopedists are doctors who are concerned with the problems that arise when the straightness of children is threatened by disease or injury or faulty habits affecting the bony framework of the body or its operation.

Bones joined together form the skeleton or inside framework of the body. The principal mechanical function of this framework is to support the weight of the body above the ground against the pull of gravity and to protect the soft structures of the body.

To permit motion the skeleton must be jointed. The principal function of the muscles attached to bones (voluntary muscles) is to move the bones by furnishing motive power at appropriate points.

Bone Architecture

Good framework material combines strength and durability with lightness. Bone is a material of this kind. It consists of a compact ivorylike outer shell with an inner lacelike structure in which innumerable tiny tubes cross and recross each other like miniature beams along the lines of the normal stresses for each particular bone. The walls of these tiny tubes are composed of concentric layers of a complex compound of calcium, phosphorus, and small amounts of other mineral salts. Embedded

393

in the mineral walls in a spiral pattern are fibers of collagen,[1] the chief organic constituent of bone.

Blood vessels run through the bony tubes. They are connected by delicate channels with the bone cells which live between the concentric layers of bone. The bone cells build and repair bone with material brought to them by the blood. The work of the bone cells makes possible the repair of a fractured bone. The blood vessels enter the bone from a thin membrane called the periosteum (from the Greek, meaning "around bone") which forms its outer covering.

The long, heavy-duty bones of the arms and legs have very thick outer shells. The shafts of these long bones are hollow and filled with yellow marrow consisting primarily of connective tissue and fat. The ends contain red bone marrow. It is in the red marrow located in the ends of the shafts of the long bones and to a greater extent in the ribs, breastbone, vertebral bodies of the spine, and the loose bony tissue between the inner and outer layers of the bones of the skull that the red cells of the blood are manufactured (see Blood and Its Composition, in Chap. 4).

The shapes of the various bones are adapted to the work they are called upon to do. If protection is the main job of the bone, its form is comparatively flat like that of the shoulder blades, the breastbone, and the bones of the cranium, or brain case. If the bone must act as a lever when moved by the muscles, it is long like those of the arms, legs, and fingers. If flexibility in a group of bones is necessary, the individual bones tend to be short like those of the wrist and ankle, or irregular like those of the spine.

Joints

The meeting places of the various bones that form the skeleton are called joints or articulations. Some joints are not movable, as in the cranium; some are only slightly movable, as in the spinal column; but the greater number are freely movable, as in the shoulders, elbows, fingers, hips, and knees.

Joints are classified according to the shape of the articulating surfaces. The four most important types of joints in the human body are the ball-and-socket (at the shoulders and hips) which permits movement in all directions; the saddle (between the vertebrae of the spine) which permits movements backward, forward, and sidewise; the hinge (for example, between the bones of the fingers) which permits movement in only one direction; and the rotary (usually combined with a hinge joint, as in the

[1] Collagen is a gelatinous protein substance which can be changed by boiling into glue or gelatin.

elbow) which allows the bones to rotate at the joint like a corkscrew or a key in turning a lock.

The articulating surfaces of all movable bones are protected with pads of elastic cartilage, and the bones are held in place at the joint by ligaments, that is, bands made up of tough fibers. Nearly all movable joints are enclosed in a capsule of very tough material strengthened by ligaments and lined with a membrane that secretes a thick fluid like white of egg. This fluid acts as a lubricant to reduce friction between the articulating surfaces. In addition the joint capsule is padded with small sacs filled with fluid called bursae. These little "water cushions" are also interposed beneath and between muscles, tendons, or other structures at places where friction would otherwise develop. Chronic irritation of the bursae causes the painful inflammatory condition called bursitis.

The Skeleton

The skeleton is composed of more than 200 separate bones and is divided into two main parts: (a) the axial skeleton, consisting of the spine and its immediate outgrowths, the head, ribs, and sternum (breastbone); and (b) the appendicular skeleton, consisting of the supporting framework for the limbs (the shoulder girdle and the pelvic girdle) and the bones of the arms and legs themselves.

Some knowledge of the way in which the skeleton is put together and moved, and of the functions of its various parts under normal conditions, will be helpful to the teacher in recognizing deviations from normal in posture and gait, and in dealing with bone injuries.

The Axial Skeleton

The Spinal Column. The spinal column is the mainstay of the body. All the rest of the skeleton is directly or indirectly attached to it.

The spine is made up of 33 (or 34) vertebrae which are piled on top of one another to form a strong hollow column. The vertebrae are bound firmly together by strong ligaments, and between each two is placed a pad of tough elastic cartilage. These pads act as shock absorbers and allow free movement of the neck and trunk.

The vertebrae differ in size and shape, but except for the top two, they are built very much alike. Seen from above, as in Figure 76A, a typical vertebra consists of a solid disk, or body, with an arch of bone extending from it. Spinous processes project sideways and backward from the roof of the arch. The "spines" give the spinal column its name. We see and feel as rounded knobs the "spines" that project backward (Fig. 76B).

The spinal cord passes through the hollow column formed by the arches of the superimposed vertebrae much as the string passes through

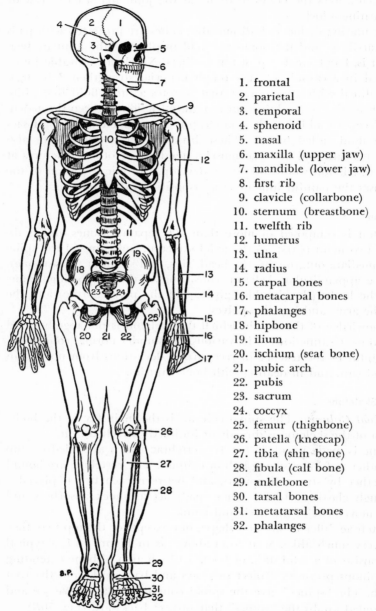

1. frontal
2. parietal
3. temporal
4. sphenoid
5. nasal
6. maxilla (upper jaw)
7. mandible (lower jaw)
8. first rib
9. clavicle (collarbone)
10. sternum (breastbone)
11. twelfth rib
12. humerus
13. ulna
14. radius
15. carpal bones
16. metacarpal bones
17. phalanges
18. hipbone
19. ilium
20. ischium (seat bone)
21. pubic arch
22. pubis
23. sacrum
24. coccyx
25. femur (thighbone)
26. patella (kneecap)
27. tibia (shin bone)
28. fibula (calf bone)
29. anklebone
30. tarsal bones
31. metatarsal bones
32. phalanges

FIG. 74. The skeleton of a fifteen-year-old boy, front view.

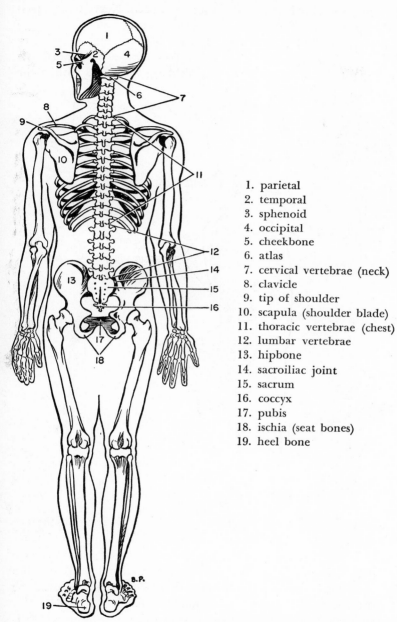

1. parietal
2. temporal
3. sphenoid
4. occipital
5. cheekbone
6. atlas
7. cervical vertebrae (neck)
8. clavicle
9. tip of shoulder
10. scapula (shoulder blade)
11. thoracic vertebrae (chest)
12. lumbar vertebrae
13. hipbone
14. sacroiliac joint
15. sacrum
16. coccyx
17. pubis
18. ischia (seat bones)
19. heel bone

FIG. 75.   The skeleton of a fifteen-year-old boy, back view.

the hollow centers of spools strung together (Fig. 76C). Nerve trunks pass out from the spinal cord between each two vertebrae.

.The first two vertebrae differ from the rest because they must carry the head. The top vertebra is called the atlas because it supports the head as the giant Atlas was fabled to uphold the heavens. Unlike the

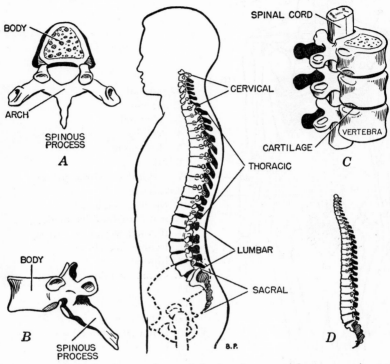

FIG. 76. The spinal column of an adult showing normal curves. *A*, vertebra viewed from above. *B*, vertebra viewed from left side. *C*, spinal cord passing through vertebral arches. *D*, spine of a ten-year-old child.

others it has no body but consists of a bony ring with cups on the top surface into which knobs of the occipital bone of the skull (see further on) fit. This makes it possible to move the head backward and forward like a rocking chair. A bony peg rising from the second neck vertebra (the axis) forms a pivot around which the atlas rotates like a revolving platform when the head is turned from side to side.

Viewed from front or back the spine is seen to be a column which is narrower at the top than at the base. The vertebrae at the upper levels of the column are small and light because they do not have so much to carry. The vertebrae at the base of the column are large and stout because they must carry the accumulated weight of all parts above them.

Viewed from the side, the part of the spinal column toward the front of the body is curved like the letter S. This long S-curve makes it possible to distribute body weight properly in the upright position (see Posture, further on).

The Sternum (Breastbone) and Ribs. The sternum is a plate of bone about six inches long situated in the middle of the front wall of the thorax. It provides points of attachment for the collarbones and ribs (Fig. 74).

The ribs are semiflexible arches of bones enclosing the thoracic cavity. At the back the 12 pairs of ribs are attached by strong ligaments to the 12 thoracic vertebrae which form the upper outward curve of the spinal column. In front the first seven pairs of ribs are attached to the sternum by means of elastic cartilages. Each of the next three pairs is attached to the cartilage of the pair immediately above. The front ends of the last two pairs hang free, and so they are called floating ribs.

The cagelike arrangement of bone and cartilage enclosing the chest is an admirable compromise between stability and mobility. The heart and lungs must be protected; yet they cannot be shut up in a rigid box as the brain is, since the lungs must expand in breathing and the heart must beat. The mobile elastic chest cage is more readily influenced by exercise and the deep breathing that goes with it than is any other part of the skeleton. In boys and girls who engage in athletics, the circumference of the chest is larger than in those who have little physical exercise.

The Skull. The skull rests upon the top of the spinal column. It is divided into two parts: the cranium, or brain case, and the face.

The eight immovable interlocking bones of the cranium (Figs. 74 and 75) form a firm case for the brain. Four of these bones (the occipital, two parietals, and the frontal) are typical flat bones, composed of two dense layers—the outer one thick and tough, the inner one thinner and more brittle—with loose bony material sandwiched between. Hence they are admirably fitted to protect the delicate brain from ordinary bumps and blows.

Blood vessels and nerve trunks pass in and out of the brain through openings at the base of the cranium. The largest opening is an outlet for the constricted part of the brain where it narrows down to join the spinal cord.

The very hard temporal bones, one on each side of the cranium, are hollowed out in a series of very small peculiarly shaped cavities to contain, in addition to the organs of hearing, the organs of equilibrium, which record where we are in space and the direction in which we are moving (see The Balancing Apparatus, further on).

In front of the opening in the occipital bone through which the spinal cord passes downward from the brain, the irregular wedge-shaped sphenoid bone rises steeply. At the top of this declivity is the tiny saddle-shaped fossa, or ditch, in which the pituitary gland (see Observations Related to Endocrine Activity, in Chap. 3) is lodged. The sphenoid bone and the sievelike ethmoid bone in front of it separate the brain cavity from the face.

The olfactory bulbs of the brain rest on a ridge of the ethmoid bone. From these bulbs the olfactory nerves (nerves of smell) pass downward into the nasal cavity through openings in the bone. It was once believed that the mucus, which we know as a secretion of glands in the mucous membrane of the nose lining, was a secretion of the brain. Excessive secretion of mucus, as in a head cold, was considered to be the means by which the brain cleansed itself of noxious "humors."

The face extends from the eyebrows to the chin (Fig. 74). The 13 immovable bones of the face form the bony settings of the eyes, nose, and mouth. The only movable one is the lower jawbone (mandible) which moves up and down and sidewise on sliding hinge joints in speaking and chewing.

Eye Sockets. Above and on either side of the mid-line of the face are the bony orbits, or sockets, for the eyeballs and their related structures. The promontories represented by the bones of the cheek and upper nose guard the eyes against blows. Lacrimal ducts, through which tears drain into the nose (see Fig. 62), pass for part of their distance through canals in the lacrimal bones located in the inner walls of the eye orbits.

Head Sinuses. Above each eye in the frontal bone, on each side of the nose in the maxillae, and in the sphenoid and ethmoid bones in the floor of the cranium there are air-containing sinuses or cavities. Reference has been made to the troubles caused by the swelling shut of the very narrow openings through which the sinuses lead into the nose (see Respiratory Infections in Particular, in Chap. 5).

The Nose. The upper part of the bridge of the nose is formed by two small bones placed side by side. The lower part of this bridge is made of cartilage. The nasal bones are rather easily broken by a direct blow.

A thin bone shaped somewhat like a plowshare (the vomer) forms part of the septum, or wall, which divides the nose into two corridors. Sometimes it deviates, that is, bends to one side or the other, thus making the nasal corridors of unequal size. The inferior turbinates are thin, scroll-shaped bones situated in the outer wall of each nostril. They overhang the corridors below and help to increase the area over which the air passes as it flows through the nose (see Fig. 38). A deviated septum and enlarged inferior turbinates cause some of the more common nose troubles, largely owing to their interference with the ventilation and drainage of the nasal passages and sinuses.

The Jaws. The two maxillae meet in the mid-line of the face to form the whole of the upper jaw. Together with the palatine bones, they form part of the floor of the eye orbits, the floor and sides of the nose cavities, and the roof of the mouth.

The mandible, or lower jawbone, is shaped like a horseshoe. It is the largest and strongest bone of the face. The curved portion forms the chin, and the two perpendicular portions are joined by sliding hinge joints to the temporal bones of each side of the cranium just in front of the ears. Fractures and dislocations of the lower jawbone are quite common injuries. Sockets in the lower rims of the maxillae and the upper rim of the curved portion of the mandible hold the teeth.

The Hyoid Bone. The base of the tongue is supported by a small U-shaped bone called the hyoid bone (*hyoeides* in Greek means "U-shaped"). This bone also furnishes attachments for some of the tongue's muscles. The hyoid bone may be felt in the neck, just above the Adam's apple.

The Appendicular Skeleton

In human beings a more or less complete division of labor with regard to the two important activities, locomotion and grasping, is reached by the assignment of locomotion to the legs and feet and of grasping to the arms and hands.

Arms and legs are essentially much alike—one long strong bone nearest to the trunk, then two bones, then several little bones, forming in the arm the wrist and hands, and in the leg the ankle and foot. However, legs are not nearly so flexible as arms. Sturdy support for the body's weight with a reasonable degree of movability is all that is required of legs. The series of bony levers making up the arms and legs are attached to the trunk by a supporting framework consisting of two girdles—the shoulder girdle and the pelvic girdle.

The Shoulder Girdle. This girdle is composed of the two long double-curved collar bones (clavicles) and the two flat triangular shoulder blades (scapulae). Each clavicle is attached at one end to the sternum and at the other end to a scapula (Figs. 74 and 75). Each scapula is a large, flat triangular bone placed point down over the upper ribs at the back of the thorax. Folded back across its upper portion is a prominent ridge of bone which ends in a projection (the tip of the shoulder) to which the outer end of the clavicle is attached.

The Arm. The bone of the upper arm (the humerus) has a rounded head, or knob, at the top which fits into a shallow cuplike depression in the scapula, forming a ball-and-socket joint. The shoulder joint is the most freely movable joint in the body and is quite easily dislocated. The curved lower end of the humerus fits into a big notch at the upper end of the large bone of the forearm (the ulna) to form the elbow joint. The lower end of the ulna articulates with a disk of cartilage which separates it from the wrist.

The other bone of the forearm (the radius) is shorter and smaller than the ulna, to which it is attached near both ends. The lower end of the radius articulates with the top row of bones forming the wrist.

The Wrist. The wrist is composed of eight small irregularly shaped bones (the carpals) united by ligaments. They are arranged in two rows of four bones each and articulate with one another as well as with the bones of the forearm and hand, thus permitting a wide range of motion.

The Hand. The five bones of the palm (metacarpals) articulate at their bases with the lower row of wristbones and at their heads with the first row of finger bones (phalanges). The 14 finger bones (three in each finger and two in each thumb) give the hand its extraordinary flexibility. The hands are the copartners of the brain in performing all acts of manual dexterity and skill. The thumb is the most important "finger." A good thumb and only one finger make a far more useful hand than four fingers minus a thumb.

The Pelvic Girdle. The two hipbones are joined together in front by a narrow bridge of bone. They form, with the sacrum and coccyx behind, the basin-shaped ring of thick, heavy bones known as the pelvic girdle (Figs. 74 and 75). This girdle with its attached muscles forms the floor of the abdominal cavity and also serves to attach the lower limbs to the trunk.

The broad, flaring upper portion of each hipbone (the ilium) forms the prominence of the hip. It is joined tightly at the back with the sacrum to form the strong sacroiliac joint. The sacroiliac joints permit little motion in the lower back region but are subjected to very great pressure from the weight of the trunk. One of the common causes of low-back pain is strain of the sacroiliac joints caused by improper lifting of too-heavy objects or by poor distribution of body weight in walking or standing. The ischium is the lowest and strongest portion of the hipbone, while the pubis is the narrow portion which curves around to join its mate on the other side in front to form the pubic arch.

The Thighs. In the outer surface of the hipbone, at the junction of its three portions, there is a deep socket into which the round head of the femur, or thighbone, fits, forming a ball-and-socket joint. The femur is the largest and strongest bone in the skeleton. Its lower end is wider than its upper end and is divided into two large knobs which articulate with the tibia, or shin bone, and the patella, or kneecap, to form the knee joint. The head of the femur is not so easily dislocated as is the less tightly fixed head of the humerus but is much more difficult to put back into its socket.

The Knee. The knee joint is a strong hinged joint which is protected by the patella, or kneecap. The patella is a small triangular bone situated in the tendon of the big muscle (the gastrocnemius) which is used in kicking.

The Leg. Anatomically speaking, the word leg is used for that portion of the lower limb between the knee and the ankle. It contains two bones, the tibia and the fibula.

The lower end of the tibia, or shin bone, is much smaller than its upper end and is prolonged downward to form the inner rounded prominence of the ankle. The fibula, or calf bone, is attached at the top to the tibia. The lower end is prolonged downward to form the outer pointed prominence of the ankle. The fibula is smaller than the tibia and in proportion to its length is the most slender of all the long bones. It is more often fractured alone than is the tibia, but fracture of both bones is a common injury.

The Ankle, Foot, and Toes. The ankle joint is formed by the junction of the lower ends of the tibia and fibula with the talus (one of the tarsals). The seven tarsals, or anklebones, are firmly bound together by tough ligaments. They are larger and more irregularly shaped than are the wristbones. The heel bone is the largest and strongest, as it must transmit the weight of the body to the ground and form a lever for the muscles of the calf of the leg in walking.

The shape of the foot is roughly like that of a triangle, with the apex at the point where the leg bones fit over the talus. The long arch, or instep, of the foot is formed by five bones (the metatarsals) which extend from the ankle to the base of the toes. The phalanges forming the toes are similar in number and arrangement to the phalanges forming the fingers.

Muscles

The word muscle comes from the Latin *musculus* meaning "little mouse," because the spindle shape of the muscles that move bones resembles that of a running mouse. Each skeletal muscle is a bundle of muscle fibers running lengthwise, and its surface is covered with a protecting sheath.

The fibers of these bone-moving muscles, which are under the control of the will (voluntary muscles), are striped crosswise or striated, whereas those of the involuntary muscles, which bring about movements in the large organs of the interior (the viscera) are smooth. The action of smooth muscle is slow and rhythmical, like the movements of an earthworm, while that of striped muscle is swift.

The special characteristic of muscular tissue which enables it to do its work is the ability to contract—become shorter—and then to relax so that it can be stretched—made longer. Voluntary muscles work in pairs; when one of the pair contracts, its opposite relaxes. Although we think of this action as entirely voluntary, we merely establish the conditions that make alternate contraction and relaxation possible when we command movement in arms or legs or other parts of the body. After these conditions have been set up, movement "happens," just as it rains or snows when the conditions are right.[2]

Each voluntary muscle is attached by one end to a bone and by the other end to an adjoining bone or to skin or cartilage or some special organ like the eyeball. The ends of muscle fibers that connect muscle with bone have become coarse and hard, forming tough white cords called tendons. Some tendons run through a sheath of dense strong tissue lined with membrane which secretes a lubricating fluid like that which "oils" the joints.

The Mechanics of Muscle Contraction. It is easy to see how voluntary muscles bring about movement. When a muscle attached at one end to one part and at the other end to another part becomes shorter and thicker (contracts) it is bound to pull the two parts toward each other in the direction permitted by the joint. This may be demonstrated by lifting the hand to the shoulder. The bulge of the contracting biceps pulling the forearm toward the upper arm is clearly seen. While this contraction is taking place the muscle at the back of the arm (the triceps) is stretched. The tension set up in the stretched muscle produces a tendency to contract and reverse the movement, that is, to extend, or straighten out the arm. The continuous alternating contraction and relaxation (stretching) of thousands upon thousands of muscle fibers in paired muscles produce movements of infinite variety in all activities such as walking, running, jumping, climbing, and riding a bicycle.

Muscle Tone. No healthy muscles are ever completely relaxed. Reflex action keeps them always in a state of mild steady contraction like that of a violin string that is correctly tuned. This state is called muscle tone. Its purpose is to make the muscles springy and ready for instant action

2 TODD, MABEL ELLSWORTH, "The Thinking Body," p. 7, Hoeber, New York, 1937.

when impulses demanding movement come from the brain. If our muscles had to take up slack, so to speak, before starting to pull on the parts to which they are attached, they would use up about a fifth more time and energy in performing their tasks. Muscle tone also has a steadying effect, much as a firm hold on a steering wheel helps to steady a vehicle. When the muscles that work against the pull of gravity are completely relaxed, as in fainting, for example, the body collapses.

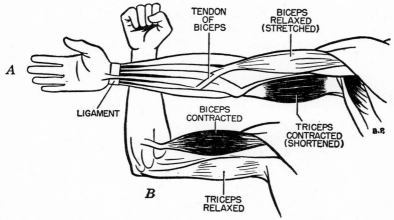

FIG. 77. Diagram showing alternate contraction and relaxation in paired voluntary muscles.

Muscle tone varies according to the general condition of the body. This can readily be observed especially in the face. In healthy rested children the skin of the face is tight and firm. When children are tired or ill, the tone of the facial muscles is decreased and their faces look weary. The slumping or sagging of the body associated with fatigue posture (see further on) is also due partly to a decrease in muscle tone.

The Chemistry of Muscle Contraction. It has been demonstrated in recent years that a powerful chemical called acetylcholine is liberated from the muscle terminals of motor nerves. Acetylcholine serves as a transmitter of the nerve impulses to muscle fibers and so makes them contract. The energy for contraction is obtained through a series of highly complicated chemical reactions, involving the breaking down and rebuilding of various substances present in muscle. Free oxygen is not required in the first stage when the muscle actually contracts. It is necessary only in the recovery stage to rewind the chemical clockwork so that the muscle can contract again.

Toward the end of the contraction stage, the muscle fuel glycogen breaks down into lactic acid. Lactic acid is a waste substance in the sense that it must be quickly eliminated or changed. At the beginning of the recovery stage, part of this lactic acid is oxidized, with the result that carbonic acid (CO_2 plus H_2O) is formed. The carbonic acid diffuses into the blood and is carried to the lungs for removal from the body in the form of carbon dioxide and water. The energy obtained from burning a portion of the lactic acid is used to change the remainder back into glycogen.

Even when a muscle is completely at rest, glycogen is being broken down into lactic acid. This happens so slowly that the lactic acid can be removed as quickly as it appears. During strenuous muscular activity, however, lactic acid is formed faster than it can be partly burned and partly changed back into glycogen. The accumulation of excess lactic acid would force the muscles to stop working in a very few minutes if nothing were done about it.

The temporary measure that allows us to continue strenuous exercise for more than a few minutes is called "muscle buffering." It consists in the neutralization of excess lactic acid by the alkaline salts dissolved in the blood and body fluids.

Why Muscles Get Tired. By the mechanism of buffering we are able to keep on working in spite of the fact that lactic acid is being produced in far greater quantities than there is oxygen available to remove it. But as soon as the muscle buffers are exhausted and the reaction of the muscle reaches a certain acidity as a result of the formation of lactic and other acids, further contraction becomes impossible. This is the condition known as muscular fatigue. Once a muscle is fatigued a rest interval is necessary for its complete recovery.

The capacity of the muscle buffers varies in different individuals. It is well known that some people can work harder and longer without fatigue than others can. Knowing when to stop before the muscles become exhausted is an important part of the hygiene of physical exercise. Not only do exhausted muscles cause pain and discomfort, but also chemical injury may be done by the piling up of lactic acid. Such muscles may become overtense and unable to relax, or they may lose tone and become flabby. If muscles are allowed to rest when they begin to slack off in their work, they "come back" far more quickly than when they are driven to the point of giving up completely.

WHY MUSCLES CAN WORK TOGETHER IN MOVING AND BALANCING THE BODY

In discussing sensations (see Chap. 3) reference was made to the somatic sensations that make us aware of the movements and relative positions of our limbs and other parts of the body. Sensory receptors in skeletal muscles and in the tendons and joints and the organs of equilibrium in the skull furnish us with this information.

Muscle Coordination

The term "kinesthetic" (from two Greek words meaning "to move" and "sensation") is used in referring to the group of receptors in muscles, tendons, and joints which transmit and receive the impulses calling for muscular coordination. The sensory receptors involved are stimulated by pressure or stretch. The strains and stresses set up in muscles, tendons, and joints during muscular contraction provide this stimulation. As a result of reports received in the central nervous system from these receptors, individual muscles and groups of muscles are guided in working together to produce smooth, finely adjusted, and effective movements. Such coordinated movements would be impossible without this guidance.

The Balancing Apparatus

The feeling of equilibrium or balance is derived from sensations that arise in special organs lodged in three tiny tunnels—the semicircular

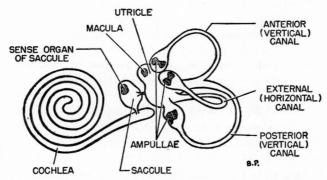

FIG. 78. The organ that makes it possible for us to keep our balance (the semicircular canals) is shown at the right, the organ of hearing (the cochlea), at the left.

canals—in each temporal bone near the inner ear. These tunnels are no bigger than capillaries. Because of their complicated windings, they are called labyrinths, and keeping our balance is referred to as the labyrinthine function. Lodged in each bony labyrinth is a membranous labyrinth. The membranous labyrinth is filled with fluid, and a similar fluid lies between it and the walls of the bony labyrinth.

The semicircular canals lie in planes that are approximately at right angles to one another (Fig. 78). The one toward the outside of the head is the horizontal canal; and the ones toward the front and back are the vertical canals. The planes in which they lie correspond to the three dimensions of space: length (backward and forward), breadth (from side to side), and height (upward and downward).

At one extremity of each canal there is a bulblike arrangement (ampulla) which contains a sense organ (crista) consisting of a gelatin-covered mound of sensory hair cells for the reception of messages about body movement. Both extremities of each canal open into a roundish chamber called the vestibule. In the vestibule two fluid-filled sacs—the utricle and the saccule—are situated. The openings of the semicircular canals lie in the utricle, which also communicates with the saccule by a small canal (Fig. 78). The utricle contains a sense organ (macula) for the reception of messages about body position. It consists of a gelatin-covered plaque of sensitive hair cells upon which are situated tiny concretions of lime. These curious crystals are the otoliths (called ear stones or ear dust). The layer of gelatinous material upon which they are situated is the otolith membrane. The saccule also contains a sense organ which is similar in construction to that of the utricle.

Now, how does this miniature balancing apparatus work? The fluid flowing past the sensitive hair cells in the ampullae of the semicircular canals when the head is moved provides the stimulus that provokes the sending of impulses about body movement. Response is made only to the change in velocity (speeding up or slowing down) of forward or backward movement or to changes in direction of movement, that is, curving from a straight line to one side or the other, upward or downward.

Because of the shifts in current in the fluid of the semicircular canals and their influence on the hair cells, we can tell when we move forward or backward, when we start or stop, when we slow down or speed up, when we deviate to the right or left, when we are going upward or downward. And with this awareness of the direction and speed of our movements, we automatically make the compensatory *movements* of our eyes and limbs required to maintain our equilibrium.

The sense organs in the vestibules of the semicircular canals are responsible for the muscular reactions resulting from the *position* already induced by stimulation of the hair cells in the ampullae of the canals. When the head is in the erect position, the otolith membrane exerts an even pressure on the hair cells. But when the head is tipped one way or another, the otolith membrane is pulled by gravity to the inclined side away from the hair cells. This stimulation sets up reflexes which exert a tonic effect on the muscles and reflexes responsible for a return to the upright position from an inclined position (righting reflexes) and for the compensatory positions of the eyes.

Dizziness

Dizziness, or vertigo, is a common sensation. We may deliberately make ourselves dizzy by spinning around several times, as children do in playing certain games.

In rapid rotation the brain becomes confused. It is accustomed to associate a displacement of fluid in the semicircular canals in one direction with a movement in the opposite direction. For example, when we go forward, the fluid in the horizontal canals bends the hair cells backward. This gives the sensation of going forward. When we spin round and round in an erect position, the fluid in the horizontal semicircular canals bends the hair cells backward, just as if we were going forward, but on stopping the fluid in the canals bends the hair cells in the opposite direction. This gives us the feeling of revolving in the opposite direction. However, our legs and our common sense tell us that we are standing still. We solve that problem by assuming that it is the world and not ourselves that is spinning about us in the reverse direction. That is, we are "dizzy." To keep from falling, we sway to one side or the other, or backward or forward, depending upon the position of the head during rotation.

Vertigo arises from many other causes besides rotation, for example, alcoholic intoxication, seasickness, swinging, gastrointestinal upsets, infections, and high blood pressure. Often people complain of feeling dizzy when they are nauseated or very tired or about to faint. Unusual or abnormal actions of the eye muscles also produce vertigo. Just as the semicircular canals influence eye movements, so eye movements influence the semicircular canals. Dizziness is therefore a common effect of eye fatigue or of watching the landscape from a rapidly moving vehicle, such as an automobile or train. Eye movements also play a part in motion sickness.

Whatever may be the precipitating cause of dizziness, the sensation arises immediately as a result of excitation of the semicircular canals or of their connections in the brain or spinal cord.

The Cerebellum

Incoming impulses from the muscles of the face, limbs, and trunk, and from the organs of equilibrium, are routed to a part of the brain called the cerebellum. This "little brain" (cerebellum is the diminutive for cerebrum) lies just below the cerebrum and is shaped somewhat like a moth, that is, it has a long narrow body and two "wings" spread out over the medulla oblongata. Through its connections with motor nerve centers in the brain and spinal cord the cerebellum sends the outgoing impulses based on "information received" which either decrease or increase the tone of the muscles. These finer adjustments of tone and the distribution of tone between various groups of muscles, depending upon conditions existing at the moment, are essential for maintaining posture and for performing complicated and precise voluntary movements. "In other words, upon the general background of tonus established through connections in the cord and brain, the cerebellum makes the final delicate adjustments which enable the various muscle groups to act smoothly and harmoniously, i.e., as a cooperative whole, in a given movement." [3]

When the cerebellum is damaged by disease or injury these nice cooperative actions are impossible. As a result voluntary movements become jerky and irregular. This condition is called ataxia. It is thought to be largely due to weakness and loss of tone of the muscles themselves rather than to failure of coordination.

POSTURE AND ITS APPRAISAL

It is customary to think of posture as meaning the general impression of body carriage conveyed to the beholder when one is stationary. The familiar command "straighten up" is associated with this conception. To "straighten up" somehow implies ramrod stiffness—the disciplining of a body that has fallen into bad habits.

Actually, good posture means much more than "standing straight." It is the use of all parts of the body to maintain balance with ease and grace. It involves constant shifts in position of various parts of the body in relation to other parts at all times and under all circumstances. These shifts are the reactions of the muscles within to physical forces acting upon the body from without. The primary force is gravity. Like all other objects on the earth's surface the body is continuously subject to a pull toward the earth's center and must incessantly meet it.

The center of gravity of any body is the center of its mass or weight. In the upright human body, this is located in the back wall of the pelvis in line with the spinal column. When the center of gravity is "supported" —that is, when a line dropped from it passes through the base of any body—that body is in equilibrium and will not fall. The base of the upright human body is represented by the feet and the area between them.

When body weights are distributed too far to one side or the other, or too far to the front or back of the spinal column, the center of gravity is thrown off center. In that case, the body is off balance and compensat-

[3] BEST, CHARLES HERBERT, and NORMAN BURKE TAYLOR, "The Physiological Basis of Medical Practice," p. 928, Williams & Wilkins, Baltimore, 1945.

ing shifts of weight must be made to withstand the pull of gravity. The muscles are called upon to bear the burden of these off-center weights. Yet the bones properly are the weight bearers, and the main job of the muscles is to move the bones. They should not be called upon unnecessarily for the support of off-center weights in order to maintain equilibrium. Not only does an unbalanced adjustment of weights strain the muscles, which must contract against the pull of gravity, but also the bones themselves must suffer.

The three principal segments of body weight are the head, the thorax, and the pelvis. The weight of the head rests on top of the spinal column and the combined weights of the head, thorax, and pelvis are supported on the heads of the powerful thighbones. Gravity pulls perpendicularly on the erect body, that is, down through the vertical axis represented by the spinal column. Body balance in the erect position, or good posture, as we are accustomed to call it, means simply that body weights are so adjusted that they stay up by themselves on the two leg props with the least possible effort on the part of the muscles to hold them in line.

The curves of the spinal column are of great assistance in this adjustment of weights. If the spinal column were straight up and down, like the pole of a clothes tree, for example, the weight of the organs of the chest and abdomen would pull the body forward out of balance, just as several heavy overcoats suspended on the hooks at the front of a clothes tree would topple it over. As it is, the four spinal curves, alternately convex and concave, not only balance each other but also divide up the weight of the three loads supported by the spinal column —the head, the chest, and the pelvis—and balance these loads as they accumulate toward the base represented by the heads of the thighbones.

It would be a mistake to think that balance is brought about in the body by opposing weight for weight at equal distances from the center line as can be done in draping clothes on a clothes tree or building a tower of blocks or a snow man. The weights are there to be supported in the positions assigned to them. And the weight bearers—the bones— have muscular attachments which can shift such burdens within limits as the need arises.

It sometimes happens, however, that for one cause or another—weak muscles, chronic fatigue, poor posture sense, or bone deformities, for example—these weights must be held out of balance more or less constantly. The essential supporting mechanism—the spinal column—must then adapt itself to these off-balance weights. It can do this because its flexibility enables it to accent or even to distort the normal curves so as to compensate for poor weight distribution. This throws extra work on the muscles and ligaments about the individual vertebrae.

Also, other muscles, those in the neck, for example, may be called upon to bear more weight than is their proper task.

Postural Characteristics According to Age

As children grow from babyhood into childhood and on into adolescence, their posture tends to change. That is why an indispensable factor in observing children for postural characteristics is the age of the child observed. It is important not to confuse real defects with conditions that children normally outgrow.

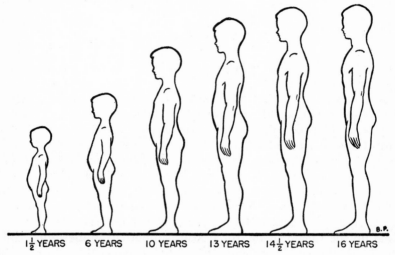

$1\frac{1}{2}$ YEARS   6 YEARS   10 YEARS   13 YEARS $14\frac{1}{2}$ YEARS   16 YEARS

FIG. 79. Postural characteristics of a boy according to age.

The characteristic changes in posture come about through skeletal growth and development and the strengthening of the child's muscles as he learns to sit up, creep, stand, and finally to walk, run, climb and take part in active play. When the child enters school the abdomen normally protrudes because of the relative weakness of the abdominal muscles. In proportion to the prominence of the abdomen the lower spinal curve (lumbar curve) normally is exaggerated (lumbar lordosis).

The muscles of the shoulders, neck, and upper trunk all help to hold the head, shoulders, and chest in position. It is normal for young children to hold their heads slightly forward and to have chests deeper in proportion to their breadth. The chest gradually becomes broader and flatter and the shoulder blades closer together during the years immediately before and after entering school. Good muscular and skeletal development makes it possible for the child of school age to carry his head, neck, chest, and shoulders in good balance.

Table 19. INFLUENCES ON POSTURE

Factors contributing to good posture	Factors contributing to poor posture
A sound body free of physical defects, deformities, or frequent or long-continued infections	Poor eyesight or hearing, which tends to make a child lean forward or sideways or cock his head or take other unnatural positions in order to see or hear better
	Deformities such as those caused by congenital defects (clubfoot, wryneck, etc.), by infections (polio, tuberculosis of bones and joints, osteomyelitis), or by nutritional deficiency (rickets)
	Chronic focal infections such as diseased tonsils or adenoids which may contribute to substandard health
Good nutrition, attained by a well-balanced diet including liberal supplies of foods that help to build bone and muscle, and supplemented by some good source of vitamin D (fish-liver oils, vitamin-D milk, etc.)	Poor nutrition caused by a diet in which overemphasis is placed on energy foods (cereals, breads, potatoes, sweets, etc.) at the expense of bone-building and muscle-building foods (milk, meat, eggs, green vegetables, fruits, etc.) or by some condition that interferes with the digestion, assimilation, or metabolism of the food eaten
Freedom from fatigue attained by plenty of sleep and rest, good nutrition, peace of mind, and keen interest in life	Overfatigue caused by too little sleep and rest, malnutrition, anxiety, or lack of interest in life
Symmetrical muscular development through varied outdoor activities and games	Lack of symmetry in muscular development through too little vigorous exercise or not enough variety in exercise
Freedom of movements made possible by wearing well-fitting, well-planned clothing and shoes which put no strain on muscles, bones, or soft tissues	Restraint of movements by clothes which are too tight or too heavy and by shoes that are not long enough or wide enough or flexible enough to fit the feet properly
Good sitting positions made possible by comfortable chairs that support the back with the feet resting firmly on the floor	Strained sitting positions caused by chairs that are so large that the back and feet are unsupported for long periods
Good sleeping positions made possible by beds of ample length, with firm, flat springs and mattresses and light nonrestricting bedclothes	Strained sleeping positions caused by sagging bedsprings, too-soft mattresses, or pillows so large that the neck is bent forward

With the increase in strength of the muscles of the abdomen and but-
tocks in the adolescent period, the abdomen flattens and the lumbar
curve straightens out so that the lower back becomes less "hollow." In
this period types of body build (see Chap. 2) become apparent, and the

General Appearance	A well-poised body giving the effect of good physical and emotional health and enthusiasm for life.	
Head	Head erect, or inclined slightly forward, with chin in.	
Shoulders	Level and down in back with flat shoulder blades. Upper outer tips curved slightly forward in front.	**Back** Normal spinal curves. Neck curves slightly inward (toward front); upper back curves outward ("dorsal prominence"); lower back curves inward ("lumbar curve"). † Buttocks curve outward.
Chest	Moderately elevated and symmetrical.	
Abdomen	Flat from the hips to the breastbone.*	
Thighs	Curved slightly backward.	
Knees	Straight, barely touching each other.	
Feet	Toes pointed straight forward, inner sides parallel, body weight carried on balls and outer sides of the feet.	

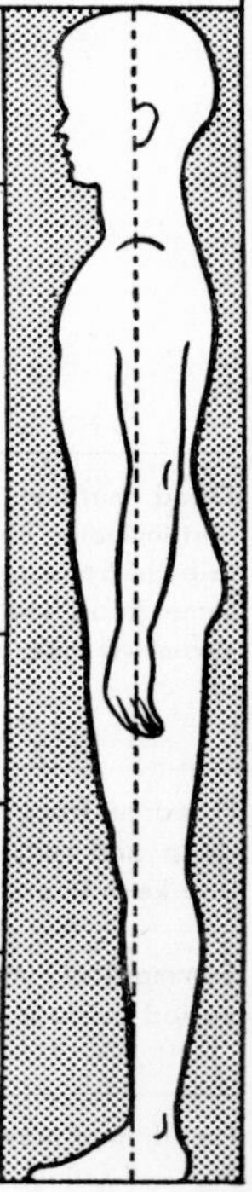

D.P.

* A protruding abdomen is normal in pre-adolescent children.
† A straight upper back and an exaggerated lumbar curve are normal in
childhood.

FIG. 80. Good posture.

posture reveals trends which become definite characteristics in adult life.

It is at this time also that posture faults are most likely to develop.
However, it may be difficult to distinguish between real defects and
temporary maladjustments or retarded development of the mature spinal
curves. For example, girls, becoming aware of their maturing breasts,
may try to conceal them by letting their shoulders droop forward, and
tall weedy boys may slouch to make their height conform more nearly
to that of their associates. Also, as has been pointed out (see Chap. 2),
rapid growth during adolescence may result in awkwardness in body

movements. On the other hand, adolescent youngsters learn that excellence in sports and games and an attractive physical appearance contribute to social success. This idea furnishes a strong incentive for efforts to correct postural defects and to develop the strong muscles that help to maintain good body balance.

General Appearance	A slumping body giving the effect of substandard health, fatigue, inadequacy for life.	
Head	Markedly inclined forward.	
Shoulders	One shoulder higher than other. In back, shoulder blades stick out.* In front, shoulders sag forward.	Back Exaggerated curvature of dorsal prominence (kyphosis, or "humpback"); extreme curvature in lumbar region (lordosis); deviation of spinal column to right or left (scoliosis, or lateral spinal curvature).
Chest	Markedly depressed or deformed ("funnel breast" or "chicken breast").†	
Abdomen	Markedly protruding and sagging.	
Thighs	Curved slightly forward.	
Knees	Slightly bent, close together.	
Feet	Toes pointed outward, ankles turned inward, body weight carried on inner sides of feet.	

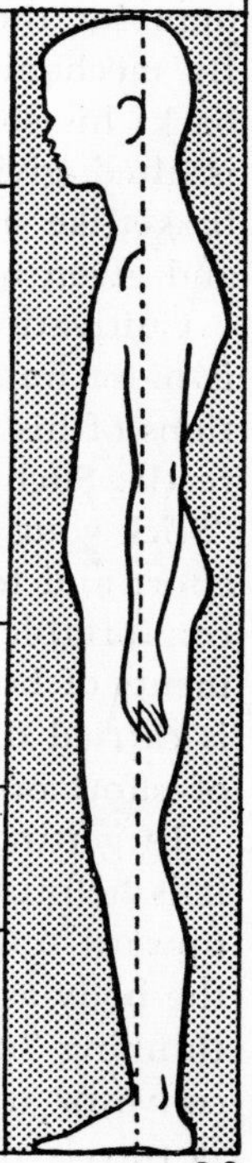

B.P.

*Slight pressure only required to place the fingers definitely under the inner border or tips of the shoulder blade.

† Funnel-like depression at the end of the breastbone or a forward bulging of the breastbone with the ribs sloping away to the sides.

FIG. 81. Poor posture.

Although various postural characteristics considered undesirable in physically mature individuals are normal in earlier stages of development, it is important to be on the lookout for conditions that persist beyond the time at which they should be outgrown. Conditions that should be referred for attention at all ages are exaggerated front-to-back (natural) spinal curves, lateral (unnatural) spinal curves (scoliosis, see further on), chest deformities, flat feet (see further on), cramped toes, and generally poor body balance due to lowered muscle tone (see also Table 21).

The "Feel" of Balance

Long before the child enters school he has succeeded in his early efforts to cope with the forces of gravity and has developed skill in maintaining the equilibrium of his erect jointed body over a small base of support. His spine has been changed from a horizontal beam for the suspension of weights, as in the all-fours, or quadruped, position, to a vertical column for the support of weights in the two-footed, or biped, position. By mechanical necessity his spine curves forward at the small of his back; his shoulders fall back and down of their own weight; his chest is lifted, giving room for lung expansion; and by a series of shelflike and basketlike arrangements, the organs of his trunk are being supported and given maximum space for full and vigorous function.

Cultivation of the child's posture sense, or over-all feeling for balance, is more important than the singling out for correction of separate portions of his anatomy which, from an adult point of view, are held incorrectly. Such commands as "Push your head up," "Hold your chin in," "Stick your chest out and up," and "Throw your shoulders back" suggest effort and tension and, in effect, are futile. Good posture is relaxed and comfortable, graceful, attractive, and efficient. When the various segments of body weight are well poised one above the other, total weight is carried directly to the seat or ground by the bones with a minimum of effort on the part of the muscles.

In getting the "feel" of balance in oneself and in observing children, it is helpful to think of the weights at the front of the body as passing upward toward the shoulders and head and the weights at the back of the body as passing downward from the top of the spine to the base. In thinking "up in front and down in back" it is useful to visualize a belt conveyor traveling upward with loaded cups and dumping the load as it travels downward. In this up-in-front–down-in-back picture of erect posture, the head, shoulders, chest, abdomen, and back have the appearance noted in Figure 80.

Standing and Walking

No one ever stands completely still. Standing, even when the body weights are perfectly balanced, requires delicately graded alternations of muscle tension which may be as tiring as walking. The entire weight of the body in standing is borne by the feet. It is the arched formation of the feet that gives them the power to absorb and distribute the crushing weight of the body. The heel bone gives one point of contact of the foot with the ground, and the heads of the metatarsal bones give the other points of contact. In proper standing the weight of the body is distributed between the heel and the ball of the foot with weight felt as falling slightly to the outside of the foot.

In walking, the motion of the ankles, feet, and toes is produced largely by the action of muscles located in the legs. These muscles are connected with the bones they move by long tendons. The muscles of the legs act as shock absorbers in walking and running. They also are largely responsible for holding the feet in proper position (see further on). These muscles are strengthened as the child learns to stand and walk. As he becomes increasingly active, they help to keep his whole body in good balance.

When the feet are used correctly in walking, the toes point straight ahead, the inner sides of the feet are parallel with each other, and the knees just miss each other. In stepping forward, the heel and the ball of the foot should strike the ground as nearly as possible at the same time, and the weight of the body should fall toward the outer edge.

Feet and Their Troubles. Babies who are learning to stand and walk are very unsteady on their feet. All toddlers have knock-knees (knees together with ankles far apart) and some degree of toeing out of the feet. At about the age of six, the knees normally become straight and the toeing out is greatly decreased. In some children, however, knock-knees and toeing out remain to become the defect known as "pronated feet."

A child with pronated feet walks with the toes pointed outward and the ankles turned inward. This position increases the strain on the ligaments and fatigues the muscles on the inner side of the foot. As a result the foot sags on the inner side below and in front of the ankle. The long arch of the foot is weakened and in severe cases "flatfoot" or "fallen arches" develop. In children with pronated feet the heels of the shoes are usually worn over on the inside (Plate 15). Often faulty weight bearing and weak or flattened arches can be corrected by special exercises for the feet.

Some foot deformities are the result of congenital conditions. One of the most common is talipes (Latin for "clubfoot"). In this condition the foot is twisted out of shape or position. Some forms of clubfoot may be acquired after birth by disease or injury. Pigeon toe (a toeing-in position of the feet) may be due to rickets (see further on).

Sitting

In sitting, the weight of the head and trunk properly falls on the rocker-like lower portions (ischia) of the hipbones (see above). For this reason the ischia are sometimes called the seat bones. It is easy to fall into bad habits of sitting because the very fact of having a seat permits almost any slumps or contortions of the body. Standing would be impossible with the spinal sag in which many people sit for much of the time. Children sit in school for a large part of the school day. It is inevitable that habits in sitting will be formed. To make possible natural comfortable sitting positions so that such positions will become habitual is the object of adjusting chairs and desks or tables to the individual child in school.

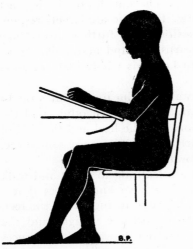

FIG. 82. Good sitting posture in school made possible by an adjustable desk top and an adjustable seat that gives proper support to the lower back and thighs.

What the seat must accomplish is to ensure that when the child relaxes in it his posture will be erect and comfortable. This means that the pelvis must sit vertically with the forward lumbar curve preserved and the shoulders hanging back freely. The points of the seat bones, the crests of the hipbones, and the shoulder tips should be in the same plane, and in this position there should be no uncomfortable pressures, strains, pushes or pulls.

One of the bad habits that are easiest to fall into in the seated position is that of sliding forward so that one sits on the end of the spine instead of upon the seat bones. In the typical stoop or slump characteristic of a tendency to slide forward on the seat or to pitch forward at the shoulders, the pelvis tips backward so that a plane passing through the seat bones and the crests of the hips would pass far behind the shoulders. Then the forward curve in the small of the back disappears and there is a single continuous outward curve from seat to neck with consequent displacement and crowding of the organs of the chest, abdomen, and pelvis.

To prevent any forward-sliding tendency, the seat should slope slightly backward. It should also provide support under the thighs when the feet are extended forward, but should not be so high or so deep, front to back, as to cause pressure under the knees when the child sits as far back as the back support permits. The seat should be just high enough above the ground to allow the feet to rest comfortably on the floor while the lower part of the back is supported by the chair back. When sitting at a desk or table it should be possible to rest the forearms on the top surface with the shoulders level and relaxed.

Posture and Fatigue

The fatigue caused by poor posture is due to the muscular and nervous strains required to balance the body when the weight masses are out of line. The fatigue associated with malnutrition, the effects of illness, a focal infection, skeletal or muscular defects, nervous strain, or emotional instability is usually reflected in poor posture. Fatigue posture in a sitting position is illustrated in Plate 16.

The tendency of the body to slump is the chief characteristic of fatigue posture. Practically all of us have experienced loss of muscle tone after a hard day's work or a period of prolonged or strenuous physical exercise. We start out feeling fresh and rested, with erect body and springy step. At the end of the day or after a long hike, for example, we have actually become smaller with rounded shoulders, perhaps, and forward-drooping head, because the tone of the muscles is decreased.

A period of rest or a good night's sleep is all that is needed to cure temporary fatigue. Even if children tend to droop at the end of the day, there is nothing to worry about if they come to school in the morning looking rested and glowing with vitality. It is only when a child seems to tire more easily than most children do or habitually slumps in his seat or moves in a listless manner that medical attention is needed to determine the cause.

CRIPPLING DEFECTS IN SCHOOL CHILDREN

Statistical reports provided to the Children's Bureau by the 53 official state agencies administering the crippled children's programs under the Social Security Act (including the 48 states, the District of Columbia, Alaska, Hawaii, Puerto Rico, and the Virgin Islands) give the most comprehensive picture of the number of children and young people who are handicapped more or less seriously by crippling impairments. Congenital malformations brought more children to the program during 1950 than any other diagnostic group (see Fig. 83). Almost as many children had conditions affecting the bones and organs of movement (excluding congenital malformations or other conditions elsewhere classified), for example flatfoot, curvature of the spine, osteomyelitis, and arthritis. Poliomyelitis and cerebral palsy (see Chap. 5) rank third and fourth as handicapping conditions.

Congenital and Prenatal Conditions

A large number of orthopedic defects are the result of congenital conditions and prenatal influence and injuries of the nervous system that occur during birth. As one would expect, congenital defects and birth injuries are responsible for the majority of orthopedic handicaps in the

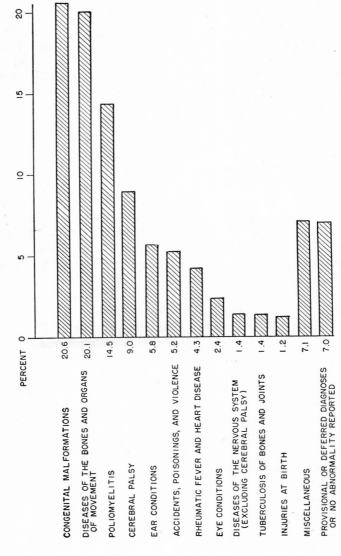

FIG. 83. The wide range of impairments included under the Crippled Children's Program in 1950. (From "Diagnosis of Children Served in the Crippled Children's Program 1950," Children's Bureau Statistical Series No. 21, United States Department of Health, Education and Welfare, 1954.)

Table 20. DIAGNOSES OF CHILDREN SERVED IN THE CRIPPLED CHILDREN'S PROGRAM 1950 *

Diagnosis †	No. of states and territories including diagnosis in definition of crippling condition	No. of children	Children who received physician's services, prevalence rate per 10,000 population
Poliomyelitis, acute and late effects..........	47–51	31,109	5.8
Cerebral palsy..........................	52	19,334	3.6
Accidents, poisoning, and violence...........	51–52	11,031	2.1
Clubfoot, congenital or unspecified..........	52	14,662	2.8
Osteomyelitis and periostitis, except tuberculous	52	3,895	0.7
Rickets, active and late effects..............	46–52	2,032	0.4
Curvature of spine except congenital or late effect of poliomyelitis or tuberculosis.......	52	5,278	1.0
Tuberculosis, except respiratory.............	51	2,910	0.5
Injuries at birth, except cerebral palsy and epilepsy..................................	48–51	2,574	0.5

Sources: Prevalence rates computed by Metropolitan Life Insurance Company.

Diagnosis—United States Department of Health, Education and Welfare, Children's Bureau Statistical Series No. 21, "Diagnoses of Children Served in the Crippled Children's Program 1950."

Population—United States Census of Population 1950 P-B 1, Table 38.

* Includes District of Columbia, Alaska, Hawaii, Puerto Rico, and Virgin Islands. Excludes Arizona, which did not participate in the Crippled Children's Program under the Social Security Act during 1950.

† Represents primary diagnosis.

early years of life. Since many of these defects can be corrected or their effects greatly minimized by early treatment, they become numerically less important in the later years of childhood, and acquired defects become numerically more important.

When uncorrected, deformities due to congenital conditions or birth injuries cause various abnormalities in posture or gait. Some of the more common are briefly described here.

A child with clubfoot may walk on the heel with the toes elevated, or on the toes or forepart of one or both feet, or on the inner borders of the feet with the feet turned outward (pronated), or on the outer borders with the feet turned upward (supinated).

In uncorrected congenital dislocation of the hips, the child may walk with a waddling gait, "duck walk," but usually he can get about with relative freedom.

In wryneck (torticollis), caused by the contraction of the muscles on one side of the neck as the result of a birth injury, the head is tilted to one side and the child looks as if he were "listening to his shoulder."

There are several other forms of wryneck other than congenital torticollis, some of which are temporary in character. Most of us are familiar with the tendency to screw the neck into the least painful position when the neck muscles feel sore and tight as a result of a cold or "a touch of rheumatism." Uncorrected hearing and visual defects often affect the position of the head. Habitually cocking one side of the head toward the speaker is a common indication of loss of hearing in one ear. A high degree of astigmatism is so closely associated with wryneck that ocular torticollis is a well-recognized condition.

Wryneck also may be a sign of hysteria or a form of tic or habit spasm in which there is spasmodic contraction of the neck muscles, producing deviations of the head.

In Erb's palsy, caused by injury at birth to the network of nerves supplying the muscles of the arms (brachial plexus), there is paralysis of one or both arms. The affected arm hangs limply at the side and is turned inward toward the body. The child, when asked to bring the palm of his hand to his mouth, will "kiss the back of the hand" instead.

Orthopedic Impairments Caused by Infections

The infections, other than poliomyelitis, that are responsible for an appreciable number of orthopedic impairments among children are osteomyelitis and tuberculosis.

Osteomyelitis. Osteomyelitis is an infection of the bone which is usually caused by staphylococci, although other bacteria—notably the streptococcus and the pneumococcus—may be responsible.. This infection occurs most frequently before the age of ten. It may be acute or chronic. Destruction of the bone takes place in both forms but is less active in chronic osteomyelitis. The long bones, especially the large bone of the leg (tibia), are most often affected.

Following a compound fracture, osteomyelitis may develop as a result of infection with staphylococci introduced from the skin. It may develop, however, without apparent injury.

The infection may remain localized at one spot or spread to the marrow and thence throughout the bone. In acute osteomyelitis there is, in addition, general poisoning by the staphylococcal toxin, and in about half the cases the staphylococci invade the blood stream.

The onset of acute osteomyelitis is usually abrupt with signs of severe illness, accompanied by pain, swelling, and redness at the site of the infection. It is extremely important to get the child under a doctor's care at once, because the use of sulfadiazine or penicillin in the early stages of osteomyelitis often averts a serious illness and extensive bone destruction with severe crippling.

Tuberculosis of the Bones and Joints. Tuberculous infection of the bones and joints was a prominent cause of disability only a generation ago. Since then it has decreased markedly in frequency and now accounts for less than 1½ per cent of all orthopedic defects among children under twenty-one. The hipbones, the knee joints, and the spinal vertebrae are the most common sites of tuberculosis of the joints and bones in the young. Tuberculosis of the spine is known as Pott's disease. With adequate treatment it may be arrested, but it frequently leaves the child with a permanent deformity.

Rickets

Rickets is the most important nutritional disease of the bones. Once a very common cause of crippling, it is now rarely encountered in our country (see Table 20). The steady rise in standards of living, rapid advances in the science of nutrition, and the wide use of scientific knowledge in child feeding as a result of public health education account for this progress in the control of rickets.

The fundamental feature of rickets is a disturbance of calcium-phosphorus metabolism, which results in the defective formation of bones. Vitamin D is essential for the proper utilization of calcium and phosphorus to form normal bone. Since the bones are relatively soft and pliable in rickets, they are easily bent and twisted by muscular action, and the natural curvatures of the long bones become exaggerated. The various bone deformities that develop include knock-knees, bowlegs, lateral spinal curvature (scoliosis), malformation of the chest (pigeon breast, chicken breast, funnel breast), narrow pelvis, soft depressible areas in the skull, and bosses or beadings on the sides and ends of bones (for example, "beading of the ribs").

Vitamin-D deficiency is a prime factor in the cause of rickets. In the absence of vitamin D, the body has difficulty absorbing adequate amounts of calcium or of phosphorus. Rickets is essentially a disease of the first two years of life, when bone formation and growth are most active. Infantile rickets seldom commences after the second year nor does it usually progress beyond that time. However, the deformities caused by it persist. Late or juvenile rickets is essentially the same as infantile rickets but occurs in older children—from four to sixteen years. Juvenile rickets is very rare in our country.

In the days before the antirachitic properties of fish-liver oil were discovered, the incidence of rickets was high in cities in the northern latitudes. There are fewer hours of sunshine annually in northern localities than in southern localities, and the sunshine in the winter months is less intense and contains a smaller proportion of the shorter ultraviolet rays. Moreover, the high content of smoke, dust, and water vapor in the atmosphere of large cities acts as a screen to keep most of the ultraviolet rays available from reaching the earth. Also children in temperate climates spend a large part of their time indoors in winter and expose less of their bodies when they are outdoors. Hence, with the discovery of the role of vitamin D in the prevention and treatment of rickets and its importance in promoting optimum growth, cod-liver oil and other fish-liver oils rich in vitamin D have been a great boon to babies and children everywhere.

Spinal Curvature

Curvature of the spine, especially lateral curvature (scoliosis), is among the leading causes of orthopedic impairment among children. There are few individuals with ideally curved spines. In observing children we are concerned only with pronounced degrees of deviation from the technically ideal form. A distinction is usually made between structural scoliosis, in which there is a true spinal deformity, and postural or functional scoliosis.

Congenital weakness of the ligamentary apparatus or muscular attachments of the spine accounts for some cases of structural scoliosis. In others, disease of the vertebrae or the supporting muscles may be to blame.

Postural or functional scoliosis in children is rare. It may result from assuming poor body positions habitually. This poor posture is usually caused by weak musculature. Postural scoliosis can be overcome voluntarily when contributing causes, such as poor nutrition, too little rest, or improper seating, have been eliminated and the child's cooperation in correcting his faulty posture, through corrective exercises, has been secured.

Other Crippling Conditions

There is a large group of miscellaneous conditions that cause crippling but are of relatively infrequent occurrence. Of these the most common are disturbances of the normal process of bone growth at the epiphyses (see pp. 33–34). The cause of such disturbances is unknown; in some cases it may be congenital. The bones most frequently affected are the upper end of the thighbone (femur) and less commonly the upper end of the large leg bone (tibia). Children from five to ten are most likely to be affected. The onset is gradual. The early sign is a limp, which may be associated with pain and tenderness.

COMMON BONE, JOINT, AND MUSCLE INJURIES

Luckily, children are not so likely to be seriously injured as a result of falls, bumps, and blows as are older people. Their bones are supple, like green sticks, and bend easily but do not readily break. The parts of children's bodies that are most likely to be injured are heads, arms and legs, and collarbones.

First-aid Supplies

In schools that do not have a special room equipped to deal with emergencies, it will be helpful to have on hand in the first-aid cabinet the following supplies for use in case of broken bones and sprains:

Splinting materials
    Splints made of yucca, basswood, wire mesh, or similar light rigid
        material
    Roller bandage or strips of cloth for fixing splints in place
    Cotton or cloth for padding splints
Triangular bandages for slings, etc.
Scissors
Safety pins

Fractures in General

A fracture is a break in a bone. There are, in general, two kinds of fractures: simple and compound. In a simple fracture there is no wound extending from the ends of the broken bone out through the surface of the skin. In a compound fracture, there is a wound made either from the inside by one or both ends of the broken bone or from the outside by the impact of whatever caused the fracture. The movements of a person with a simple fracture or careless handling by the person giving first aid may cause the sharp ends of the broken bone to pierce through the tissues and skin, thus changing the injury into a compound fracture.

Compound fractures are more serious than simple ones both because of the greater likelihood of shock (see Shock, in Chap. 4) and because of the danger of infection.

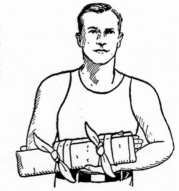

Broken Limbs

A child who has broken an arm or leg may complain of pain or tenderness in the region of the break, and the pain becomes more severe on pressure or attempts to move. Swelling is moderate to severe and appears quickly. The injured limb may look deformed because of overlapping of the broken ends of the bone, or it may be

FIG. 84. Splint for a broken forearm (*Figs. 84–86, from "First Aid," Metropolitan Life Insurance Company.*)

crooked or shorter when compared with its uninjured mate.

In a compound fracture, the broken ends of the bone may protrude through the flesh. There may be severe bleeding.

When in doubt, handle as a fracture any injury of the limbs received as the result of a fall or blow. The physician, nurse, or other person in the school authorized to give first aid should be summoned at once. In the meantime, keep the child quiet and warm. Stop severe bleeding if it is present (see pp. 179–181). Do not let him move or try to move him. If it is essential to move him before expert help arrives, splints must first be applied.

Any rigid material which is long enough to reach beyond the joints above and below the break will serve as splints. "Tailor-made" splints

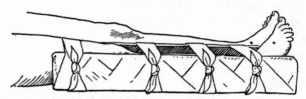

FIG. 85. Splint for a broken leg.

should be used if available. If not, splints may be improvised by using a light board, firm pillow, a thick magazine, or several layers of newspaper. The splint should be well padded with cloth or cotton on the side that goes next to the injured limb. It should be bandaged in place firmly but gently, taking care not to place bandages over the point of the fracture.

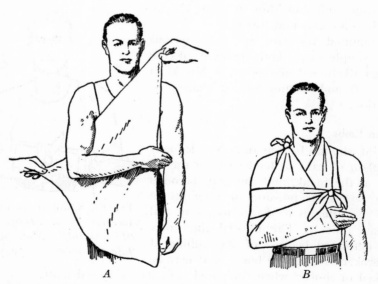

A   B

FIG. 86. A, first position for adjustment of a triangular bandage to make a comfortable sling. B, completed sling for a fractured collarbone.

Broken Collarbone

Fracture of one of the clavicles is a common injury, as these two bones are long and slender. As the injured person stands or sits with his arms hanging, the shoulder on the injured side is lower than the other shoulder and tends to droop forward. The broken ends may be felt by running the finger gently along the clavicle. Place a large pad of cotton or soft material in the armpit and between the chest and the arm so that the elbow is held away from the side of the body. Put the arm on the injured side in a large triangular bandage sling, with the hand raised to a point slightly above the elbow. Then tie the arm to the body firmly but not too tightly with a long strip of cloth (Fig. 86, *A* and *B*).

Accidental Injuries Involving the Head and Back

Injuries to the head and back sometimes result in damage to the brain or spinal cord. For that reason the right handling is extremely important.

Blow on the Head. If a child has received a severe blow on the head or has fallen on his head or has lost consciousness for even a very short time, a fracture of the skull or brain concussion should be suspected.

If a blow on the head has bruised the brain without fracturing the skull, the injury is called a "concussion."

In fracture of the skull there may be a scalp wound and a fissure or crack in the skull, or there may be a crack on the skull without a wound. There may be bleeding from one or both ears and sometimes from the mouth and nose and into the eyes.

Even though the victim of a severe blow or fall on the head is conscious and no wound or bruises or other evidence of injury can be seen, he must be handled as a case of skull fracture or concussion of the brain. The first-aid treatment for both is the same.

First send for the nurse or doctor. Then lay the child on his back with his head raised by a pillow or pad if his face is flushed; or on a level or slightly lower than his body if his face is pale. Keep him comfortably warm and quiet. Give him nothing by mouth. Check severe bleeding if it is present, by placing a gauze compress over the wound. If the child must be moved, lift and carry him in a horizontal position.

In one type of skull fracture, bleeding between the brain and skull (intracranial hemorrhage) occurs. Quite often a blow (possible from a baseball or stick) produces only a short period of unconsciousness. Following recovery a headache is the only complaint. But after a varying length of time (from a few hours to days) the child becomes confused and dopey. Gradually his somnolence deepens to unconsciousness. Immediate medical attention is necessary if the child's life is to be saved.

Injury to the Back. Wrong handling of a child who has suffered a severe back injury may result in damage to the spinal cord, thus causing permanent paralysis. If possible the child should be allowed to remain where he is and be kept warm and quiet until the doctor or nurse arrives. No attempt should be made to "straighten him out," and he should not be permitted to sit up or to lift his head even for a drink of water.

If it is necessary to move a child with a back injury, it is important to find out, if possible, what, if any, part of the spine has been injured. This information will determine the manner in which the child should be transported.

When the spinal cord is pressed, stretched, torn, or severed, paralysis of the muscles occurs below the point of the injury. If the child is conscious he may be able to tell where he has been hurt. Pain in the neck or back may be the only symptom. If the child cannot move his hands or fingers, his neck is probably broken. If he can move his fingers, but not his feet and toes, his back is probably broken. Nevertheless, the child may be able to move both his hands and feet and yet have a spinal injury.

The victim of a broken neck should be transported *face upward* on a door, a wide board 5 feet or more in length, a shutter, or a similar rigid support. If his back is broken, he should be transported on the rigid support *face downward*. If the location of the spinal injury is unknown, he should be transported face upward.

Two or more persons will be needed to place the child in the correct position onto the board or door. His body *must be moved as a unit*, with no tilting forward or backward of the head in case of neck fracture, and with no bending of the back in case of fracture of the spine below the neck. Transportation must be accomplished without jolts or jars, and the child must be kept warm during the process.

Dislocations

In a dislocation the bone at a joint is forced out of place. As a result the ligaments and cartilage at the joint and the blood vessels, tendons, nerves, and muscles in the neighborhood are usually damaged. The joints that allow a wide range of motion (the shoulder and hip joints) and those which are subject to strong muscular pulls or blows (the finger, thumb, toe, knee, lower jaw, and elbow joints) are the ones that are most frequently dislocated.

The injured joint is painful and swelling is rapid. It has a misshapen appearance when compared with a similar joint. Motion is limited or completely lost and there may be numbness due to pressure on nerves.

Have the injured person lie down and keep him quiet and comfortably warm. Support the joint in a comfortable position. Apply cloths wrung out in very cold water to relieve the pain and to contract the blood vessels, thus reducing swelling.

Amateur attempts to put back in place (reduce) dislocations are practically certain to result in further injury to the damaged tissues. For that reason the aid of a physician should be secured promptly for the proper treatment of a dislocation. The only ones that a layman may attempt to reduce in an emergency are those of the fingers, toes, first (upper) joint of the thumb and big toes, and the lower jaw.

Reducing a Dislocation of a Finger (or Toe). Face the injured person and with one hand grasp the finger firmly on each side of the dislocated joint. With your other hand pull the end of the injured finger straight toward you. At the same time gently press on the dislocated joint until the bone slips into place. *Do not try to reduce a dislocation of the joint at the base of the thumb (the joint nearest the wrist).*

Reducing a Dislocation of the Lower Jaw. When the lower jaw is dislocated the jaw sags downward, and the person is unable to close his mouth.

Place the person in a chair and have an assistant steady his head from behind. Wrap your thumbs in several thicknesses of cloth to protect them from the person's teeth. Then place your covered thumbs on the lower teeth, well back on each side, and with your fingers grasp his jaw under the chin. Press first downward and then backward with your thumbs and upward under the jaw with your fingers. As the jaw starts to close, slip your thumbs off the teeth toward the inside of the cheeks so that they will not be caught between the teeth when the jaw springs into place.

Sprains

A sprain is caused by a sudden wrench which violently stretches, twists, or actually tears the ligaments supporting a joint and the capsule that envelops it. The ankle and wrist joints are the ones most often sprained. Twisting the foot and turning the ankle in walking or some other form of exercise or in a fall are common causes of sprained ankles.

A sprained joint is very painful right after the injury. Swelling develops rapidly; discoloration develops somewhat later, as a result of ruptured blood vessels. A sprain may be only a slight injury from which recovery is rapid, or it may be very severe. What seems to be a bad sprain may be a fracture. Therefore, a physician should be consulted for a sprain unless it is very slight.

Raise the injured joint in a comfortable position so that it will get less blood. Support a sprained wrist in a large triangular sling; for a sprained ankle or knee, place pillows or folded coats under the leg. Then apply compresses wrung out in cold water. As the swelling recedes, hot applications help in hastening the return of the tissues to normal.

Strains

A strain is like a sprain but it is the muscles or tendons that are injured rather than the joint ligaments. Usually a strain is caused by over-stretching. The muscles of the back are often strained as a result of heavy lifting in an improper position. In severe strains the muscle fibers or tendons may be torn.

There is sharp pain or cramp at the time of the injury. Stiffness and soreness develop within the next few hours and movement is painful.

Rest and the application of heat give relief. Gentle rubbing helps relieve pain and is useful in stimulating the circulation. For severe strains, especially of the back muscles, a physician should be consulted.

OBSERVING CHILDREN FOR ORTHOPEDIC DEFECTS

Many children with orthopedic disabilities come to orthopedic specialists or clinics too late to have the condition corrected by the simpler forms of treatment. Defects found during the early years of life are more amenable to treatment because the body framework is then more plastic. It is believed by many persons doing orthopedic work that the ortho-pedic problem in the school could be solved by having teachers learn to discover orthopedic defects as they have learned to discover visual and hearing defects.

> In examining for orthopedic defects it would not be the function of the teacher to say why the pupil limps, or why the posture is poor or spine curved, but to select the children who have these conditions for an examination by a physician or orthopedist. The problem of discovering orthopedic de-fects and preventing increased deformity in those having them should be undertaken by the schools. As the majority of school systems have assumed the responsibility of the crip-pled child's education, vocational training and adjustment to society, so they should assume the responsibility for early detection of crippling conditions and see that children are directed to the proper places for treat-ment.[4]

At the present time, however, there are very few school systems in which teachers or nurses are trained to give screening examinations for

[4] "Orthopedically Handicapped Children," Report of the Sub-committee on Ortho-pedically Handicapped Children, Board of Education of the City of New York, p. 53, The Board, New York, 1941.

Table 21. INDICATIONS OF ORTHOPEDIC DEFECTS *

Point of observation	Deviations from normal
Gait..................	Limping
	Dragging of foot
	Spastic gait (each leg swings forward as a solid piece in a narrow arc with the feet turned inward and toes scraping along the floor; called the "scissors gait," as the legs tend to cross each other in walking)
	Waddling gait (called the "duck walk")
	Walking on the toes or heels
	Walking on the inner or outer borders of feet
Feet and toes..........	Habitually standing with toes pointed in (pigeon toes) or out
	Standing with ankles rolled inward (weak ankle posture)
	Heels of shoes worn down on the inside or outside in a short time
	Complaints of pains in the feet or legs
	Reporting of corns, bunions, blisters, calluses on balls of feet
Legs..................	Bowlegs
	Knock knees
Back and shoulders......	Upper back humped (kyphosis)
	Lower back hollow (lordosis)
	Round shoulders
	One shoulder considerably higher than the other
	Complaints of backache
Chest.................	Abnormally high
	Hollow-chested
	Narrow-chested
Arms and hands........	Limp, or flaccid
	Deformities of fingers
Head and neck.........	Head abnormally large
	Wryneck (head tilted to side)

* See also Figures 80 and 81.

orthopedic defects. To give such examinations it is necessary to remove the greater part of the clothing. However, the teacher can make valuable observations even when the child is fully clothed if she is alerted to the importance of noticing deviations from normal in gait and posture. In junior and senior high schools, where the children wear gymnasium suits while participating in physical-education activities, the physical-education teacher occupies a strategic position for observing abnormal spinal curvatures, winged scapulae, and other defects not easily detected in the fully clothed child.

In Table 21 are listed deviations from normal which teachers can observe in children dressed in ordinary clothes or which children may report to her.

The School Program for Orthopedically Handicapped Children

Not all of the deviations from normal listed in Table 21 are crippling enough to require special educational procedures. For some children, enrollment in special classes or tuition at home is necessary, but the majority of crippled children can adjust to the regular school curriculum and attend regular classes.

Practically all those who work with orthopedically handicapped children agree that such children should attend regular classes if it is at all possible for them to do so. The effects of isolation in special classes may tend to accentuate feelings of difference and inadequacy in some children. In regular classes handicapped children have an opportunity to make normal social adjustments as well as to benefit from general school activities, such as assembly and extracurricular programs.

It has already been pointed out that the teacher who has a crippled child in her class can do that child the greatest service by unobtrusively making it possible for him to become as independent as possible. Physically handicapped children have the same sort of feelings as normal children. They want to be as much like the others as possible, to have fun and companionship and a chance to excel—to amount to something in their own eyes and those of their peers. It is the teacher's privilege to set the stage for the making of good social adjustments and for successful participation in school activities.

The handicapped child's physical welfare is usually taken care of under medical supervision by the physical education department and the physical therapy department in school systems that have these facilities. Otherwise, it is necessary for the child's teacher to work in cooperation with the physician and nurse serving the school and the parents to see that the proper care is given.

If the child is already under the care of an orthopedic specialist, the school should know what treatment, such as braces or physical therapy, has been prescribed. With this knowledge, those in contact with the child in school can give the encouragement that is often needed to win his cooperation and that of his parents in following the recommendations. If the child obviously needs orthopedic care and is not getting it, the family should be given the necessary information as to the location of clinics or other facilities in the community for diagnosis and treatment.

There is another group of children found in practically every school who have no definite orthopedic defects but who show signs of poor body mechanics, poor coordination, poor nutrition, and the like. These children need careful watching and more frequent medical examinations than are given to the rest of the school population. The postural difficulties of these borderline cases may be met by a program of physical education and participation in physical activities suited to individual needs.

DO YOU KNOW?

1. Match each bone named in Group A with the part of the anatomy named in Group B which you associate with it.

Group A	Group B
Occipital bone	Face
Carpals	Chest
Humerus	Leg
Tarsals	Shoulder girdle
Vertebrae	Pelvic girdle
Sacrum	Knee
Mandible	Upper arm
Sternum	Feet
Patella	Spine
Clavicle	Ankle
Femur	Cranium
Metatarsal	Wrist
Tibia	Thigh

2. Tell the difference between

   a. Orthopedics and pediatrics
   b. Voluntary muscles and involuntary muscles
   c. Ilium and ischium
   d. Acetylcholine and lactic acid
   e. Semicircular canals and cerebellum
   f. Flatfoot and clubfoot

g. Simple fracture and compound fracture

h. Strain and sprain

3. In the following groupings of diseases and conditions one does not belong in the group. Select the one that is out of place and tell why.

a. Kyphosis, lordosis, tuberculosis, scoliosis

b. Osteomyelitis, poliomyelitis, rickets, Pott's disease

c. Erb's palsy, ataxia, talipes, congenital torticollis

SUGGESTED ACTIVITIES

1. Appraise your own standing posture. One way to do this is to stand with your left side facing a full-length mirror and then to turn your head to look in the mirror. Another way is to study full-length snapshots taken of your front and side views. Compare what you observe about your own posture with Figures 80 and 81 showing good and bad posture in a child. Are you satisfied with your posture? If not, what can you do to improve it?

2. Hold a class election by secret ballot to choose the students in the class who have the best posture. Ask those who receive the most votes to demonstrate good standing, walking, and sitting posture for the rest of the class. After the demonstrations, discuss the various factors involved in attaining and maintaining good posture (see Table 19).

3. Observe the posture and gait of the children in your class in practice or laboratory school. In checking your observations, use Figures 80 and 81, Table 21, and the information given in the text (see Posture and Its Appraisal, in this chapter) about posture characteristics according to age. Talk over with the nurse serving the school any findings that lead you to believe that particular children are in need of orthopedic examination.

4. The next time you visit the shopping center of a town or city, observe the heels of persons walking ahead of you. Keep tally of the number of individuals observed and the number with shoe heels worn over on the inside. What percentage of the persons observed have pronated feet? Compare your findings with others in the class who have carried on this activity. Discuss ways in which you would help a child known to have pronated feet because of bad habits of standing and walking.

5. The next time you visit a shoe store, unobtrusively observe the persons buying shoes. Notice their facial expressions and posture as they

walk about in the shoes selected to try out. In your opinion, who made good choices in purchasing walking shoes (not evening or party shoes) and who made poor ones? Have a class discussion on the points to consider in buying shoes for everyday wear; in buying shoes for children. How would you help a child who came to school in a pair of new shoes that obviously hurt his feet?

6. If possible, have a member, or committee, of the class visit (a) an orthopedic clinic, to observe and report on the orthopedic examination of a school child; (b) the physical therapy department of a school system, to observe and report on the measures used to correct remediable orthopedic defects. Discuss ways in which you would help (a) an orthopedically handicapped child if you had one in a class you were teaching; (b) a child who has poor body mechanics because of poor nutrition, a poorly balanced program of rest and exercise, or some remediable physical defect or condition.

SELECTED REFERENCES

AMERICAN MEDICAL ASSOCIATION: *Wonder Stories of the Human Machine: The Framework (Bones)*, Chicago, 1948. (Pamphlet 1 in a series explaining how the principal organs of the body work.)

AMERICAN MEDICAL ASSOCIATION: *Wonder Stories of the Human Machine: The Running Gear (Muscles)*, Chicago, 1948. (Pamphlet 2 in the series.)

LANE, JANET: *Your Carriage, Madam!; a Guide to Good Posture*, 2d ed. New York, John Wiley & Sons, Inc., 1947.

LASALLE, DOROTHY: *Guidance of Children through Physical Education*, New York, A. S. Barnes and Company, 1946.

LEWIN, PHILIP: *The Back and Its Disorders*, New York, McGraw-Hill Book Company, Inc., 1948. (Anatomy and physiology of the back and prevention and correction of its disorders.)

LEWIN, PHILIP: *Arthritis and the Rheumatic Diseases*, New York, McGraw-Hill Book Company, Inc., 1951.

MORTON, DUDLEY J.: *Oh, Doctor! My Feet!* New York, Appleton-Century-Crofts, Inc., 1939. (A popular presentation of the principles of foot care.)

RANEY, RICHARD B., and ALFRED R. SHANDS: *Primer on Prevention of Deformity in Childhood*, Chicago, National Society for Crippled Children and Adults, 1941. (Common childhood afflictions that may cause deformity, and simple preventive measures that may forestall serious deformities.)

TURNER, T. ARTHUR: *Microbes That Cripple,* Chicago, National Society for Crippled Children and Adults, 1944. (Deals largely with micro-organisms that permanently impair the central nervous system or the muscles, bones, or joints.)

Organizations

Institute for the Crippled and Disabled
National Society for Crippled Children and Adults

Addresses of Organizations

American Council on Education, 1785 Massachusetts Avenue, N.W., Washington 6, D.C.

American Dental Association, 222 East Superior Street, Chicago 11, Ill.

American Diabetes Association, 1 East 45th Street, New York 17, N.Y.

American Hearing Society, 817 14th Street, N.W., Washington 5, D.C.

American Heart Association, 44 East 23d Street, New York 10, N.Y.

American Home Economics Association, 1600 20th Street, N.W., Washington 9, D.C.

American Medical Association, 535 North Dearborn Street, Chicago 10, Ill.

American National Red Cross (National Blood Program), 17th and D Streets, N.W., Washington 13, D.C.

American Public Health Association, 1790 Broadway, New York 19, N.Y.

American Speech and Hearing Association, Inc., Wayne University, Detroit 1, Mich.

Child Study Association of America, 132 East 74th Street, New York 21, N.Y.

Food and Nutrition Board of the National Research Council, Washington 25, D.C.

Illuminating Engineering Society, 1860 Broadway, New York 23, N.Y.

Institute for the Crippled and Disabled, 400 First Avenue, New York 10, N.Y.

Metropolitan Life Insurance Company (Health and Welfare), 1 Madison Avenue, New York 10, N.Y.

National Association for Mental Health, 1790 Broadway, New York 19, N.Y.

National Education Association, 1201 16th Street, N.W., Washington 6, D.C.

National Epilepsy League, 130 North Wells Street, Chicago 6, Ill.

National Foundation for Infantile Paralysis (Education Service), 120 Broadway, New York 5, N.Y.

National Health Council, 1790 Broadway, New York 19, N.Y.

National Publicity Council for Health and Welfare Services, Inc., 257 Fourth Avenue, New York 10, N.Y.

National Safety Council, 425 North Michigan Avenue, Chicago 11, Ill.

National Society for Crippled Children and Adults, 11 South La Salle
   Street, Chicago 3, Ill.
National Society for the Prevention of Blindness, 1790 Broadway, New
   York 19, N.Y.
National Tuberculosis Association, 1790 Broadway, New York 19, N.Y.
NEA Service, Inc., 1200 West 3d Street, Cleveland, Ohio.
Public Affairs Committee, Inc., 22 East 38th Street, New York 16, N.Y.
Science Research Associates, Inc., 57 West Grand Avenue, Chicago 10, Ill.
Science Service, 1719 N Street, N.W., Washington 6, D.C.
United States Department of Agriculture, Bureau of Human Nutrition
   and Home Economics, Washington 25, D.C.
United States Department of Health, Education and Welfare, Washing-
   ton 25, D.C.
      Children's Bureau
      Office of Education
      Public Health Service
Volta Speech Association for the Deaf, 1537 35th Street, N.W., Wash-
   ington 7, D.C.

Visual Aids

The visual aids listed below and on the following pages can be used to supplement much of the material in this book. For the convenience of users, they have been grouped by chapter subjects, but it is recommended that each film be reviewed before use in order to determine its suitability for a particular group or unit of study.

Motion pictures and filmstrips are included in the following list, the character of each being indicated by the self-explanatory abbreviations "MP" and "FS." Immediately following this identification is the name of the producer and, if different, that of the distributor also. Abbreviations used for these names are identified in the list of sources at the end of the bibliography. In many instances the films can be borrowed or rented from local or state 16mm film libraries. (A nationwide list of these sources is given in *A Directory of 2660 16mm Film Libraries,* available for 50 cents from the Superintendent of Documents, Washington 25, D.C.) Unless otherwise indicated, the motion pictures are 16mm, sound, black-and-white; the filmstrips are 35mm, black-and-white, silent. The length of motion pictures is given in minutes (min), that of filmstrips in frames (fr).

This bibliography is a selective one, and film users should examine the latest annual editions and supplements of *Educational Film Guide* and *Filmstrip Guide,* published by The H. W. Wilson Company, New York. The *Guides,* standard reference books, are available in most school, college, and public libraries.

Chapter 1 Seeing the Child as a Whole

Body Defenses against Disease (MP; EBF; 11 min). Skin, phagocytic cells, lymphatic vessels, and blood; microphotography of phagocytosis; types of antibodies. (Supplementary filmstrip, same title, 70 fr)

The Body Fights Bacteria (MP; McGraw; 17 min). Describes various types of organisms and nature's counterbalances; indicates protective functions of body parts. (Follow-up filmstrip, same title, 30 fr)

Do You Know Your Adolescents? (FS; Meth Pub; 69 fr: 78 rpm disk, 20 min). Presents four family situations involving adolescents—choosing a vocation, puppy love, youth friendships, and Sunday school attendance—

prepared for use by parents to help them find solutions to their own similar problems.

Embryology of Human Behavior (AAMC/IFB; 28 min color). Explains that a child grows in accordance with certain universal laws and at the same time develops as an individual. Traces the patterning process of behavior.

Face of Youth (MP; Wisc U; 28 min). Story of how the parents, nurse, and teacher work together to help two boys with their problems and take the boys to a child-guidance center where, with the help of a therapist, they learn to adjust to their worlds.

Family Circles (MP; CNFB/McGraw; 31 min). Portrays, through three dramatized situations, the interplay between home and school influences and how family attitudes affect children's success in school.

Functions of the Body (MP; UWF; 15 min). Demonstrates the interdependence of body systems: skeletal, muscular, vascular, respiratory, excretory, endocrine, and nervous.

How the Organs of the Body Function (MP; Bray; 30 min). Brief presentation of how we breathe, digest our food, circulate nourishment, eliminate waste, and perpetuate life.

Nine Basic Functional Systems of the Human Body (MP; Bray; 11 min). Skeletal, muscular, excretory, circulatory, nervous, sensory, digestive, lymphatic, and endocrine.

Teacher Observations of School Children (FS; Met Life; 43 fr: $33\frac{1}{3}$ rpm disk, 18 min). Visualizations of signs of good health and of certain noticeable deviations from it.

Unity of Personality (MP; PCR; 18 min silent). Consistency of expressive movements are shown, via films made with their knowledge, of five individuals with very different personalities. Shows and explains similarities of expressive behavior characteristics, which relate to the "unity of personality."

Your Children's Play (MP; BIS/McGraw; 20 min). Gives examples of play behavior of one- to eight-year-olds, and emphasizes the need for parents and teachers to understand the reasons for such behavior patterns.

Chapter 2   The Growing Child

Adolescent Development (MP series; McGraw). Series of five motion pictures with follow-up filmstrips.

1. *The Meaning of Adolescence* (16 min). Points to the unsure status of the adolescent, neither child nor adult, and provides an over-all view of the social, emotional, mental, and physical changes occurring in the years between childhood and adulthood. Emphasizes the need to help a teen-ager adjust to five aspects of adult life: physical maturity, social living, the opposite sex, religious beliefs, and a moral code. (Follow-up filmstrip, 34 fr)

2. *Physical Aspects of Puberty* (19 min). Describes, through animation, the physiological aspects of puberty—primary and secondary sex characteristics, maturation in boys and in girls, variation among individuals, and the emotional and social effects of such variations. (Follow-up filmstrip, 34 fr)

3. *Age of Turmoil* (20 min). Portrays early adolescence, 13–15 years, and the behavior characteristics of giggling, noisiness, criticism of school, day-dreaming, and seemingly useless activities. Gives examples of different personality types and of various parent-child situations. (Follow-up filmstrip, 36 fr)

4. *Social-Sex Attitudes in Adolescence* (22 min). Portrays a boy and a girl taken through their entire adolescent experience, their early sex education, awareness of the opposite sex, dating, finding common interests, falling in love, and marrying. (Follow-up filmstrip, 35 fr)

5. *Meeting the Needs of Adolescents* (19 min). Points out, through a study of a family with a seventeen-year-old girl and a fourteen-year-old boy, what parents can do to meet the needs of their adolescents. (Follow-up filmstrip, 34 fr)

Baby Meets His Parents (MP; EBF; 11 min). Points out how differences in personality can be accounted for, not only by heredity but also by the human relationships and environmental factors experienced during the first years of life.

Child Development (MP series; McGraw). Series of eight motion pictures, five of them with follow-up filmstrips.

1. *Principles of Development* (17 min). Outlines the fundamentals of child growth and development and considers the variables which make each child different from every other one. (Follow-up filmstrip)

2. *Child Care and Development* (17 min). Explains the habits of daily physical care that ensure a happy, healthy child. Covers good habits of eating, sleeping, bathing, the wearing of proper clothing, and outdoor exercise. (Follow-up filmstrip)

3. *Heredity and Prenatal Development* (21 min). Discusses cell growth and heredity, describes fertilization of the ovum and traces development of the fetus until delivery, considers development of physical functions

of the newborn, and stresses the connection between physical and emotional sensitivity. (Follow-up filmstrip)

4. *Children's Emotions* (22 min). Discusses the major emotions of childhood—fear, anger, jealousy, curiosity, and joy—and points out what the parent can do to lessen fears and promote the child's happiness and natural development. (Follow-up filmstrip)

5. *Social Development* (16 min). Offers an analysis of social behavior at different age levels and the reasons underlying the changes in behavior patterns as the child develops. (Follow-up filmstrip)

6. *Play* (In preparation, 1955).

7. *Brothers and Sisters* (In preparation, 1955).

8. *Children and Fantasy* (In preparation, 1955).

Experimental Studies of Children's Learning (MP; Calif U; 13 min silent). Describes laboratory processes used in measuring rates of learning by children.

From Sociable Six to Noisy Nine (CNFB/McGraw; 22 min color or black-and-white). Portrays characteristic patterns of behavior exhibited by children from six to nine, and constructive efforts of parents to understand and guide these children.

The Frustrating Fours and Fascinating Fives (CNFB/McGraw; 22 min color or black-and-white). Portrays characteristic patterns of a four-year-old boy, from imaginative craftsmanship to inconsistent destructiveness, and the changes that occur as he grows into a five-year-old.

Genetics and Behavior (MP; PCR; 16 min silent color or black-and-white). Documents the thesis that the structure which limits behavior is inherited, but not behavior itself. Showings restricted to professional personnel.

He Acts His Age (CNFB/McGraw; 15 min color or black-and-white). Survey of typical behavior patterns of children from ages one to fifteen, demonstrating that as children grow, their interests, activities, and emotions change.

Individual Differences (MP; McGraw; 23 min). Differences between children, illustrated by a study of a shy, slow child contrasted with his classmates and particularly with his older brother.

Life with Baby (MP; MOT/McGraw; 18 min). How children grow, mentally and physically. Based on Gesell studies at Yale University.

Life with Junior (MP; MOT/McGraw; 18 min). Follows Junior through a typical day. Shows in some detail the work of the Child Study Association of America.

Performance Testing (MP; Minn U; 30 min silent). Use of the manikin, sequin form board, Knox cube, diamond, and memory tests with children of various chronological and mental ages.

Personality Development (MP; EBF). Series of four films with the following titles and running times:
1. *Answering the Child's Why* (13 min).
2. *Baby Meets His Parents* (11 min).
3. *Helping the Child to Accept the Do's* (11 min).
4. *Helping the Child to Face the Don'ts* (11 min).

The Terrible Twos and Trusting Threes (CNFB/McGraw; 22 min). A study of child behavior at two and three years, showing what to expect from youngsters of these ages, and suggesting how parents can deal constructively with their problems.

Your Body During Adolescence (MP; McGraw; 10 min). Portrays variations in the size and shape of teen-agers, and explains the general changes that take place during puberty.

Chapter 3   Thoughts and Feelings, Actions and Reactions

Allergies (MP; EBF; 12 min color). Explains the nature of allergies, research being carried on in this field, and tests for detecting allergies.

Angry Boy (MP; MHFB/IFB; 32 min). Tells the story of emotional disturbances engendered by family tensions. Tommy, a preadolescent boy, is caught stealing. At a child-guidance clinic, a psychiatric team traces his disturbances to its basic causes, and is able to help him.

Born in the White House (MP; NFIP; 26 min). Traces progress in the conquest of disease, with particular emphasis on recent (1954) gains in polio research and treatment.

The Brain (MP; Brandon; 75 min silent). Structure, cranial nerves, embryonic development, ventricles, fissures and convolutions, cerebral hemispheres.

Breakdown (MP; CNFB/McGraw; 40 min). Case study of a young woman who has a schizophrenic breakdown. Follows the course of her treatment from a mental-health clinic to a state hospital, and concludes with her discharge from this institution to complete her rehabilitation as a member of her family.

Emotional Health (MP; McGraw; 20 min). Frequency of emotional upsets; when professional care and treatment are necessary; basic techniques of psychiatry. (Follow-up filmstrip, 25 fr)

Farewell to Childhood (MP; MHFB/IFB; 23 min). Dramatized story of a teen-age girl, full of the swift emotions typical of adolescence and the longing for and fearing of the privileges of adulthood. Portrays the adolescent moods of rebellion and trust, anger and irresolution, self-pity and idealism, and the parents' bewilderment and confusion.

Fears of Children (MP; MHFB/IFB; 30 min). Parent-child situation in which the mother tends to coddle her five-year-old son and the father expects too much of him. Explains how the conflict magnifies the child's fears.

Functions of the Nervous System (MP; PCR; 13 min). Describes the central nervous system; cranial, cervical, thoracic, lumbar, and sacral connections; sympathetic ganglia; sense organs; and the mechanism of muscular coordination.

His Fighting Chance (MP; BIS; 11 min). Explains the physiotherapy and modern treatment (1949) of poliomyelitis. Approved by American College of Surgeons.

Introduction to Clinical Neurology (MP series; USPHS/PCR). Series of four films, all silent, with the following titles and running times:

1. *General Neurological Examination and Clinical Signs of Disorders of the Pyramidal System* (19 min).

2. *Disorders of the Extra-pyramidal System and the Posterior Columns* (20 min).

3. *Cerebellar Disorders, Disorders Involving the Lower Motor Neurones, and Convulsive States* (17 min).

4. *Functional Syndromes with Pronounced Physical Symptoms* (17 min).

Judging Emotional Behavior (MP; Churchill; 20 min). A motion-picture test designed to measure the sensitivity of individuals to the emotions of others. Ten sequences are shown in which two people react as if certain events described by a narrator were happening to them.

Mental Mechanisms (MP series; CNFB/McGraw). Series of five films portraying, through dramatized case studies, certain mental-health problems of young adults, and tracing their roots back through adolescence to childhood and infancy.

1. *The Feeling of Rejection* (23 min). Documentary-dramatic study of a young woman whose feelings of rejection are manifested in maladjustment and physical illnesses. Traces, through flash backs, her feelings of rejection to childhood origins and, through psychiatric help, shows her beginning to understand her problem.

2. *The Feeling of Hostility* (27 min). Documentary-dramatic study of Clare, a young woman apparently successful in her profession but a failure in personal relationships. Traces, through flash backs, her hostility to childhood experiences and shows how psychiatric treatment helps her direct her hostility into constructive efforts.

3. *Overdependency* (32 min). Dramatized story of a young married man whose inability to face the ordinary problems of life, including vague physical ailments and vocational maladjustment, stems from a childhood too dependent upon his mother and sister.

4. *Feelings of Depression* (30 min). Dramatized case study of how and why feelings of depression shadow the business and home life of John, a conscientious young married man. Explains how psychiatry could help him understand himself and the reasons for his feelings.

5. *To Serve the Mind* (25 min). Case study of a doctor who suffers a schizophrenic breakdown, showing the various forms of treatment that gradually lead to his recovery and return to work.

Nervous System (MP; EBF; 11 min). Structure of the nervous system, pathways and connections, nerve impulses, reflexes, sensory integration, and activity of the cerebrum.

Personal Problems of Adolescent Youth (FS; OSU; 43 fr, with script and bibliography). Explains generally the behavior and problems of high-school students.

Personality and Emotions (MP; EBF; 13 min). Illustrations of behavioral expressions of emotions and an explanation of their relationship to individual personalities.

Shyness (MP; CNFB/McGraw, 23 min). Portrays the lonely existence of a shy adult, and illustrates the causes of shyness through studies of three children. Explains the reasons for shyness and how this problem may be overcome.

Testing Intelligence with the Stanford-Binet (MP; Ind U; 18 min). Gives an overview of the types of items on an intelligence test and the method of administering the test.

Unconscious Motivation (MP; Assn; 38 min). Demonstrates how unconscious motives can influence and direct everyday thoughts, feelings, and actions; and explains how psychological techniques can be used to detect the presence of troublesome, repressed ideas.

Chapter 4   What to Know about the Heart, Blood, and Lymph

Care of the Cardiac Patient (MP; USOE/UWF; 33 min). Nursing care given a cardiac patient, including comfort, rest, sleep, diet, feeding, elimination, cleanliness, and diversional and occupational therapy. (Supplementary filmstrip, 77 fr)

Circulation (MP; UWF; 16 min). Systemic and pulmonary circulation of the blood; structure and functions of the heart, lungs, arteries, veins, and capillary networks.

Congenital Malformations of the Heart (MP series; Wash U). Three color films with the following subtitles:
   Part 1. *Development of the Normal Heart* (17 min).
   Part 2. *Acyanotic Congenital Heart Disease* (16 min).
   Part 3. *Cyanotic Congenital Heart Disease* (31 min).

Control of Body Temperatures (MP; EBF; 11 min). Phenomena associated with changes in body temperature, the blood stream as the distributor of heat, and the hypothalamus as the controller.

The Crippled Heart (FS; AHA; 76 fr color: $33\frac{1}{3}$ rpm disk; 15 min). Case history of a ten-year-old boy illustrating the St. Louis rheumatic-fever program. Includes drawings and clinical photographs of the heart.

Guard Your Heart (MP; Bray; 27 min). How the heart works and what changes take place in major heart diseases. Animation and live-action photography. Produced in cooperation with the American Heart Association.

The Heart—How It Works (MP; McGraw; 11 min). Shows by animation the heart, the flow of blood through it, and the functions of its parts. Explains methods of testing the heart, facts about its work load, and ways of maintaining a healthy heart.

Heart and Circulation (MP; EBF; 11 min). Mechanics of pulmonary and systemic systems; microscopic scenes of capillary action; and the significance of blood pressure. (Supplementary filmstrip, same title, 73 fr)

Heart Disease—Its Major Causes (MP; EBF; 11 min). Over-all view of three major diseases—high blood pressure, hardening of the arteries, and rheumatic fever.

Jimmy Beats Rheumatic Fever (FS; Met Life; 80 fr: $33\frac{1}{3}$ rpm disk; 15 min). The story of an eight-year-old boy's successful battle with rheumatic fever.

Pump Trouble (MP; AHA; 14 min color). Animated cartoon deprecating exaggerated fears of heart disease, and emphasizing the importance of having a thorough medical examination.

Report on the Living (MP; USPHS; 27 min). Documentary story of the recovery of Richard Wood, age ten, from rheumatic heart disease following his treatment with ACTH, the adrenocorticotrophic hormone compound.

Stop Rheumatic Fever (MP; AHA; 12 min). Emphasizes that rheumatic fever can be prevented by prompt treatment of its forerunners, streptococcal infections.

Taming the Crippler (MP; RKO/McGraw; 16 min). Describes the various efforts to control poliomyelitis, including physical therapy, gamma globulin, and the Salk vaccine.

Valiant Heart (MP; AHA; 28 min). Explains the facts about rheumatic fever, its treatment and prevention, through a case history of an eight-year-old boy.

Wonder Engine of the Body (MP; Bray; 10 min). Explains the anatomy, physiology, and proper care of the heart. Short version of *Guard Your Heart.*

Chapter 5 On the Air Route

Articulatory Movements in the Production of English Speech Sounds (MP; USVA):

Part 1. Consonants (25 min color). Through the use of animated drawings of the breathing process and direct photography of the movements of the laryngeal and articulatory structures in a patient with extensive loss of facial tissue, illustrates the production of speech. Movements of the lips, mandible, tongue, velum, and pharyngeal constrictor muscles are shown in illustrations of oral continuant consonants, nasal continuants, plosives, and affricatives commonly present in American speech.

Part 2. Vowels and Glides (26 min color). Through live-action photography of the movements of the laryngeal and articulatory structures in a patient with extensive loss of facial tissue, illustrates the production of vowels and their movements with glide sounds. Shows the importance of resonance as a factor in speech intelligibility, through samples of connected speech.

Artificial Respiration (MP; USCG; 11 min). Explains and demonstrates two new methods of artificial respiration adopted by the U.S. Coast Guard

—the Holger-Nielsen, or back-pressure, arm-lift method, and the Emerson, or back-pressure, hip-lift method.

Billion Dollar Malady (MP; Bray; 17 min). Stresses the economic importance of colds, explains what is known about colds, and suggests methods for their cure and prevention.

Coming Home (MP; Nat TB; 15 min). Story of a family and their fight against tuberculosis; discovery, treatment, and cure.

Escape the Cold Wave (FS; Zurich; 100 fr: 33⅓ rpm disk; 15 min). How to prevent the spread of colds.

How to Catch a Cold (MP; Assn; 10 min color). Walt Disney cartoon showing how colds are spread and what one should do when he "catches a cold."

Human Throat (MP; Bray; 12 min). Describes the throat, pharynx, and larynx, from functional and anatomic aspects.

Ka-choo (FS; Zurich; 100 fr: 33⅓ rpm disk; 15 min). Colds and their prevention.

Mechanisms of Breathing (MP; EBF, 11 min). Gaseous exchange in lungs and body tissue cells; factors affecting rate and depth of breathing.

Movements of the Tongue in Speech (MP; IFB; 14 min). Movements of the human tongue and lips during speech. Slow-motion photography.

The Nose, Structure and Function (MP; EBF; 11 min color or black-and-white). Covers the function of the nose, physiology of the nasal cavity, and nasal hygiene.

Nose, Throat, and Ears (MP; McGraw; 10 min). Structures and functions. Animated diagrams. (Follow-up filmstrip, 28 fr)

Sneezes and Sniffles (MP; McGraw; 10 min). How colds are spread by sneezing, coughing, and careless handling of infected things; and precautions to prevent the spreading of colds.

Speech Defects (FS series; SVE). Three color filmstrips with the following titles:
   1. *Nature of Speech Defects* (55 fr).
   2. *How Speech Defects Develop* (49 fr).
   3. *What Speech Clinics Are Doing* (48 fr).

TB—Everybody's Problem (FS; Nat TB; 48 fr color). Pictorial explanation of tuberculosis, its cause, spread, treatment, control, and prevention.

Tuberculosis (MP; EBF; 11 min). Nature, transmission, diagnosis, and treatment of pulmonary tuberculosis.

Chapter 6   Along the Alimentary Route

Come Clean (MP; ADA; 8 min color or black-and-white). Humorous character by the name of Adolphus narrates his experiences in the care of his teeth. Story shows the behavior changes that may be brought about through proper instruction.

Digestion (MP; UWF):
  Part 1. (15 min). Mechanical and muscular processes involved in the digestion of food; animated diagrams.
  Part 2. (18 min). Chemical changes involved in the digestion of carbohydrates, proteins, and fats.

Digestion of Foods (MP; EBF; 11 min). Digestive process in the mouth, stomach, and small intestine; secretions, enzymes, and relation of circulatory and nervous systems to digestive process. (Supplementary filmstrip, same title, 86 fr)

Elimination (MP; UWF; 12 min). Describes the four methods of elimination from the human body—skin, kidneys, lungs, and colon. (Supplementary filmstrip, same title, 33 fr)

Foods and Nutrition (MP; EBF; 11 min). Metabolic processes showing body's use of carbohydrates, fats, proteins, minerals, and vitamins. (Supplementary filmstrip, same title, 86 fr)

Fundamentals of Diet (MP; EBF; 10 min). Gives a functional classification of foods, and depicts experiments with animals illustrating the results of food deficiencies.

Human Digestion (MP; Athena; 10 min). Principal steps of the digestive process.

Kidneys, Ureters, and Bladder (MP; Bray; 11 min). Anatomic features; animated drawings describe functional relationships.

Obesity (MP; EBF; 12 min color or black-and-white). Explains the physiology of fat formation in the body, the dangers of being overweight, and ways to control one's diet.

Save Those Teeth (MP; EBF; 11 min). Emphasizes the importance of proper cleansing in the care of teeth, and explains the reasons for tooth decay.

The Teeth (MP; EBF; 11 min). How teeth develop and grow; proper foods; how to brush teeth; dentist care. (Supplementary filmstrip, same title, 82 fr)

Tooths and Consequences (MP; ADA; 10 min color). Explains the importance of giving adequate care to a child's temporary teeth.

Work of the Kidneys (MP; EBF; 11 min). Function of the kidneys; structure and processes.

Chapter 7   The Body's Envelope

The Human Hair (MP; Bray; 11 min). Growth of hair within the follicle, individual duration, renewal, and relation to sebaceous gland.

Human Skin (MP; Bray; 12 min). Functions and structure of the skin. Photography and animated drawings.

Scrub Game (MP; MTP; 30 min). Function and structure of the skin; care and prevention of blackheads, ringworm, lice, itch, and boils.

Your First Defense (FS; Zurich; 100 fr: 33⅓ rpm disk; 15 min). Discusses the function and care of the skin, including how to avoid occupational dermatosis.

Chapter 8   Stop! Look and Listen

The Deaf Post-rubella School Child (MP; Lex Sch Deaf; 12 min). Capacities and behavior, during their first two years of school life, of two groups of children born deaf as a result of maternal rubella.

Ears and Hearing (MP; EBF; 11 min). Describes the physiology and operation of the human ear by means of animated drawings and close-up photography of the ear as it is functioning. (Related filmstrip, same title, 70 fr)

The Embryology of the Eye (MP; AMA; 43 min color). General picture of the development of the ocular structures. Prepared by the American Academy of Ophthalmology and Otolaryngology.

Experimental Psychology of Vision (MP; IFB; 16 min silent). Phenomena and techniques of research in visual perception.

Eyes and Their Care (MP; EBF; 11 min). Physiology and hygiene of the eye; structure and function; eye movements, field of vision, visual defects (nearsightedness and farsightedness). (Supplementary filmstrip, same title, 78 fr)

Factors in Depth Perception (MP; PCR; 14 min silent). Illustrates the cue factors in perceiving depth, including interception, interposition, distinctness of objects, and relative motion.

Johnny's New World (MP; NSPB; 16 min color). Illustrates the eye care given to a young school child by teacher, school nurse, mother, and eye specialist. Explains common eye conditions such as myopia, hyperopia, strabismus, etc.

The Magic Pathway (MP; Movies; 21 min color). Dramatizes the highlights of vision, uses cartoon treatment to explain the complex structure of the eyes and the intricate brain and eye coordination necessary to vision, and emphasizes the need for periodic eye check-ups.

More Than Meets the Eye (MP; Am Opto; 26 min color). How we see and how vision is corrected.

Out from Silence (FS series; SVE). Three color filmstrips with the following titles:
1. *Nature of Hearing Loss* (48 fr).
2. *Safeguarding Your Hearing* (44 fr).
3. *Rehabilitation of the Hard-of-Hearing* (48 fr).

Your Children's Ears (MP; BIS; 15 min). Explains by animated diagrams the physiology of the ear, and shows the close relationship between the nose and throat.

Your Children's Eyes (MP; BIS; 20 min). Explains the structure of the eyes and illustrates common eye defects, diseases, and injuries and their treatment. Models and diagrams are used.

Your Future Is in Sight (FS; Zurich; 100 fr: 33⅓ rpm disk; 15 min). The importance, function, care, and protection of the eyes.

Chapter 9   On Growing Straight

As Others See You (FS; McGraw; 33 fr). How to stand and walk; good grooming habits.

Care of the Feet (MP; EBF; 11 min). Structure of the foot; causes of structural foot ailments, remedies, and treatment. (Supplementary filmstrip, same title, 85 fr)

First as a Child (MP; Va Health/IFB; 22 min). Case history of a crippled child from the public health nurse's first visit to his home through diagnosis, treatment, and aftercare. Points out the necessary consideration given to the child's emotional troubles.

Human Skeleton (MP; UWF; 11 min). Animation and x-ray photography explains the structure, parts, and functions of the human skeleton.

Muscular System (MP; UWF; 11 min). Explains the action of muscles in maintaining body posture; arm movements through the action of biceps, triceps, and related muscles; and the relation of muscles to bones and joints.

Our Feet (MP; Bray; 11 min). Functioning and construction of the foot; skeleton, ligaments, and muscles; longitudinal and transverse arches.

Posture and Exercise (MP; EBF; 11 min). Muscle activity and physiology of exercise; relation of nervous system to skeletal muscles.

The Skeleton (MP; EBF; 12 min). Illustrates the formation, growth, development, and functions of the human skeleton.

The Walking Machine (MP; Am Foot; 14 min). Emphasizes the importance of foot care, illustrates the basic items in foot hygiene, and shows methods for selecting footwear.

Your Body Speaks (MP; Col U; 20 min). Explains the basic factors which make for good and bad posture, including state of mind, personality, and general health.

SOURCES OF FILMS LISTED

AAMC—American Association of Medical Colleges, 185 N. Wabash St., Chicago 1.

ADA—American Dental Assn., 222 E. Superior St., Chicago 11.

AHA—American Heart Assn., 44 E. 23rd St., New York 10.

AMA—American Medical Assn., 535 N. Dearborn St., Chicago 10.

Am Foot—American Foot Care Institute, Inc., 1775 Broadway, New York 19.

Am Opto—American Optometric Assn., 4030 Chouteau Ave., St. Louis 10.

Assn—Association Films, Inc., 347 Madison Ave., New York 17.

Athena—Athena Films, Inc., 165 W. 46th St., New York 19.

BIS—British Information Services, 30 Rockefeller Plaza, New York 20.

Brandon—Brandon Films, Inc., 200 W. 57th St., New York 19.

Bray—Bray Studios, Inc., 729 Seventh Ave., New York 19.

Calif U—University of California, Educational Film Sales Dept., Los Angeles 24.

Churchill—Churchill-Wexler Film Productions, 801 N. Seward St., Los Angeles 38.

CNFB—Canadian National Film Board, 1270 Avenue of the Americas, New York 20.

Col U—Columbia University Press, Center for Mass Communication, 413 W. 117th St., New York 27.

EBF—Encyclopaedia Britannica Films, Inc., 1150 Wilmette Ave., Wilmette, Ill.

IFB—International Film Bureau, 57 E. Jackson Blvd., Chicago 4.

Ind U—Indiana University, Audio-Visual Center, Bloomington, Ind.

Lex Sch Deaf—Lexington School for the Deaf, 904 Lexington Ave., New York 21.

McGraw—McGraw-Hill Book Company, Inc., Text-Film Dept., 330 W. 42nd St., New York 36.

Meth Pub—Methodist Publishing House, 810 Broadway, Nashville 2, Tenn.

Met Life—Metropolitan Life Insurance Co., 1 Madison Ave., New York 10.

MHFB—Mental Health Film Board, Inc., 166 E. 38th St., New York 16.

Minn U—University of Minnesota, Minneapolis 14.

MOT—March of Time, Forum Films, 364 Lexington Ave., New York.

Movies—Movies, U.S.A., 729 Seventh Ave., New York 19.

MTP—Modern Talking Picture Service, Inc., 45 Rockefeller Plaza, New York 20.

Nat TB—National Tuberculosis Assn., 1790 Broadway, New York 19.

NFIP—National Foundation for Infantile Paralysis, 120 Broadway, New York 5.

NSPB—National Society for the Prevention of Blindness, 1790 Broadway, New York 19.

OSU—Ohio State University, Teaching Aids Laboratory, Columbus.

PCR—Psychological Cinema Register, Pennsylvania State University, University Park, Pa.

RKO—RKO Radio Pictures, 1270 Avenue of the Americas, New York.

SVE—Society for Visual Education, Inc., 1345 W. Diversey Parkway, Chicago 14.

USCG—U.S. Coast Guard, Washington 25.

USOE—U.S. Office of Education, Washington 25.

USPHS—U.S. Public Health Service, Washington 25.

USVA—U.S. Veterans Administration, Central Film Library, Washington 25.

UWF—United World Films, Inc., 1445 Park Ave., New York 29.

Va Health—Virginia Department of Health, Richmond, Va.

Wash U—University of Washington, Seattle.

Wisc U—University of Wisconsin, Bureau of Visual Instruction, 1312 W. Johnson St., Madison 6.

Zurich—Zurich Insurance Companies, 135 S. La Salle St., Chicago 3.

Index

A

Abdomen, muscles of, 255, 260, 412, 414
 organs of, 113, 411, 418
  circulation in, 156–157
  sensitivity of, to pain, 261–262
 pain in, 262, 266, 267, 271, 272
 posture and, 412, 414–416
Abrasions, first-aid treatment for, 344
Abscess, in middle ear, 377
 in outer ear canal, 377
 in tooth, 285
Absences from school, chief causes of, 17–20
 encouragement of, in early signs of illness, 220, 224
 records of, in determining causes of illness, 16
 studies of, 16
Acarina, 340
Acceleration in school, 69–70
Accident-proneness, 117, 148
Accidents, as cause, of child deaths, 14
 of orthopedic defects, 420
 of school absences, 20
 prevalence of, 421
Accommodation of eye, 360–361
 in farsightedness, 362–364
 in nearsightedness, 362–364
Acetylcholine, 405
Acne, adolescent, 322–324
Acromegaly, 35
ACTH in treatment, of psoriasis, 319
 of rheumatic fever, 162
Adam's apple, 195, 401
Adenitis (swollen glands), 176, 212, 213
Adenoids, enlarged, in mouth breathing, 222
 (*See also* Tonsils and adenoids)
Adipose tissue, 36–37, 289–290
 (*See also* Subcutaneous fat)
Adolescence, 78–80
 acne in, 322–324
 awkwardness in, 73, 414–415
 dementia praecox in, 141
 depression in, 145
 dreaminess in, 120

Adolescence, early, 73
 emotional problems of, 41, 42, 78–79
 growth spurt in, 40, 41, 79
 late, 73
 posture in, 412, 414–415
 ringworm of scalp and, 338
 simple goiter in, 96
 spiritual needs in, 81
 voice changes of boys in, 79, 232, 234
Adrenal cortex, hyperfunction of, 35
 hypofunction of, 35
 influence of, on skeletal growth, 34
 secretion of, 34, 94
Adrenal glands, 93
Adrenal medulla, secretion of (adrenaline), 94–95
 teamwork of, with sympathetic nervous system, 95–96
Adrenaline, action of, 95–96
Aerosols, 222
Age, chronological, and attitudes, 79
 and averages for height and weight, 41, 43, 44
 and body dimensions, 41–42
 and mental age, 42, 65n.
 and physical growth, 31, 39–42
 mental, 64–65
  in relation to chronological age, 42, 65n.
 physiological, 79, 80
Aggressiveness, excessive (overaggressiveness), 118, 119, 142, 146–147
 dealing with, by teacher, 119
 after illness, 217
 in nail biting, 325
 normal, in latent period, 73, 78, 119, 146
Airborne infections (*see* Respiratory infections)
Alhazen, 360
Alimentary canal, diagram of, 251
 divisions of, 250
 muscle of, 251–252
 sphincters of, 250–251
 stations in, of autonomic nervous system, 256

Allergens, 106–109
    in bronchial asthma, 218, 219–220
    in hay fever, 218–219
    in skin allergies, 330–331
    in wheal formation, 320
Allergic reactions, 106–109
Allergic rhinitis, 107, 218
Allergy, 106
    acquired, 107–108
    bacterial, 110
    emotional, 110
    familial, 107, 108, 218
    mechanism of, 108–109
    respiratory, 218–220
    skin, 320–321, 329
    tests for, 108, 219, 330–331
    treatment of, 109, 218, 219
Alveoli, 192, 193
    in pneumonia, 210
American Academy of Pediatrics, Com-
        mittees on School Health and Rheu-
        matic Fever of, 162–164
American Hearing Society, 385n., 388n.
American Heart Association, Committee
        on Prevention of Rheumatic Fever,
        162
American Public Health Association, 339n.
Amino acids, absorption of, 254
    breakdown of (deaminization), 290, 302,
        304
    as products of protein digestion, 253,
        254, 290
    use of, in body, 290
Ammonia, change of, to urea, 304
    in saliva, 282
Ampullae of semicircular canals, 408
Anal canal, in defecation, 255
    pinworms in, 272
    sphincters of, 250–251, 255
Anal period of child development, 73
Anemia, in hookworm infestation, 274
    iron-deficiency, 171, 299–300
    in malaria, 183
    pernicious, 171
    red blood cells in treatment of, 165
    types of, 171
Anger, motor reaction to, 95
    repressed, 75, 115
Ankle, 394, 401, 403, 417
    sprained, 429
    turned inward, 415, 417, 431
Anopheles mosquitoes, 183, 184, 186
Antagonism (see Hostility)
Anterior pituitary, hyperfunction of, 35
    hypofunction of, 35
    influence of, on adrenal cortex, 162

Anterior pituitary, influence of, on pu-
        beral cycle, 40
    on skeletal growth, 34
    secretion of, 94
Antibiotics, 15, 17, 130, 178, 335, 378
    action of, on disease agents, 197–198
    definition of, 197n.
    medical uses of, 131, 205, 210, 266, 267
Antibodies, allergic, 106–109
    bacterial and viral, 106, 107, 110
    formation of, 103–104
    in gamma globulin, 106, 128, 164, 200,
        290
    Rh factor and, 169, 170
Anticonvulsants in epilepsy, 134
Antigen-antibody reactions, 103–104
Antigens, 103–104, 106–107
Antihistamine drugs, 219
Antisocial tendencies, 146–147
Antitoxin, in passive immunization, 104–
        106
    from diphtheria, 105, 106, 205
    from tetanus, 105, 345
    production of, 106, 345
    in treatment of tetanus, 345
Anus (see Anal canal)
Anxiety, of adult, effect on child, 80
    signs of, 95, 120, 137
        falsetto voice as, 232, 234
        reading difficulty as, 366
        stuttering as, 243, 244
    unconscious conflicts and, 77–78, 116
Anxiety hysteria, 137–138
Aorta, 155–157
Aphasia, 229
    types of, 239–240
Appendicitis, 270–271
    as cause of death in school children, 14,
        19
    character of pain in, 271
    pinworms and, 272
    progress in control of, 19
    vomiting in, 260, 271
Appendix, vermiform, 250, 251
    inflammation of, 102, 270
    pinworms in, 272
Appetite, abnormal, 274
    loss of (anorexia), 261
        in intestinal worm infestation, 272
        in psychogenic reactions, 114, 261
        in rheumatic fever, 163
        in stomach upsets, 257, 261
        in tuberculosis, 214
    stimulation of, 261

Aptitudes, 64
  detection of, 66, 68
Arch (instep) of foot, 403
  fallen, 417
Arms, bones of, 394, 395, 401, 402
  first aid, for bleeding from, 179, 181
  for fractures of, 425–426
  orthopedic defects of, Erb's palsy as, 422
    indications of, 431
Arterial blood pressure, 158
  high (see Hypertension)
  measuring of, 158–160
Arteries, bleeding from, 179
  blood pressure in, 158–160
  pulsing of, 157
  tree of, 156, 158
  walls of, 157
Arterioles, 157
  autonomic control of, 87, 89, 95, 110–111, 158
  influence of, on blood pressure, 158, 159
    on skin color, 326–327
    on wheal formation, 319
Arthropoda, 340
Artificial respiration, back-pressure–arm-lift method, 225–227
  prone-pressure method, 225
Arytenoid cartilages, 229–230
Ascorbic acid (see Vitamin C)
Asphyxia, 225
  artificial respiration for, 225–227
  in choking, 196
Asthma, bronchial, 95, 107, 109, 218–220
Astigmatism, 364–365
  detection of, 372
  wryneck and, 422
Ataxia, 136, 410
Athetosis, 135
Athlete's foot, 336–337
Atlas, 397, 398
Audiometers, obtaining of, 385–386
  phonograph, 384
  pitch-tone, 385
Auditory acuity, testing of, 384–388
Auditory (hearing) center, 87
  in aphasia, 239
  in central deafness, 383
  in speech, 238
Auditory nerve, 382
  lesion of, in central deafness, 383
    in speech disorders, 229
Auditory strings, 379, 380
  vibration of, 382
Aura, epileptic, 134
Aureomycin, 15, 197n., 198, 267, 275
Auricles of heart, 155, 157

Authority, adult, abuse of, 78, 80, 147
  children's reactions to, 74, 76, 114–115, 118, 119, 147
  stuttering as, 243
Autonomic nervous system, 87–89
  controlling influence of, 94–96, 110–111, 114, 137, 158, 251–252, 256, 304, 355
Avenzoar, 340
Axis (vertebral), 398

B

Baby talk, 229, 240
Bacilli, as cause of respiratory infections, 197–199
  microscopic pictures of, 198
Back, first aid for injuries of, 427–428
  in good posture, 414, 416
  pain in, 203, 402
  in poor posture, 415, 431
  stiffness of, 124
  strained, 430
  support for, in sitting, 418
Backache, 203, 431
Backward children, 65
  education of, 70–71
  identification of, 70
  problems of, 71, 144
Bacteria, acid-forming, 281–283
  as antigens, 103–104
  body defenses against, 101–104
  destruction of, in lymph nodes, 175
    by phagocytes, 101, 102, 167–168, 176, 334–335
    in tonsils, 177
  in feces, 255
  hypersensitivity to, 110
Bacterial flora, of colon, 255
  of nasopharynx, 197
  of skin, 329
Ball-and-socket joint, 394, 402, 403
Banting, Sir Frederick, 98
Basilar membrane, 379, 380
  vibrations of, 381–382
BCG vaccination, 217
Bed wetting (enuresis), 137, 305
Behavior, attacking, 118–119, 146–147
  after recovery from illness, 217
  signs of, 142
  changes in, as danger signal, 144–145, 163
  childish, versus adult, 7, 75
    regression to, 138
  hearing loss and, 382–384
  nutritional status and, 297

Behavior, withdrawing, 119–121, 146
  after recovery from illness, 217
  in schizoid states, 141
  signs of, 142
Behavior patterns, development of, 86,
  114, 118, 121, 137, 141, 143
Behavior problems, identification of, 141–
  148
  mental-hygiene clinics and, 148
  school and, 148
  teacher and, 119–121, 141, 143, 148–149
Behavior reactions, to frustration, 118–121
  to hostility, 115–117
  to overdirection, 118
Belching, 258
Bell, Alexander Graham, 385
Beriberi, 292–293
Biceps, 404, 405
Bicuspids, 278, 279
Bile, in digestion of fats, 253, 254, 262
  and excretion of bilirubin, 262
Bile duct, obstruction of, 263
Bilirubin, 262, 263
Binocular (two-eyed) vision, 357–358
Birth injuries, 419–422
Birthmarks, moles as, 321
Bites, animal, first-aid treatment for, 345
  insect, first-aid treatment for, 347
Black eye, 350–351
Blackheads (comedomes), 320
  in acne, 322, 323
Bladder, urinary, functions of, 304
    pleasure in, 73, 76
    psychosomatic mechanisms and,
    114–115
  nervous control of, 304, 305
  pinworms in, 272
Bleeding (see Hemorrhage; Wounds,
  bleeding from)
Blepharitis marginalis, 350
  in vitamin deficiencies, 300, 301
Blindness, in corneal injury, 354
  hysterical, 138
Blinking, 115, 142, 365, 374
Blisters, 320
  in athlete's foot, 337
  fever (herpes simplex), 275
  first-aid treatment for, 346
Blood, acid-alkali balance in, 291, 406
  arterial, 156, 157
  circulation of (see Circulation)
  color of, in anemia, 171
    in cyanosis, 160–161
    factors influencing, 327
    in leukemia, 171
  composition of, 164–170

Blood, disorders of, 170–173
  exchanges of, with body cells, 154, 157–
  159
  oxygenation of, 156, 157
    skin color and, 160–161, 327
  venous, 156, 157
Blood cells (see Red blood cells; White
  blood cells)
Blood clotting, 101, 291
  elements of, 165
  process of, 166, 168
Blood grouping, 168–170
Blood groups, 168–170
  Rh factor in, 169–170
Blood plasma, amino acids in, 290
  antibodies in, 104, 164, 200, 290
  composition of, 164–166
  filtering of, in kidneys, 302, 303
  fractionation of, 164, 166
  gamma globulin in, 164, 200
  as origin of tissue fluid, 173–175
  in treatment of shock, 165, 166
Blood platelets (thrombocytes), 165
  in blood clotting, 168
  origin of, 168
  reduction of, in leukemia, 171
    in purpura, 173
Blood poisoning (septicemia), 335
Blood pressure (see Arterial blood pressure)
Blood tests, 170
Blood transfusions, 168–170
  Rh factor in, 169–170
  universal donors in, 168
  universal recipients in, 169
Blood vessels, arrangement of, 156
  (See also Arteries; Arterioles; Capillaries; Veins; Venules)
Blueness (cyanosis), 160–161, 327
  in breath holding, 161
  in chilling, 111, 161, 327
  in choking, 196
  in epilepsy, 134, 161
Blushing, 88, 92, 327
Bodian, David, 125
Body balance, good posture as, 410, 411
  semicircular canals and, 407–408
  weight distribution and, 410–412
Body build, emergence of, 414
  identification of (Wetzel's grid), 49
  influence on, of endocrine hormones,
  34–36, 93
    of heredity, 33
    of muscles, 53
    of skeleton, 33, 44, 53
    of subcutaneous fat, 53

Body build, variations in, 33, 44
Body heat, conservation of, 111
  production of, 110, 157, 289
  removal of excess, 110–111, 289, 302, 312, 316
Body measurements, school recording of, 43, 44n., 53, 58–59, 62–63
  selected percentiles for, 54–57
  value of, to parents, 63
    to physician in appraising health status, 42–44, 49, 53, 59, 62–63
    to teachers in health education, 63
Body movements, coordination of, 407–408
Body resistance against infection, 200
  lowering of, by fatigue, 200
    by focal infections, 285
    by malnutrition, 200
    by protein deficiency, 299
  role of amino acids in, 290
Body size, chronological age and, 41
  terminal, 39
  unusual, as problem, 41–42
  (See also Height; Weight)
Body temperature, in fever, 111–112, 318
  normal, 6, 110
  regulation of, 110–111, 289, 312, 318
Body types (see Body build)
Boils (see Furuncles)
Bone marrow, red, formation in, of blood platelets, 168
    of red blood cells, 166–167, 394
    of white blood cells, 168
  yellow, 394
Bones, articulations of, 394–395
  broken, first aid for, 425–427
  calcification of, 33–34, 291, 293
  circulation in, 394
  growth of, 34, 40, 394
    effect on, of diet, 33
      of growth-controlling hormones, 34–35, 40
      of nutritional deficiency, 34, 293–294, 299, 301, 423–424
      of poor posture, 34, 411, 424
  infection of, 422–423
  shapes of, 394
  structure of, 393–394
  (See also Orthopedic defects; Skeleton)
Bonomo, Cosimo, 340
Bow legs, 34, 299, 423
Bowel (see Colon)
Bowel function, pleasure in, 73, 76
  psychosomatic mechanisms and, 114–115
Bowel movement, involuntary, 134
  (See also Defecation)
Bowman, Sir William, 302

Bowman's capsule, 302, 303
Brain (cerebrum), 87–88
  areas of, 87, 239
  cerebellum and, 409–410
  concussion of, 427
  confusion of, in dizziness, 409
  head injuries and, 378, 427
  hearing and, 382, 383
  organic disturbances of, 121–122, 132–133, 135, 136, 239–240
  pain and, 113
  speech and, 238
  vision and, 356–357
  (See also Cerebral cortex)
Brain stem, 91, 135
Brain waves, 132–133
Breastbone (see Sternum)
Breathing, difficult, 160, 178, 210, 218–219
Bright's disease, 306
Bronchial tubes, 95, 192, 193, 197
  in allergic reactions, 109, 219–220
  inflammation of, 102, 207–208
Bronchioles, 192, 193
Bronchitis, 102, 207–208
Bruce, Sir David, 269
Brucella melitensis, 267, 269, 270
Brucellosis (see Undulant fever)
Bruises, black eyes as, 350
  first aid for, 346
  subcutaneous bleeding in, 346, 351
Bullying, 119, 147
Burns, as cause, of blisters, 320
  of pain, 112, 113
  first-aid treatment for, 346
Bursae, 395
Bursitis, 395

C

Cabot, Richard C., 100n.
Calciferol (vitamin D₂), 294
Calcium, body's need for, in blood clotting, 168
  in bone formation, 33, 291, 393, 423–424
  in tooth building, 291
  daily requirements of, 295
  dissolving of (decalcification) in dental caries, 281
  effects of deficiency of, 34, 299, 423
  food sources of, 296, 299
Calmette, Albert, 217
Calories, 289, 290
  daily requirements of, 295
  effects of slow intake of, 297
  food sources of, 296

Cancer, 20, 171–172
Canker sores, 275
Cannon, Walter B., 99
Capillaries, 156
　bleeding from, 179
　in dermis, 314, 315, 326–327
　　rupture of, in bruises, 346, 350
　　as shock tissue in allergic skin reactions, 107, 329–331
　in exchanges between blood and tissues, 157–159, 173–174
　in lungs, 157, 192
　reaction of, in infection, 101–102
　　in shock, 166, 178–179
　　in vitamin-C deficiency (scurvy), 293, 301
　　in wheal formation, 319–320
Carbohydrates (sugars and starches), 249, 289
　calorie value of, 289
　and dental caries, 281, 282, 283
　digestion of, 250, 253, 254, 289
　effects of deficiency of, 299
　food sources of, 299
　oxidation of, 289
　　thiamine and, 292
Carbon dioxide, action of, on respiratory center, 194
　excretion of, 157, 192, 289, 302, 406
　formation of, in oxidation, 157, 289, 302, 406
Carbon monoxide asphyxia, 225
Carbonic acid, 302, 406
Carbuncles, 334, 342
Carotene, 292
　food sources of, 296, 300
Carpal bones, 396, 402
Carriers, of diphtheria, 204
　of malaria, 185
　of meningococcal meningitis, 131–132, 203
　of poliomyelitis, 125
　of streptococcal sore throat, 204, 212
　of typhoid fever, 265, 267
Cartilage, at joints, 395, 398, 399, 402, 428
　of larynx, 195
　of nose, 400
　ossification centers in, 33
Cecum, 250, 270
　pinworms in, 272
Cellulose, 294
　as aid to elimination, 264, 294
　in feces, 255, 264
Cementum of teeth, 279, 280
Central nervous system, 86–88
　infection of, 121, 136

Central nervous system, infection of, in encephalitis, 132
　in meningitis, 130–132
　in poliomyelitis, 122
　in rabies, 345
　in tetanus, 344
　injury of, 121, 136, 419, 427–428
　and intelligence, 64
　and muscle coordination, 407
　and referred pain, 113
　(See also Autonomic nervous system; Brain; Cerebral cortex; Spinal cord)
Cerebellum, 239, 409
　function of, 410
Cerebral cortex, areas of, motor, 87, 239
　　sensory, 87
　as seat of thought and voluntary action, 86, 92
　sensation and, 90–92
　(See also Brain)
Cerebral palsy, 135–136
　and orthopedic defects, 419, 420
　prevalence of, 421
Cerebrum, 87, 409
　(See also Brain; Cerebral cortex)
Chapping, 321–322
Cheeks, color of, 7, 315, 328
Cheilosis, 275, 293, 300
Chemotherapeutic drugs, 178, 272
Chemotherapy, 198
Chest (thorax), bones of, 397, 399
　"cold" in, 208
　deformities of, 415, 423, 431
　development of, 412, 416
　examination of, in tuberculosis, 216
　movements of, in respiration, 193, 399
　pain in, 161, 210
　　referred, 113
　position of, in good posture, 414, 416
　　in poor posture, 415, 418
　as segment of body weight, 411
Chest circumference, in athletes, 399
　measurements of, 54–61
Chicken breast, 415, 423
Chickenpox, 104, 222, 320
　attack of, 202
　school absences and, 18, 19
　virus of, 197, 202
Chiggers (harvest mites), 341
Chilblains, 322
Child-health problems, emotional and social, 141–148
　physical, 13–20
Chill (chilliness), in malaria, 184–185
　mechanics of, 111
　in pneumonia, 210

Chill (chilliness), in symptom complex, 112, 124, 221, 267
Chilling of body, effects of, on respiratory mucous membranes, 200–201
  pneumonia and, 209
  poliomyelitis and, 126, 127
Chloramphenicol, 267
Chloromycetin, 197*n*.
Choking, first aid for, 196
Cholera, 264, 265
Cholesterol, 294
Chorea, 115
  Sydenham's (St. Vitus's dance), 162
Choroid coat of eye, 354, 360, 361
Cilia, 196
  effect on, of cold, 201
Cilial escalator, 196, 201, 210
Ciliary body, 354, 360
Ciliary muscle, 360, 361, 368
Ciliary processes, 360, 361
Circulation, in abdominal organs, 156, 157
  to arms, 156
  arterial, 156–158
  in bones, 394
  in brain, 399
  capillary, 156–159
  in dermis (skin), 160, 314–315, 326–328
  disorders of, 159–164
  in eyeball, 353, 354
  to head, 156
  through heart, 155
  in kidneys, 156, 157, 302–303
  through lungs, 155
  in nose, 196, 200–201
  pulmonary, 157
  purpose of, 154, 158–159
  scheme of, 156
  in shock, 178
  systemic, 157
  in teeth, 280, 284
  venous, 156–157
Clavicle (collarbone), 396, 399, 401
  broken, 427
Cleft-palate speech, 229, 237–238
Clinics, child-guidance, 68, 139, 148
  mental-hygiene, 139, 148
  orthopedic, 430, 433
  speech, 228, 244
Clothing, body lice in, 343
  disinfestation of, 272, 343
  dry, in preventing colds, 224
  pinworm eggs in, 272
  posture and, 413
Clubfoot (talipes), 413, 417, 421
  prevalence of, 421
Coccyx, 396, 397, 402

Cochlea (inner ear), 376, 407
  organ of hearing in, 380
  structure of, 378–381
  transmission of sound in, 381–382
Cohn, Edwin J., 166
Cold sores (herpes simplex), 275
Colds, chemotherapy in prevention and treatment of, 201
  chilling of body and, 200–201
  chronic (catarrh), 202, 207
  contagiousness of, 221
  effect of, on eyes, 352
    on hearing, 377
    on voice, 236
  herpes simplex and, 275
  recurrences of, as diagnostic aid, 163, 178, 211
  research on, 206
  school absences and, 17
  secondary infections in, 176, 202, 207–208, 210
  signs and symptoms, mechanics of, 201
    similarity of, to those of other conditions, 219, 221
  virus of, 197, 202
Collagen, 394
Collarbone (*see* Clavicle)
Colon (large intestine), 250, 251, 258, 270
  effect on, of purgatives or laxatives, 263
    of irregular toilet habits, 264
  in elimination of waste products, 254–256, 302
  misbehaving, 264
  nervous control of, 256
  stimulation of, 255, 256, 264, 294
Comedomes (*see* Blackheads)
Communicable-disease control, methods of, for gastrointestinal infections, 266–267
  for insect-borne diseases, 183, 186–188
  for respiratory infections, 202–203, 205, 220
  progress in, 7–8, 14–15, 264, 265
  school and, 10
    in gastrointestinal infections, 265
    in poliomyelitis, 130
    in respiratory infections, 220–224
    in ringworm of scalp, 339–340
  teacher and, in impetigo, 333–334
    in insect-borne diseases, 183–184, 188
    in poliomyelitis, 130
    in respiratory infections, 220–221
    in ringworm of scalp, 339–340
Complexion, in acne, 323
  influence on, of skin pigment, 315, 328
    of skin's blood supply, 328

Compulsion neurosis, 138
Conduction, 110
Conflict, unconscious, 77–78
    expressions of, 95, 115–116, 119, 138
    psychotherapy and, 139
Congenital defects, of heart and blood vessels, 159, 160
    influence of, on physical growth, 33
    orthopedic, 419–422
    as result of German measles in pregnancy, 19
Conjunctiva of eye, 351
    inflammation of, 102
    causes of, 353
        in eye fatigue, 353, 365
    inspection of, for foreign body, 356
    jaundice and, 262, 263
Conjunctivitis (pinkeye), 353
Conscience, 72, 77, 78, 115
Consciousness, loss of, in epilepsy, 133–134
    in fainting, 182–183
    in head injuries, 427
Constipation, 5, 124, 272, 274, 300
    causes of, 263–264
    furred tongue and, 257
    psychogenic, 115
Constitution, definition of, 71
Convection, 111
Conversion hysteria, 138
Convulsions, 121
    epileptic, 133–134
Cornea, 353–354, 360
    in astigmatism, 364
    inflammation of, 354
    riboflavin and, 293, 301
Cortisone, in psoriasis, 319
    in rheumatic fever, 162
Cough, in bronchial asthma, 219–220
    in bronchitis, 208
    in colds, 201, 207
    as protective reflex, 100
    in symptom complex, 112, 202, 210, 215, 221
Coughing, technique of, 223
    typical, in whooping cough, 204–205
Cranial division, autonomic nervous system, 89
Cranium, bones of, 394, 399–401
Cretinism, 35
Crippled children (see Handicaps)
Crippled Children's Program of Children's Bureau, 419, 421
Crystalline lens of eye, 354, 360
    in astigmatism, 364

Crystalline lens of eye, changes in, during accommodation, 360–361
    suspensory ligament of, 354, 360, 361
Curriculum enrichment for gifted children, 70
Cuspids, 278, 279
Cuticle, care of, 325
Cuts, infected, 103
    first aid for, 344
Cyanosis (see Blueness)
Cycloplegic, 368
Cycloserine, 218

D

Dandruff, infectious, 335–336
    simple, 325
Daydreams, 120, 141
DDT, 186, 342, 343
Deafness, forms of, 382–383
    hysterical, 138
Death rates, from accidents, 14
    from appendicitis, 14, 19
    from common childhood diseases, 14
    from diabetes, 98
    from influenza, 208, 209
    from pneumonia, 14, 208, 209
    from poliomyelitis, 123
    from rheumatic fever and organic heart disease, 14, 18, 161
    of school-age children, by age group, 13
    decline of, 13–15
    from tuberculosis, 14, 18, 213
    from typhoid fever, 15, 265
    of United States population, 167
Decibels, 385, 386
Defecation (bowel movement), 255–256
    in constipation, 263–264
    in diarrhea, 264
    establishing habit of, 263–264
    voluntary control of, 250–251, 255, 263
Delinquency, 142, 147
Dementia praecox, 141
Dental caries, cause of, 281, 282
    detection of, 287, 288
    halitosis and, 257–258
    incidence of, 281, 284, 287
    malocclusion and, 285
    nutritional status and, 281
    prevention of, by dentifrices and mouth washes, 282, 283
        by sodium fluoride, 283–284
        by temperance in use of sweets, 282
        by toothbrushing, 282–283
    results of, 284–285
    variations in susceptibility to, 281, 282

Dental defects, prevalence of, 20, 279, 280, 287
  school absences and, 17
Dental examinations, 11, 287–288
  x-rays in, 285, 287
Dental hygienist, 11, 287–288
Dentine, 279, 280, 284
Depression, in infectious hepatitis, 267
  in manic-depressive illness, 140
  in young people, 140, 145–146
Dermatitis, allergic, 108–110, 330
  in chapping, 321
  in pellagra, 293, 301
  in skin infestations, 341, 342
  vesicle formation in, 320
Dermatologist, 321, 338
Dermis, 316, 317, 320, 333, 335, 346
  in allergic reactions, 109
  circulation in, 314–315, 326–328
  structure of, 313–314
Development, emotional and social, 71
  (See also Personality development)
  physical, 31
    determining levels of (Wetzel's grid), 49, 52, 53
    speed of (Wetzel's grid), 52
    (See also Growth, physical)
Diabetes, cause of, 97
  detection of, by urinalysis, 97, 303, 307
  insidious development of, 4
  juvenile, 97–99
  urination in, 97, 305
  weight loss in, 37, 97
Diabetic coma, 99
Diaphragm, 251, 255, 260
  in respiration, 193
Diarrhea, 264
  in symptom complex, 124, 266, 268, 272–274
Diastole, 155
  and blood pressure, 158
Diet, daily, for school children, 296
  influence of, on muscular growth, 36
    on skeletal growth, 33–34
    on weight, 38
Diethylstilbestrol in prevention of mumps orchitis, 205, 278
Digestion, absorption of products of, 254
  chemical, 252–254
  disturbances of, 257
    psychogenic, 256–257
    school absences and, 17, 19
    (See also Gastrointestinal disorders)
  effect of, on blood pressure, 158
  excretion of waste products of, 254–256

Digestion, mechanical, 250–252
  nervous control of, 256–257
Digestive juices, action of, 253–254
  secretion of, nervous control of, 87, 91
    psychic control of, 256
Digestive tract, 87, 95, 159
  (See also Gastrointestinal tract)
Diphtheria, 204–205
  bacillus of, 199, 204
  immunization from, 15, 104–106, 205
Dislocations, 402, 403, 428–429
  of finger or toe, reduction of, 429
  of lower jaw (mandible), 401
    reduction of, 429
Dizziness, 409
  in symptom complex, 121, 182, 272, 365
Docility, 142, 146
Donders, Franz Cornelius, 367, 368
Double vision (see Vision, double)
Dramamine, 261
Dreaminess, 120, 142, 146
Droplet nuclei, 221, 224
Drowsiness, 99, 112, 121, 124, 132, 266, 327
Ductless glands (see Endocrines)
Duodenum, 250, 254, 256
Dwarfism, 35
Dysentery, amebic, 265
  bacillary (shigellosis), 265, 266, 268
    bacilli of, 265, 266
    detection of, 268
    diarrhea in, 264, 266, 268

E

Ear, bleeding from, 427
  cocking of, 383, 413
  range of auditory response in, 385
  rubbing of, 374
  running, 377–378
  stuffiness in, 374, 377, 383
  (See also Cochlea; Eardrum; Middle ear; Outer ear canal)
Ear examinations, medical, 387, 388
Ear wax, 374, 375
Earache, 377
  in symptom complex, 112, 177, 221
Eardrum, 374
  equalizing air pressure on both sides of, 375–377
  in middle-ear infection, 377
  prevalence of defects of, 384
  vibrations of, in transmitting sound, 375, 381, 382
Eczema, 106, 107, 109, 110, 330–331

Edema (dropsy), 174–175
  in hookworm, 274
  in kidney disease, 174, 306
  in wheal formation, 320
Ego, formation of, 71–72
  strengthening of, 74, 80, 81
  in unconscious conflicts, 77–78, 115–116, 137–139
Elbow joints, 394–395, 402
Electric shock, 193, 225
Electroencephalograph, 132–133
Electroshock therapy, 140
Emetics, 260
Emotional disturbances, bronchial asthma and, 220
  epilepsy and, 133
  fear of heart trouble and, 161
  hearing loss and, 382
  poor nutrition and, 297n.
  prevention of, in school, 148–149
  in rheumatic children, 164
Emotional health, role of teacher in developing, 148–149
Emotional needs of children, 80–81
Emotional problems, of adolescents, 79–80
  of backward children, 71
  forms of, 141–148
  of gifted children, 68–69
  solution of, by repression, 77
Emotions, effect of, on appetite, 114, 261
    on autonomic nervous system, 95–96, 137
    on blood pressure, 158
    on cutaneous blood vessels, 327
    on digestion, 256–257
    on eye pupils, 355
    on heart rate, 158
    on vomiting reflex, 260
  learning to control, 75
  stuttering and, 241–244
Emulsification, 329, 332
Enamel of tooth, 278–280
  differences in solubility of, 281
  dissolving of, in dental caries, 281, 282
  mottling of, 283
  protection of, by sodium fluoride, 283–284
Encephalitis, epidemic ("sleeping sickness"), 132
Endemic disease, definition of, 186
Enders, John F., 128
Endocrines, 93–94
  disturbances of, 96
    in diabetes, 97
    in functioning of intelligence, 66, 70
    in growth control, 35

Endocrines, disturbances of, in nutrition, 297n.
    in reading difficulties, 366
    in simple goiter, 96
    in voice disorders, 232, 234
  effect of emotions on, 88, 95
  functions of, 94
    growth-controlling, 34, 37, 40
  interrelationships of, 96
Endolymph, 380, 381
Energy as mechanical equivalent of heat, 157
Energy metabolism (see Metabolism, energy)
Environment, 22
  influence of, on functioning of intelligence, 66–67
    on growth, 33
    on personality development, 22, 71
  interactions with, 22–23, 64, 77, 118
Enzymes, action of, 252–253
    in digestion, 250, 253–254
    in energy metabolism, 289
  amino acids in, 290
Epidemic disease, definition of, 186
Epidemics, of dysentery, 265
  of encephalitis, 132
  of infectious hepatitis, 267, 270
  of influenza, 208–209
  of meningitis, 131–132, 203
  of mumps, 277
  of ringworm of scalp, 337
  school procedures during, 221
    in ringworm of scalp, 339–340
  of streptococcal sore throat, 204, 212
  of typhus, 186, 342
  of warts, 321
Epidermis, 312–313
  in allergic reactions, 108, 109, 330
  in growth, of hair, 317
    of nails, 318
  horny layer of, 312–313
    in blister formation, 320, 346
    scaling of, 329, 332
      in psoriasis, 319
      in simple dandruff, 325
  in impetigo, 333
  itch mites in, 341
  nourishment of, 314
  pigmentation of, 314, 315
  warts and, 320
Epiglottis, 195, 229
Epileptic children, in school, 135
  teacher and, 135
Epilepsy, 132–135
  famous people and, 133

Epiphyses, 33–35, 40, 424
Equilibrium (see Body balance; Semicircular canals)
Erb's palsy, 422
Erythrocytes (see Red blood cells)
Esophagus, 194, 195, 250, 251
  sphincter of, in swallowing, 258–259
  stimulation of, by acid, 258
    by heat and cold, 262
    in nausea, 260
Ethmoid bone, sinuses in, 207, 401
Eustachian tubes, 177, 194, 195
  function of, 375–376
  swelling of, during a cold, 376–377
Eustachio, Bartolomeo, 375
Excretion, 249
  of metabolic wastes, 302
  of waste products of digestion, 254–256
Exercise, muscular, effect of, on heart rate, 101, 158
    on respiration rate, 101, 194
  heat production in, 110, 327, 328
  lactic acid production in, 406
  loss of muscle tone in, 406, 419
Expiration, 193
Eye examinations, medical, 354, 369
  instruments for, 367–368
  subjective, 367
Eye fatigue, 365
  astigmatism and, 365
  dizziness and, 365, 409
  farsightedness and, 362, 363
  nearsightedness and, 364
  in vision testing, 372, 374
  in vitamin-A deficiency, 301
Eye socket, 349, 400
Eye specialist, 359, 366, 367, 369
Eyeball, 349
  coats of, 353–354
  conjunctiva of, 351
  development of, 363
  in farsightedness, 362, 363
  muscles of, 357
    in squint, 358, 359
  in nearsightedness, 362, 363
Eyebrows, 349
  hair of, 317
Eyeglasses, for correction, of errors of refraction, 361–363
  of squint, 359, 360
  data on, for vision-test records, 374
  education regarding, 366–367
  supervision of children wearing, 367
Eyelashes, 349
  hair of, 317
  infection of, 350

Eyelid margins, dried secretions on, after sleep, 350
  inflammation of (blepharitis marginalis), 350
  in eye fatigue, 350, 353, 365
  in vitamin deficiencies, 300, 301
Eyelids, 349
  bruising of (black eye), 350–351
  conjunctiva of, 351
    inflamed, 352–353
  puffiness of, 351, 352
  stuck-together, 350
  twitching of, 121
Eyes, bleeding into, 427
  bloodshot, 352–353
  circles under, 327, 351
  color of, 6, 355
  connection of, with nose, 351, 352, 400
  equilibrium and, 408, 409
  focusing of, 357
    during accommodation, 360–361
    in errors of refraction, 361
    in squint, 358
  foreign body in, 356
  inflamed (red), 112, 220, 352, 353
  refracting media of, 360
  rubbing of, 350, 353, 365
  sensitivity of, to light, 350, 364, 365
  size of, 349
  structure of (see Eyeball)
  in vision (see Vision)
  vitamin-A deficiency and, 292, 300
  watering (running) of, 112, 218, 221, 352, 365, 374
    as protective reflex, 100
  white of, 353
Eyesight, conservation of, 369
  posture and, 413
  (See also Vision)

F

Face, appearance of, in anterior-pituitary hyperactivity, 35
  in good health, 7, 405
  in poor health, 7, 64, 297, 405
  bones of, 400
  flushed, 215, 221
  twitching of, 115, 121, 142, 162, 242
Facial expression, 7, 9, 297, 405
  in poor hearing, 383
Fainting, 182–183, 409
  hysterical, 138
Falsetto voice, 232, 234

Farsightedness (hyperopia), 362, 363
    astigmatism and, 364–365
    changes in incidence of, by age, 364
    correction of, by glass lenses, 363
    reading difficulties and, 366
Fatigue, causes of, 297, 351
    effect of, on appetite, 261
        on digestion, 256
        on facial expression, 405
        on posture, 297, 405, 411, 413, 419
        on resistance to infection, 126, 127,
            200, 215
        on skin beneath eyes, 351
        on vomiting reflex, 260
    of eyes (see Eye fatigue)
    of muscles, 406
        temporary, 419
    as sign, in intestinal worm infestation,
        272–274
        in nutritional deficiency, 297, 299, 300
        in poor hearing, 389
        in rheumatic fever, 163
        in tuberculosis, 215
Fats in food, 249, 289
    calorie value of, 289
    digestion of, 250, 253, 254
    food sources of, 299
    results of insufficient intake of, 299
Fatty acids, oxidation of, 289, 302
    as product of digestion, 253, 254
    storage of, 289–290
Fear (see Anxiety; Emotions)
Feces, composition of, 255
    in diarrhea, 264
    excretion of, 255–256
    intestinal parasites in, 273
    playing with, 73
    retention of, in constipation, 263–264
Feebleminded children, 136
Feet, in anterior-pituitary hyperfunction,
        35
    bones of, 401, 403
    defects of, clubfoot as, 417, 421
        flatfoot as, 415, 417
        indications of, 431
        pigeon toe as, 417, 431
    hookworm and, 273, 274
    position of, in good posture, 414, 416–
        417
        in poor posture, 415, 431
        in walking, correct, 417
        incorrect, 417, 431
    ringworm infection of (athlete's foot),
        336–337
Femur (thighbone), 396, 403, 411, 424

Fever, 111–112
    characteristic, in typhoid fever, 267
        in undulant fever, 267, 269
    effect of, on heart rate, 101, 158
        on respiration rate, 101, 194
    indications of, 112
        flushing as, 111, 215, 221, 328
    in inflammations, 102
    low-grade, in mild meningitis, 131
        in rheumatic fever, 112, 161, 163
        in tuberculosis, 112, 215
    as protective device, 111
Fibrin, 165
    in blood clotting, 166
Fibrin film, 165
Fibrin foam, 165
Fibrinogen, 165
    in blood clotting, 166
Fibula (calf bone), 396, 403
Finger sucking, malocclusion and, 286
    in oral period, 73, 75, 76
    psychogenic, 114, 137, 142
Fingernails, 318
    defects of, 325
Fingerprints, 314
Fingers, bones of, 394, 402
    joints of, 394
        reducing dislocation of, 429
First-aid supplies, for fractures and
        sprains, 425
    for skin injuries, 343–344
Flatfoot, 415, 417
Flushing, in fever, 111, 215, 221, 328
    normal, 327
Focal infections, 285, 413, 419
Folliculitis, 342
Food-borne diseases, control of, 264–265,
        266n.–267n.
Food elements, 249
    (See also Nutrients, specific)
Food infections (salmonellosis), 266, 268
    staphylococcal, 266, 269
Food and Nutrition Board, National Re-
        search Council, 291n., 295
Food poisoning, 268, 269
Foodstuffs, classes of, 249
    oxidation of, 110
Foreign body, in ear, 374–375
    in eye, 356
    swallowed, 259n.
Fractures, 425
    of collarbone, 426–427
    compound, infection of, 422
    of limbs, 425–426
    of skull, 427
Francis, Thomas, Jr., 129

Freckles, 6
  formation of, 314
Freud, Sigmund, 71
Frontal bone, 396, 399
  sinuses in, 207, 400
Frostbite, 322
  first-aid treatment for, 346
Frustration, anxiety and, 137
  guilt and, 77, 143
  overcoming, in personality development,
    74–75
  reactions to, 95, 114–115, 118–121, 241
Functional illness, definition of, 100
Fundus of eye, 367, 368
Fungi, ringworm, animal, 336, 338
    human, 336, 338
    transmission of, 338–339
  skin-dwelling, 329
Fungicides, 338
Furuncles, 334–335

G

Gait, deviations from normal in, 431, 432
  in cerebral palsy, 136
  in congenital hip dislocation, 421
Gall bladder, location of, 251
Gamma globulin, antibodies in, 106, 164,
    200, 290
  in control, of infectious hepatitis, 128,
    165, 267
    of measles, 106, 128, 165, 202
    of mumps, 205, 278
    of poliomyelitis, 128–129
  as fraction of blood plasma, 164, 165
  protein in manufacture of, 290
Gangrene, prevention of, in frostbite, 346
Garrison, Fielding H., 171
Gas on stomach, 258
Gastric juice, acidity of, 251, 258
  as defense against infection, 101
  enzymes of, in protein digestion, 353
  psychic secretion of, 256
Gastric ulcer, 95
Gastrocnemius muscle, 403
Gastrointestinal tract, in allergic reactions,
    107
  disorders of, as cause of school absences,
    19
    in conversion hysteria, 137
    in niacin deficiency, 301
    signs and symptoms of, 257–264
  infection of, 265–270
    as cause of school absences, 19
    progress in control of, 15, 264–265

Gastrointestinal tract, in poliomyelitis,
    125
Genital organs, playing with, 73, 76
German measles (rubella), 202
  danger of, in pregnancy, 19
  school absences and, 18, 19
  swelling of cervical lymph nodes in, 175
  virus of, 196, 202
Germs (see Bacteria; Fungi; Viruses)
Gifted children, educational opportunities
    for, 69–70
  identification of, 67–68
  problems of, 68–69, 144
Gigantism, 35
Gingivitis, 286, 287
Glomeruli, 302, 303
  inflammation of, 305, 306
Glossitis, 276, 293, 300
Glottis, 229–230
Glucose (simple sugar), chemical formula
    of, 289
  as end product of carbohydrate diges-
    tion, 250, 253, 254
  oxidation of, 289, 302
    insulin and, 97
  storage of, as glycogen, 289
Glycerin, 253, 254, 289
Glycogen, as muscle fuel, 405, 406
  storage of, 289
Goiter, simple, 96–97, 300
Gonads (see Sex glands)
Goose flesh, 111, 113, 317–318
Graefe, Albrecht, 368
Grand mal, 133–134
Grasping, 401
Gravity, body balance and, 410–411, 416
  center of, in body, 410
  pull of, on body, 393, 405, 410
Growth, emotional and social, phases of,
    73
  (See also Personality development)
  mental, 64
    factors influencing, 66–67
    measurement of, 64–65
  physical, 31
    factors influencing, 33
    measurement of (see Body measure-
      ments)
    nutrition and, 297, 299, 300
    patterns of, 31–32, 43, 49, 52–53
    relation of, to chronological age, 31,
      39, 40–42
    stages and rates of, 38–42
    (See also Height; Weight)
  skeletal (see Bones, growth of; Skeleton)

Guidance of school children, 11, 12, 118
  meeting need for, 148–149
Guilt, aggressiveness and, 119, 147
  frustration and, 143
  hostile impulses and, 76, 77, 115–116
Gumboil, 285
Gums, 279, 280
  bleeding of, in vitamin-C deficiency,
    286, 293, 301
  inflammation of, 286, 287
  inspection of, 8
  in trench mouth, 276

H

Habit acts, 92
Habit tics, 115–116
  wryneck as, 421
Hair, 316–317
  color of, 318, 324
  dryness of, 324
  falling out of, 324
  lice in, 342–343
  life span of, 318, 324
  oiliness of, 324–325
  shape of, 318, 324
  texture of, 318, 324
  vitamin-A deficiency and, 300
Hair bulb, 317
  pigment in, 318
  in ringworm infection, 338
Hair follicles, 316, 317
  hair shape and, 318
  in ringworm infection, 338
Hair-raising muscles, 316, 317, 322
Hair shaft, 317
  air bubbles in, 318
  pigment in, 318
Halitosis (bad breath), 257–258
Hammond, William McD., 128
Hand washing, in compulsion neurosis,
    138
  in control of infection, 126, 127, 221,
    224, 265, 267n., 270, 272, 273
  facilities for, in school, 223
Handedness, 238–239
Handicaps, adjusting to, 16, 81, 388–389,
    432
  cultivating right attitudes toward chil-
    dren with, 130, 135, 136, 244, 432
  loss of hearing as, 382, 388
  orthopedic, 419
  speech defects as, 228
Handkerchief, proper use of, 223

Hands, in anterior-pituitary hyperactivity,
    35
  bones of, 401, 402
Hangnails, 325
Hard-of-hearing children, 388–389
Harelip, 229, 235, 274
Harvey, William, 164
Hay fever, 107, 109, 218–219
Head, growth of, 32
  injury of, 378, 427
  noises in, 383
  position of, in eye testing, 373
    in good posture, 414
    in poor hearing, 413, 422
    in poor posture, 415
    in poor vision, 413, 422
    in squint, 359
    in wryneck, 421
    in young children, 412
  as segment, of body height, 32
  of body weight, 411
Headache, in eye fatigue, 365
  fever and, 112
  after head injury, 427
  at onset of respiratory infections, 221
  in organic disorders of nervous system,
    121
  psychogenic (nervous), 92, 113–114, 137
  in sinusitis, 207
Health education, in control of gastro-
    intestinal infection, 265
  in nutrition, 298, 301–302, 422
  in school health service, 10, 12, 16
Hearing, colds and, 377
  organ of, 380
  psychogenic disturbances of, 115
  sensation of, 90, 91, 381–382
Hearing aids, 388
Hearing loss, detection of, by hearing
    tests (see Hearing tests)
  by teacher's observations, 4, 383–384,
    388
  forms of, 382–383
  as handicap, 382, 388
  middle-ear infection and, 377, 378
  posture and, 413
  prevalence of, 384
  referral for medical examination in, 383,
    387, 388
  signs of, 383–384
  speech disorders and, 229
  supervision of children with, 388–389
  treatment of, 388
Hearing tests, audiometric, 384–385
  preparation for, 385–386
  retesting in, 386

Hearing tests, audiometric, routine, 384
  recording results of, in decibels, 385, 386
    as fraction of norm, 387
    in sensation units, 384
  watch-tick, 387–388
  whisper, 386–387
Heart, 154–155
  disorders of, functional, 161
    organic, 159–160
      in rheumatic fever, 161–164
  innervation of, 87, 89
  referred pain in, 113
Heart murmurs, 159
Heart rate, 155
  autonomic control of, 87, 95, 137, 158
  effect on, of emotions, 95, 137, 158
    of exercise, 101, 158
    of fever, 101, 158
  functional disturbances of, 161
Heartbeat, 155
  effect of, on arterial blood pressure, 158
  mineral salts in regulation of, 291
  rate of (see Heart rate)
Heartburn, 258
Heel bone, 397, 403, 416
Height (stature), 43
  at birth, 38
  components of, 32, 38
  influence on, of endocrine disturbances, 35
  measurements of, 41, 43–62
    in classroom, 62–63
  range of, 6, 41
  rate of gain in, 32, 39
  sex differences in, 40–41
Height-age curves, construction of, 44
  normal variations from, 44–48
  use of, 49
Height-weight-age-body-build tables, 44
Height-weight-age tables, 43–44
Helmholtz, Hermann, 368
Hemoglobin, affinity of, for carbon monoxide, 225
  breakdown of, 262
  deficiency of, in anemias, 171–173
  as oxygen carrier, 166, 224, 327
Hemolysins, 199
Hemophilia, 165, 166
  antihemophilic globulin in treatment of, 165
Hemorrhage (bleeding), 165, 171, 179
  control of (see Nosebleed; Wounds, bleeding from)
  intracranial, 135, 427
  subcutaneous, in bruises, 346, 351
    in purpura, 171

Hemorrhage (bleeding), subcutaneous, in scurvy, 293
Hepatitis, infectious, 263, 267, 270
  gamma globulin in control of, 128, 165, 267
Heredity, 21–22
  constitution and, 71
  dental caries and, 281
  in determination, of eye color, 355
    of hair color, 318
    of shape of jaw, 285
  in development, of diabetes, 97
    of epilepsy, 132
    of familial allergy, 107
    of psoriasis, 319
    of rheumatic fever, 161
  hemophilia and, 165, 166
  influence of, on growth pattern, 33, 42
    on intelligence, 64
    on skeletal growth, 33
  personality and, 21–23
Herpes simplex (cold sores), 275
Hinge joints, 394, 400
Hip width, measurements of, 54–61
Hipbones, 396, 397, 402
  in sitting, 417, 418
Hips, congenital dislocation of, 421
  joints of, 394
Histamine, in allergic reactions, 109
  in sunburn, 314
Hives (urticaria), 107, 109, 329, 331
Hoarseness, 207
Holger Nielsen method of artificial respiration, 225–227
Hookworm (ancylostomiasis), 273–274
Hormones, 92–95
  of adrenal cortex, 34, 94, 162
  of adrenal medulla (adrenaline), 94–95
  amino acids in manufacture of, 290
  of anterior pituitary, 34, 94
  female (estrogens), 94, 278
  gonadal, 34, 40
  of islands of Langerhans (insulin), 94, 97
  of thyroid (thyroxine), 34, 94, 96, 291
Horstmann, Dorothy M., 125
Hostility, behavior reactions to, 115–116, 119, 147
  in reading difficulties, 366
  in stuttering, 242, 243
  and guilt, 76, 77
Humerus, 396, 402, 403
Hunger, 261
  in diabetes, 97
  in insulin reaction, 99
Hydraulic pressure of blood, 173–174
Hydrochloric acid in gastric juice, 258

Hyoid bone, 401
Hyperopia (see Farsightedness)
Hypersensitivity in allergy, 107
Hypertension, 95, 159–160
Hypoproteinemia, 165
Hysteria, anxiety, 137–138
  conversion, 137
  fainting and, 137
  wryneck and, 422

I

Id, 71, 72
Ileum, 250
Ilium, 58, 396, 402
Immunity, 104
Immunization, 104–106
  active, 104
    in poliomyelitis, 129
  in communicable-disease control, 8, 106
  passive, 104, 106
    in poliomyelitis, 128–129
  in schools, 11, 220
Immunization timetable, 105
Impetigo contagiosa, 333–334, 343
Impulse, nerve, 90–91
Inadequacy, feelings of, 119, 147
Inattentiveness, in hearing loss, 4, 383
  in petit mal, 133
Incisors, 278, 279
Incus, 376, 381
Indigestion, 257
  acid, 258
  nervous, 114, 256
  as symptom, 137, 271, 274
Infection, 340
  inapparent (mild), in bacillary dysentery, 268
  in influenza, 208
  in meningococcus meningitis, 130–131
  in poliomyelitis, 125
  in undulant fever, 269
  observing children for signs of, 220–221
  reaction of body to, 101–104
Infestation, 340
  with intestinal worms, 271–274
  with skin parasites, 340–343
Inflammation, 101–102
Influenza, epidemic, 208–210, 221
  bronchitis and, 207
  epidemic encephalitis and, 132
  pneumonia and, 208–210
  recurrences of, 211
  vaccines against, 208–209
  virus of, 197, 208, 209

Inner ear (see Cochlea)
Insecticides, 186, 187, 343
Insects, bites of, 347
  as disease carriers, 132, 183–188
Insecurity, feelings of, 80, 119
Inspiration in breathing, 193
Instinctual drives, 71, 72, 74, 77, 78, 137–138
Insulin, 97–99
Insulin reaction, 99
Intelligence, factors influencing use of, 66–67
  inferior, 70–71
  measuring, 64–65
  normal range of, 65
  superior, in epileptic children, 134
    identification of, 67–68
    problems of, 68–69
    in withdrawn children, 146
  variations in, 64
Intelligence quotient (see I.Q.)
Intelligence tests, 64–65
  administration of, 68
Intestinal juice, 253, 254
Intestines, effect on, of emotions, 95, 256, 257
  parasitic infestations of, 271–274
  (See also Colon; Small intestine)
Iodine, deficiency of, in simple goiter, 96–97, 300
  food sources of, 96, 300
  need for, by thyroid, 96, 291
  requirements for, 291n.
Iodized salt, 96, 291n., 300
I.Q. (intelligence quotient), body size and, 42
  computation of, 65n.
  high, 65, 66
  low, 65, 66, 70
  normal range of, 65
Iris, 354, 355
Iron, daily requirements of, 295
  deficiency of, in nutritional anemia, 171, 172, 299
  food sources of, 296, 299–300
  in red blood cells, 167, 291
Iron lung, 124
Irritability, 77, 124, 163, 272, 365
Ischia (seat bones), 397, 402, 417, 418
Islands of Langerhans, 93, 94, 97
Isoniazid, 218
Itch, the (scabies), 340–341
Itching, 114
  in allergic reactions, 109, 218, 330–331
  of eyes, 350, 353

Itching, in reaction to specific irritants, 272, 274, 322, 333, 336, 341–343
Ivy poisoning, 320

J

Jaundice, 262–263
  in infectious hepatitis, 267, 270
  (*See also* Hepatitis, infectious)
Jaws, 401
  reducing dislocation of lower, 429
Jealousy, 115
Jenner, Edward, 104
Joints, 394–395
  dislocations in, 428–429
  lubrication of, 395, 404
  pain in, in meningitis, 131
    in rheumatic fever, 161, 163
    in undulant fever, 267
    in vitamin-C deficiency, 301
  pain receptors in, 112
  sacroiliac, 397
    strain of, 402
  sprains of, 429
  tuberculosis of, 175, 422–423
    as cause of orthopedic defects, 420
    prevalence of, 421

K

Keratin, 313
Keratitis, 293, 354
Kidneys, 302–304
  adrenal glands and, 93
  circulation in, 156, 157, 302
  in excretion of metabolic wastes, 159, 290, 302, 304
  inflammation of, 305–306
  innervation of, 87, 89
Knee joint, 394, 403
Knees, in good posture, 414
  in poor posture, 415
  in sitting, 418
  in walking, 417
Knock-knees, 34, 417, 423
Koch, Robert, 217
Kyphosis (humpback), 415, 431

L

Labyrinth (*see* Semicircular canals)
Lacrimal ducts, 352, 400
Lacrimal glands, 351, 352
  effect on, of vitamin-A deficiency, 292

Lactic acid, 405–406
Lactobacilli, 281, 282
Landsteiner, Karl, 168
Large intestine (*see* Colon; Intestines)
Laryngitis, 207
Larynx (voice box), 195–196
  descent of, in adolescent boys, 232, 234
  inflammation of, 207
  and pharynx, 193–195
  and speech, 229–230, 238
Lassitude (languor), 112, 203, 327
Latency, period of, 73
  behavior characteristics in, 78, 146
  teacher and, 78
Laxatives, 263, 271
Left-handedness, 238–239
  observation of, 6
  and reading difficulties, 365
Legs, aching of, 114, 221
  bones of, 394, 401, 403
    first aid for fractures of, 425–426
  circulation to, 156
  measurements of girth of, 54–61
  muscles of, in walking, 417
  and stature by age, 32
Length of life, of red cells of blood, 167
  of United States population, 167
Lens of eye (*see* Crystalline lens of eye)
Leukemia, 171–172
  purpura in, 173
Leukocytes (*see* White blood cells)
Lice, body, 186, 342
  head, 342–343
  pubic, 342
Ligaments, 395, 403, 411, 417
  in dislocations, 428
  in sprains, 429
Light, refraction of, by glass lenses, 361–363
    by media of eye, 360
  sensitivity to, in blepharitis, 350
    in eye fatigue, 301, 365
    of iris, 355
    in nearsightedness, 364
  stimulation of retina by, 355–357
Limbs, aching or pain in, 112, 163
  first aid, for bleeding from, 179, 180–181
    for broken, 425–426
  supporting framework for, 395
Limp, 424, 431
Lip reading, 388
Lips, disorders of, 274–275
  healthy, 274
  and speech, 229–232, 235, 238
Lisping, 229, 235–236
Liver, circulation in, 156, 157

Liver, excretion of bilirubin by, 262, 263
  formation of urea in, 290, 304
  innervation of, 89
  location of, 251
  secretion of bile by, 253, 254, 263
  stored sugar (glycogen) in, 289
    release of, 94–95
  stored vitamin A in, 292
Lockjaw (see Tetanus)
Locomotion, 401
Lordosis, 412, 415, 431
Lump in throat, 258–259
Lungs, circulation through, 156, 157
    effects of interference with, 160–161
    exchange of respiratory gases in, 157,
      159, 192, 210
    excretion of end products of oxidation
      by, 157, 289, 302, 406
    expansion of, 193, 399
    infection of, in pneumonia, 210–211
      in tuberculosis, 215n.
    innervation of, 87, 89
Lying, 115
Lymph (tissue fluid), 154, 173
  circulation of, 175
  exchanges of, between blood and tissues,
    173–174
Lymph nodes, 175–176
  infection of, 176–177
Lymphatics, 175

                          M

Macula, of eye, 354
    in squint, 358
  of utricle, 407, 408
Maladjustment, emotional and social,
    manifestations of, in behavior, 119,
    142
    somatic, 76, 115, 142
  school acceleration and, 69
  teacher's attitude toward, 141
  (See also Behavior problems)
Malaise (feeling ill) in symptom complex,
    99, 131, 203, 221, 267, 327
Malaria, 183–186
  blood test for, 186
  control of, 183, 186
  prevalence of, 183, 185
  Sporozoa of, 183, 184
Malleus, 376, 381
Malnutrition, 4
  and lowered resistance to infection, 200,
    215
  prevalence of, 20

Malnutrition, signs and symptoms of, 297–
    298
  (See also Nutrition, poor; Nutritional
    deficiency)
Malocclusion, 285–286
  mouth breathing and, 222
  speech difficulties and, 235, 236
Mandible (lower jawbone), 396, 400, 401
  reducing dislocation of, 429
Manic-depressive illness, 140
Massachusetts Vision Test, 372
Mastication, 274, 278
Mastoid bone, 376–378
Mastoiditis, 378
Masturbation, 73, 76–77, 79
Matrix of nails, 318
  injury of, 325
Maturity, in personality development, 72,
    80, 119–120
  physical, as end of growth process, 32,
    36, 39, 41
  sexual, progress toward, 77, 79
Maxillae (upper jawbones), 396, 401
  sinuses in, 207, 400
Measles (rubeola), 202
  effect of, on eyes, 202, 352
    on middle ear, 377
  gamma globulin in prevention and
    treatment of, 18–19, 128, 165, 202
  school absences and, 19
  ultraviolet irradiation and, 222
  virus of, 197, 202
Medical examinations, cardiac, 159, 161
  of ears, 387, 388
  of eyes, 354, 367–369
  nurse and, 12–13
  orthopedic, 430
  parents and, 5, 12, 13
  physician and, 3, 5, 11–13
  school, 10–13
  teacher and, 5, 11–13
  teeth inspection in, 287, 288
  urinalysis in, 97
  use of height-weight measurements in,
    44, 49, 53, 59, 62–63
  weight reduction and, 38
Medulla oblongata, 87, 89, 239, 409
  in bulbar poliomyelitis, 124
  defecation center in, 255
  respiratory center in, 126, 193, 255, 259
  vomiting center in, 255, 259–260
Meninges, inflammation of, 131
Meningitis, 131
  meningococcal, 131–132, 203
  tuberculous, 214

Meningococcus (*Neisseria meningitidis*), 131–132, 198, 203
Menstruation, 73
    herpes simplex and, 275
Mental-hygiene movement, 139–140
Mental illness, neurotic, 137–138
    prevention of, 139, 148–149
    psychogenic versus organic, 136–137
    psychotic, 137, 140–141
    treatment of, 139–140
Meredith, Howard V., 44–48, 53, 59
Metabolism, 111, 249
    definition of, 288–289
    diabetes as disease of, 97
    energy, 34
        excretion of waste products of, 157, 289, 302
        protein, excretion of waste products of, 302
Metacarpal bones, 396, 402
Metatarsals, 396, 403, 417
Microorganisms (*see* Bacteria; Fungi)
Microsporum audouini, 337–338
    lanosum, 338
Middle ear, 375, 376
    air pressure in, 375–377
    connection of, with nasopharynx, 194, 375, 376
    infection of (*see* Otitis media)
    transmission of sound by, 381, 382
Migraine, 107, 133
Milk, contaminated, in spread of infection, 177, 204, 212, 265–267, 269
    pasteurization of, as preventive measure, 177, 203, 205, 266n., 269, 270
Miller, W. E., 281
Mineral salts, 249
    body's use of, 291, 406
    food sources of, 291
    (*See also* Calcium; Iodine; Iron; Phosphorus)
Mites, harvest (chiggers), 341
    itch, 340–341
Molars, 278, 279
    decayed, 377
Moles (nevi), 321
Mononucleosis, infectious, 176
Mosquitoes, in spread of encephalitis, 132
    in spread of malaria, 183, 184
Motion sickness, 260–261, 409
Mouth, bleeding from, 427
    as division of alimentary canal, 250, 274
    mucous membrane of, healthy, 275, 328
        inflamed, 275–276
    preoccupation with, 73
    in psychosomatic mechanisms, 114

Mouth, secretion of saliva in, 253
    effect on, of emotions, 88, 137, 256
    and vowel sounds, 230, 233
Mouth breathing, 222–223
    as diagnostic aid, 177
Mucopus, 207
Mucous membrane, 315
    allergic reactions in, 106, 107, 109
    respiratory (*see* Respiratory mucous membranes)
Mucus in nose, 101, 196, 400
Mumps (infectious parotitis), 204–205, 277–278
    complications of, after puberty, 19, 205, 277, 278
    earache and, 377
    school absences and, 19
    virus of, 197, 204, 277
Murine typhus, 187
Muscle buffering, 406
Muscle contraction, chemistry of, 405–406
    mechanics of, 404, 405
Muscle coordination, 407
    cerebellum and, 410
    effects of lack of, 135–136
Muscle tone, 404–405
    cerebellum and, 409–410
    lowering of, in fatigue, 405, 419
    in poor posture, 411, 416
Muscles, 403–404
    of alimentary canal, 251–252, 256
    ciliary, 360, 361, 368
    of eyeball, 357
    hair-raising, 316, 317, 322
    of heart, 154
    of leg in walking, 417
    pain receptors in, 112
    of respiration, 193, 194
    smooth (involuntary), 404
        autonomic control of, 87, 251–252
    striated, 403–404
    voluntary, 393, 403–404
        body dimensions and, 36, 53
        in cerebral palsy, 135
        control of, by motor area of cortex, 87, 239
        fatigue of, 406
        growth and development of, 36
        pain in, in symptom complex, 124, 131, 163, 267
        in poliomyelitis, 123–124
        posture and, 411–412, 416
        in St. Vitus's dance, 162
        in tetanus, 344
Myopia (*see* Nearsightedness)
Myxedema, 35

N

Nail biting, 325
  psychosomatic, 114, 142
  in spread of pinworms, 272
Nasal allergy, 218–220
Nasal sinuses (see Sinuses)
Nasality, 229, 236–237
Nasopharyngitis, 212
Nasopharynx, 194
  adenoids in, 177, 178
  bacterial flora of, 197
  connection of, with middle ear, 194, 375
  as reservoir of infection, 131, 197, 199,
    201, 212
National Foundation for Infantile Paral-
    ysis, 127, 128
National Society for the Prevention of
    Blindness, 361
Nausea, 260
  and dizziness, 409
  psychosomatic, 137, 261
  in symptom complex, 99, 112, 124, 184,
    204, 221, 266, 267, 271, 272
  and vomiting, 259, 260
Nearsightedness, 363–364
  astigmatism and, 364–365
  correction of, by glass lenses, 362
  development of, 4, 363, 364
Neck, abnormal positions of, 421–422
  broken, 428
  stiffness of, 124
  vertebrae of, 397, 398
Negativism, 118, 144
Nephritis, acute glomerular, 306
  chronic (Bright's disease), 306
  after streptococcal infection, 18, 203n.,
    212, 306
  tubular, 306
Nephrons, 302–303
  inflammation of, 305, 306
Nephrosis, 306
Nerve cells (neurons), 88, 90, 92
  motor, destruction of, in poliomyelitis,
    123–124
Nerve fibers, 88–90
Nerve impulse, 90–91
Nerve-muscle coordination (see Muscle co-
    ordination)
Nerve sheaths, pain receptors in, 112
Nervous system (see Autonomic nervous
    system; Central nervous system)
Neuritis, 102
Neuroses, patterns of, 137–139
  helping children to avoid, 139
  psychotherapy for, 139

Niacin (P-P factor), body's need for, 293
  crystals of, 293
  daily requirements of, 295
  effects of deficiency of, 293, 301
  food sources of, 296, 301
Nielsen, Holger, 225, 227
Nielsen method of artificial respiration,
    225–227
Night blindness, 292, 300
Nitrogen in amino acids, 290
Nitrogenous wastes, 302, 304
Nits, 8, 342–343
Nocturnal emissions in boys, 73
Normality, conception of, 6–7
Nose, 194
  as air-conditioning system, 194, 196, 222
  blowing of, 223
  bones of, 396, 400–401
  connection of, with eyes, 351, 352, 400
  discharge from, 8, 9, 103, 112, 126, 201,
    221
  mucous membrane of, in allergic re-
    actions, 107, 109, 218–219
    effect on, of chilling, 200–201
    (See also Respiratory mucous mem-
      branes)
  obstruction of, in colds, 201, 236
    in mouth breathing, 222–223
    in speech difficulties, 229, 236
  and speech, 230–232, 236
Nosebleed, 179, 182
  in rheumatic fever, 163, 179, 182
Nursing, pleasure in, 72, 73, 75
Nutrients, specific, daily requirements of,
    295, 298
    effects of insufficient intake of, 297–
      302
    food sources of, 296, 299–301
Nutrition, education in, of school children,
    298, 301–302
  of teachers, 298
  good, and posture, 413
    signs of, 297, 328
    yardstick of, 295
  poor, and eye circles, 351
    and posture, 413
    signs of, 297
  progress in science of, 423
Nutritional anemia, 171, 299–300
Nutritional deficiency, 297–298
  results of, 297–301, 316, 325, 350, 353,
    354, 423–424
  (See also Malnutrition; Nutrition, poor)
Nutritional (or health) status, appraisal
    of, by body measurements, 42, 43, 49–
    51, 53

Nutritional (or health) status, physical signs related to, 297–298
    subjective estimates of, 63–64

O

Observation of health status of children, practice of, by teacher, 6–7
    time and place of, in school, 7–9
    value of, by parents, 2–5, 9–10
        in communicable-disease control, 220, 224
    by physician, 3
    by teacher, 2–5
        in communicable-disease control, 220–221
Occipital bone, 397–400
Oedipus complex, 73, 76–77
Olfactory nerve, 257, 274, 276, 400
Ophthalmic examination, 354
    (See also Eye examinations, medical)
Ophthalmologists, 366
Ophthalmoscope, 355, 367–368
Optic nerve, 356
Oral period in emotional and social growth, 73, 75
Orchitis, 277, 278
Organ of Corti, 380
Organic illness, 100
Organs of equilibrium, 399–400
    (See also Semicircular canals)
Orthodontist, 286
Orthopedic defects, 393
    causes of, 419
        congenital conditions as, 419–422
        infections as, 422
        rickets as, 423–424
        spinal curvature as, 424
    Crippled Children's Program and, 419, 421
    indications of, 431
    observing children for, 430, 432
    posture and, 413
    prevalence of, 420, 421
    school and, 432–433
Orthopedics, 393
Orthopedists, 393
Orthoptics, 359–360
Osmosis in food absorption, 252
Osmotic pressure, in fluid exchanges between blood and tissues, 173–174
    lowering of, in nephritis, 306
Ossicles, 378, 381
Ossification centers (epiphyses), 33, 34, 40
Osteomyelitis, 413, 422

Osteomyelitis, prevalence of, 421
Otitis media, 102, 208
    acute, 377–378
    chronic, 378
        hearing loss and, 383
    prevalence of, 384
    scarlet fever and, 212
Otoliths, 408
Otological examination, 388
Otologist, 388
Outer ear canal, 374, 376
    discharge from, 8, 103, 377–378
    foreign body in, 374–375
Oval window of ear, 376, 380, 381
Ovaries, 93, 94
    inflammation of, in mumps, 205, 277
Overactivity, 142
Overdependence, 116, 120, 142, 146, 147
    dealing with, by teacher, 121
Overdirection, 118
Overeating, 114
Oversubmissiveness, 116
Overweight, 4, 37, 38, 43, 44, 97, 327
    reduction of, 38
Oxidation, 289
    excretion of end products of, 157, 192, 289, 302, 406
    formation of water in, 289, 294–295, 302, 406
        of carbon dioxide in, 157, 289, 302, 406
    insulin and, 97
    in muscle contraction, 405–406
    production of body heat in, 110, 157, 289, 302
Oxygen, in atmosphere, 192, 224–225
    body's need for, 192, 224–225
    exchanges of, between blood and tissues, 159, 160, 167, 327
        between lungs and blood, 157, 159, 160, 167, 192, 210
    increased usage of, 101, 194
    in muscle contraction, 405
    transport of, to tissues, 157, 166, 171
    (See also Oxidation)

P

Pain, 112–113, 261–262
    in appendicitis, 271
    dealing with complaints of, 113–114
    effect of, on vomiting reflex, 260
    psychogenic, 113
    referred, 113, 262
    as sign of inflammation, 101–102

Pain, in sinusitis, 207
  as somatic sensibility, 91
Palate, 236
  hard, 195, 236
    cleft in, 229, 237
  soft, 195, 236
    in speech, 232, 236–237
Pallor, in anemia, 172–173
  in fainting, 182
  natural, 315
  in nausea, 260
  psychogenic, 88, 113, 327
  in shock, 178
  in symptom complex, 163, 183, 272
Palpitation of heart, 161
Pancreas, islands of Langerhans in, 93–94, 97
  secretion of pancreatic juice by, 253
Pancreatic juice, in digestion, 253, 254
  psychic secretion of, 256
Papillae, of dermis, 314, 326–327
  of hair, 317, 318
  in ringworm of scalp, 338
Paraaminosalicylic acid (PAS), 218
Paralysis, in beriberi, 293
  in birth injury, 419
  in Erb's palsy, 422
  hysterical, 138
  in poliomyelitis, 122–124
  in spinal-cord injury, 427, 428
Parasympathetic division, autonomic nervous system, 89
Parathyroids, 93
Parietal bones, 396, 397, 399
Parotid gland, 251
  discovery of duct of, 277
  infection of, in mumps, 204, 277–278
Pasteur, Louis, 104, 345
Pasteurization of milk, 177, 203, 205, 266n., 267, 269, 270
Patella (kneecap), 396, 403
Pellagra, 293, 301
Pelvic girdle, 395, 401
  bones of, 402
Pelvis, of kidney, 304
  of skeleton, in body balance, 411
    in poor sitting posture, 418
    in rickets, 423
  (See also Pelvic girdle)
Penicillin, action of, on bacteria, 197–198
  medical uses of, 15, 19, 164, 203, 206, 212, 271, 276, 335, 378, 422
Percentile rank, definition of, 59n.
  determination of, in body measurements, 58, 59
Perilymph, 380, 381

Periodontal membrane, 279, 280
  infection of, 287
Periosteum of bone, 394
Peristalsis, 251–252
  in defecation, 255
  nervous control of, 256
  reverse, 252
    in belching, 258
    in furred tongue, 257
    in vomiting, 260
Peritonitis, 271
Pernicious anemia, 171
Personality, 20–21
  changes in, 121, 132, 144–145, 163
  disruption of, 136, 141
  mature, 72
  psychopathic, 146
  uniqueness of, 21–23, 86
Personality development, 71–72
  basic needs in, 80
  influences on, of environment, 22, 71, 77
    of heredity, 20–21, 71
    of hormones, 93
    of individual, 22–23
    of speech difficulties, 228
  phases of, 72–80
    child observation and, 143
Perspiration, 316
  acidity of, 329
  (See also Sweat)
Pertussis (see Whooping cough)
Petit mal, 132–133
Phagocytes, in antigen-antibody reactions, 103, 104
  in lymph nodes, 176
  protein in formation of, 290
  in pus formation, 102–103, 335
  in tonsils, 177
  white blood cells as, 167–168
    mobilization of, 101, 102, 168, 334–335
Phagocytosis, 102, 167–168, 334–335
Phalanges, 396, 402, 403
Phallic (genital) period in social and emotional growth, 73, 76
Pharyngitis, streptococcal, 212
Pharynx (throat), 193
  connections of, 194, 195
  in speech, 230, 237, 238
  tonsils in, 177
  (See also Nasopharynx; Throat)
Phoria, 359
Phosphorus, 291, 393, 423
Physical activity, influence of, on growth and development, 36, 399
  on posture, 413, 415
  postural difficulties and, 433

Physical activity, restriction of, 164, 217
  (*See also* Exercise)
Physical defects, influence of, in accident-
      proneness, 148
  in functioning of intelligence, 66
  in skeletal growth, 34
  prevalence of, 20
  (*See also* Orthopedic defects)
Physical therapy, 124, 432
Pigeon toe, 417, 431
Pigment, in bile, 262, 263
  in hair, 318
  in hemoglobin, 167, 262
  in middle coat of eyeball, 353
  in moles, 321
  in skin, 314, 315
    effect on, of sunlight, 314
Pilosebaceous glands, 316, 317, 322, 324
  (*See also* Sebaceous glands; Sebum)
Pimples, 103, 320, 334
  in acne, 322–323
Pineal gland, 93, 94
Pinel, Phillipe, 140
Pinkeye (conjunctivitis), 353
Pinna, 374
Pinworms (enterobiasis), 271–273
Pirquet, C. von, 106
Pituitary, 93, 400
  (*See also* Anterior pituitary)
Plasma (*see* Blood plasma)
Plasmodium, 183–184
Pneumococcus (pneumococci), 198–199
  in nasopharynx, 197, 199
  in osteomyelitis, 422
  in pneumonia, 199, 210
Pneumonia, pneumococcal, 15, 198–199,
      210
  chemotherapy in treatment of, 15, 210
  death rate from, 208
    in school children, 14
  precursors of, 210
  vaccines against, 210–211
  virus, 211
  antibiotics in treatment of, 198, 211
Poliomyelitis, 122–130
  abortive, 122, 123
  bulbar, 124, 193
  immunization from, 127–130
    active, 128–130
    passive, 128–129
  inapparent, 122
  incidence of, 122
    of paralytic type, 123
  incubation period of, 125
  infection, mode of, 125
  nonparalytic, 123, 124

Poliomyelitis, orthopedic defects and, 413,
      419, 420
  paralytic, 123–124
    aftereffects, treatment of, 124–125
  period of communicability of, 125
  precautions against spread of, 126, 127
  signs and symptoms of, at onset, 124
  teacher and, 130
  transmission of, 125, 127
  vaccine, search for, 129
  virus, effect of, on motor neurons, 123–
      124
    spread of, in body, 127–128
    types of, 122, 127
Pollens in allergic reactions, 107, 108, 218–
      219
Polymyxin, 197*n.*
Polyneuritis, 292–293
Pores, in acne, 322, 324
  in oily skin, 322
Posture, body balance and, 410–412
  characteristics of, by age, 412, 414–415
  effect on, of fatigue, 297, 413, 419
    of nutrition 297, 413, 419
    of physical deformities, 413, 419–422,
      431
  good, cultivating sense of, 416
    factors influencing, 297, 410, 411, 413,
      415
    signs of, 414
  influence of, on skeletal growth, 34
  observation of, 9, 20, 129, 297, 430
  poor, factors influencing, 297, 411, 413,
      419
    signs of, 415
  sitting, 417–418
  standing, 416–417
  walking, 417
Pott's disease, 423
Prenatal conditions as cause of orthopedic
      defects, 419
Pressure bandage, 179
Pressure points, 179, 180–181
Problem children, 118
Proteins, 249
  in allergic reactions, 107, 330
  in blood plasma, 164–166
  body's use of, 290
  calorie value of, 290
  digestion of, 250, 253–254
  effects of deficiency of, 297, 299
  food sources of, 296, 299
  in red blood cells, 167
  requirements of, 295
  in resistance to infection, 200, 290

Prothrombin, 166, 168
Protoplasm, 290, 313
Protozoa, 198
Psoriasis, 319
Psyche, 100, 113
  and soma, 88
Psychiatric services for school children,
    139, 148–149
Psychiatrist, 118, 139, 243, 244
Psychogenic manifestations, 88
Psychologist, 11, 118
Psychology, 148
Psychoses, 137
  patterns of, 140–141
Psychosomatic, definition of, 88
Psychosomatic mechanisms, 114–115
Psychotherapy in treatment, of neuroses,
    139
  of psychoses, 140
  of speech difficulties, 234, 243–244
Ptyalin, 253
Puberal cycle, 37, 39–41
Puberty, growth spurt in, 34, 39, 40, 79
  mumps and, 19, 205, 277, 278
  physical and psychic changes in, 73, 79
  tuberculosis and, 215
Pubic arch, 396, 402
Pubis, 396, 397, 402
Pulmonary artery, 155
Pulmonary tuberculosis (see Tuberculosis,
    pulmonary)
Pulmonary veins, 155
Pulp of tooth, 279, 280
  destruction of, in dental caries, 284–285
Pulse, 157–158
  taking, 158
  (See also Heart rate)
Pulse rate in shock, 178
Punishment as atonement for guilt, 116,
    117
Pupil of eye, 354–356
  and crystalline lens, 360
  effect on, of emotion, 95, 355
    of light intensity, 91, 355
  in nearsightedness, 364
Purpura, 173
Pus, formation of, 101–103
  in conjunctivitis, 353
  in furuncles, 334–335
  in middle-ear abscess, 377
  in pyorrhea, 287
  in sinusitis, 207
  in sties, 350
  in tooth decay, 285
  in stools, 268

Pustules, 320
Pyelitis, 305
Pyorrhea, 287

Q

Quarantine in poliomyelitis, 125
Quarrelsomeness, 119, 142, 147

R

Rabies, 345
Radiation, 110
Radium in removal of adenoid tissue, 178
Radius, 396, 402
Rash, 328
  in allergic reactions, 106, 329
  in German measles, 202
  inspection for, 8
  in measles, 202
  in scarlet fever, 203, 211–212
Rat fleas (Xenopsylla cheopis) in spread
    of endemic typhus, 184, 187
Rats, control of, 187
  and endemic typhus, 184
  and Salmonella, 266, 268
Reading, acquiring art of, 238
  difficulties in, in aphasia, 239–240
    in left-handedness, 365
    psychogenic, 115, 142, 366
    teaching methods and, 366
    in visual defects, 363–365
Reality, learning to meet, 74–75
  retreat from, in schizoid states, 140–141
    in withdrawing behavior, 120, 137,
      146
Rectum, 250, 251, 302
  pinworms in, 272
  stimulus of, in defecation, 255–256
    effect on, of irregular toilet habits,
      263–264
Red blood cells, 166–167
  anemia and, 171, 172–173
  in blood clotting, 166
  destruction of, 167, 262, 263
    in malaria, 183
  life span of, 167
  manufacture of, 167, 394
  number of, 167
  as oxygen carriers, 166–167, 327
  proportion of, to white cells, 165, 167
  in urine, 306, 307
  (See also Hemoglobin; Iron)
Reflex, defecation, 255–256

Reflex, scratch, 114
  vomiting, 259, 260
Reflexes, conditioned, 92
  unconditioned, 91–92
    in maintaining equilibrium, 408
      muscle tone, 404–405, 408
    as protective measures, 99, 100, 112–113, 349
    in urination, 304
Refraction, 360
  errors of, 361
    correction of, by glass lenses, 361–363
    detection of (see Vision tests)
  media of, 360
Renal tubules, 302–304
  inflammation of (nephrosis), 305, 306
Repression, 74, 75, 77
Resentment, behavior reactions to, 118–119
  psychosomatic, 115, 256
Residual whisper, 386
Respiration, mechanics of, 193
  nervous control of, 193–194
Respiration rate, 194
  factors influencing, 101
Respiratory center, 193–194
  in bulbar poliomyelitis, 124, 193
  paralysis of, in electric shock, 193, 225
Respiratory infections, causative agents of, 197–199
  control of, 211
    in schools, 220, 221–224
  middle-ear infection and, 377
  resistance to, 200
  rheumatic fever and, 162, 164, 211
  school absences and, 17–18
  signs and symptoms of, 220–221
    mechanics of, 201
  transmission of, by respiratory-tract discharges, 18, 202–205, 220, 222
Respiratory mucous membranes, air-conditioning functions of, 196
  allergic reactions in, 107, 109, 218–220
  circulation in, 196, 200–201
  mucous blanket of, 196, 201, 210
  as reservoir of infection, 197, 222
  resistance of, to infection, 197, 200, 211
    lowering of, 200–201, 210
Respiratory tract, 192–193
  diseases spread by discharges from, 201–218
Restlessness, in fever, 112
  psychosomatic, 115
  in symptom complex, 124, 131, 163, 203, 272, 273

Resuscitation in asphyxia, 225–228
Retina, 354–356
  focusing of light waves on, 356–357, 362
    during accommodation, 360–361
    in errors of refraction, 361–364
  stimulation of, 356–357
  visual purple in, 292
Retinoscope, 368
Rh factor, 169–170
  in pregnancy, 170
Rheumatic fever, 161–164
  heredity in, 161
  insidious onset of, 4, 112, 163
    signs and symptoms during, 163
  and organic heart disease, 159, 161–164
  death rate from, 14, 161
  recurrences of, 162–164
  research in, 162
  school and, 162–164
  streptococcal infections and, 18, 161, 203n., 212, 213
Rheumatism, 106
Riboflavin, body's need for, 293
  crystals of, 293
  daily requirements of, 295
  effects of deficiency of, 275, 293, 300–301
  food sources of, 296, 300
Ribs, 394–396, 399, 401
  beading of, in rickets, 423
Rickets, 423–424
  as cause of bone deformities, 34, 413, 417, 423
  prevalence of, 421
  vitamin-D deficiency and, 34, 293–294, 301, 423
Ricketts, Howard Taylor, 186
Rickettsiae, 186–187
Ringworm, of body, 336
  of feet, 336–337
  of scalp, animal-type, 338
    human-type, 337–338
      control of, 339–340
      signs of, 338
      transmission of, 338–339
      treatment of, 338
Robbins, Frederick C., 128
Rocky Mountain spotted fever, 183–185, 187–188
Romance in Oedipus complex, 73, 76
Rotary joints, 394
Roughage, as aid to elimination, 264, 294
  food sources of, 294, 296
Round window of ear, 376, 380, 381
Roundworms (ascariasis), 272–273

S

Saccule of labyrinth, 407, 408
Sacral division, autonomic nervous system, 89
Sacroiliac joint, 397
  straining of, 402
Sacrum, 396, 397, 402
Saddle joints, 394
St. Vitus's dance, 162
Saliva, animal, rabies virus in, 345
  human, as defense against infection, 101
    as digestive juice, 253, 274
    as factor in dental caries, lactobacilli in, 281, 282
    variations in composition of, 282
  secretion of, 277
    psychic, 256
Salivary glands, 251, 277
  infection of, in mumps, 204, 221, 277–278
  secretion of (see Saliva)
Salk, Jonas E., 129
Salmonella, 265, 266, 268
  typhosa, 265, 267, 268
Sanitary measures, in control, of gastrointestinal disease, 15, 264–265, 266n.–267n.
  of intestinal parasites, 272–274
  of trench mouth, 276
Scabies, 340–341
Scala media, 379–381
  tympani, 379–381
  vestibuli, 379–381
Scalp, dryness of, 324, 325
  hair of, 317
  infections of, in infectious dandruff, 335
    in ringworm, 336–340
  oiliness of, 325
  pediculosis and, 342
  psoriasis and, 319
  in simple dandruff, 325
  wound of, 427
Scapulae (see Shoulder blades)
Scarlet fever, 203, 211–213
  complications of, 18, 161, 163, 176, 203n., 211, 306, 377
  hemolytic streptococci as cause of, 199, 203, 211
  protection against, 18, 203, 212
  school absences and, 18
Scheinfeld, Amram, 21, 22
Schizoid states, 141
Schizophrenia, 137, 141
School absences (see Absences from school)
School cleaning, 224

School dental health program, 287–288
School health education, 10, 12, 16
School health examinations, 10
  health education and, 12
  interim, 12
  periodic, 11–12
  role in, of nurse, 12
    of parents, 12
    of teacher, 4, 9, 11–12
School health inspection, 7
  in epidemics, 221
  formal, 8
  informal, 9–10
School health service, 10–13
  activities of, 10–11, 16
  nurse in, 4, 9, 11–13
  physician in, 4, 9, 11–13
  teacher in, 4, 5, 9, 10–13
School program for orthopedically handicapped children, 432–433
Schoolwork, deterioration of, in adolescent depression, 145
  in rheumatic fever, 163
  overindulgence in (studiousness), in withdrawing behavior, 120, 142
Sclera (white of eye), 353, 354
Scoliosis, 415, 424
Scratches, first-aid treatment for, 344
Scratching, 114
  in impetigo, 333
  marks of, 8, 114, 341
  in pediculosis, 342–343
  in scabies, 341
Scurvy, 173, 293, 301
Seasickness, 260–261, 409
Seat bones (see Ischia)
Seating, school, in control of airborne infection, 223
  posture and, 418
Sebaceous glands, 316
  increased activity of, during puberty, 322, 338
  in warm weather, 321
  infection of, in boils, 334
    in infectious dandruff, 335
    in sties, 350
  secretion of (see Sebum)
Sebum, acidity of, 329
  formation of plugs of, 320
  secretion of, 316, 317
    decreased, in dry hair, 324
      in dry skin, 316, 321
    increased, in acne, 322–324
      in oily hair, 324–325
      in oily skin, 316, 322
Secondary sex characteristics, 40, 73

Security, need of, in childhood, 80, 120, 139
  threats to, 76
Semicircular canals (organs of equilibrium), 407–408
  stimulation of, in dizziness, 409
    in maintaining equilibrium, 408
    in motion sickness, 260–261, 409
Semipermeable membranes, 174
  of small intestine, 252
Sensations, 88, 90–91
  somatic, 91, 406–407
  unpleasant, as symptoms, 100
Sense organs, 86–87, 91
  receptors of, 90
Sensitiveness, 142, 146
Sensory receptors, 88, 90–91
  kinesthetic, 407
  of pain, 112–113
  in skin, 111, 114, 312
  of sound (auditory), 380, 382
  of vision (in retina), 356–357
Septum of nose, 194, 400
  deviated, 222
Serum albumin, in blood plasma, 165
  in treatment of shock, 166
  in urine, 306
Sex, attitudes toward, in adolescence, 79, 145
  curiosity about, 73, 119
  emergence of differences in, 40, 73
  influence of, on body dimensions, 40–41
  interest in opposite, 73, 79
  interest in same, 73, 78
Sex glands (gonads), 32, 93, 94
  inflammation of, in mumps, 19, 205, 277, 278
  influence of, in puberal cycle, 40
    in sexual development, 79
    in skeletal growth, 34
  maturation of, 73, 76
Sexuality, 72, 75–76, 79
Shigella group, 265, 266
Shivering, 111, 112, 318
Shock after injury, 178
  prevention and treatment of, by blood derivatives, 165, 166
  in first aid, 178–179
Shock tissue in allergic reactions, 107, 109
  of skin, 330–331
Shoes, dry, in preventing colds, 224
  posture and, 413
  pronated feet and, 417
Shoulder blades (scapulae), 394, 397, 401, 402
  in good posture, 414

Shoulder blades (scapulae), in poor posture, 297, 415
  in young children, 412
Shoulder girdle, 395
  bones of, 401
Shoulder joints, 394, 402
Shoulders, position of, in good posture, 414, 416, 418
  in poor posture, 297, 415, 418, 419
Sight (see Eyesight; Vision)
Signs and symptoms, 100
  of common childhood diseases, 221
  as diagnostic aid, 3
  inspection for, in school, 8–9
  of malnutrition, 297, 298
  mechanics of, in gastrointestinal disorders, 257–264
  in respiratory infections, 201
  physiological background of, 22
  psychogenic, 88, 114–115
Sinuses, nasal, 194, 207, 400
  inflammation of (see Sinusitis)
  in voice production, 236
Sinusitis, 207
  middle-ear infection and, 377, 378
Skeleton, 393, 395–397
  appendicular, 395, 401–403
  axial, 395, 398–400
  body build and, 33, 44, 53
  growth of, influences on, 33–36, 40
  pattern of, 32
  joints of, 394–395
  measuring stockiness of, 53, 58
  (See also Bones)
Skin, 312
  appearance of, in health, 314, 315, 328
    in illness, 314, 327–328
    in old age, 314, 315, 328
  circulation in, 110–111, 160, 314–315, 326–328
  disorders of, allergic, 106, 108–110, 329–331
    infectious, 329, 332–340
      school absences and, 20
      staphylococcal food infections and, 266, 269
    nutritional, 292, 293, 300, 301, 316, 328–329
    structural and functional, 319–324
  dryness of, 316
    in chapping, 321–322
  effect on, of emotions, 95
  infestations of, 340–343
  injuries of, 343–347
  innervation of, 111, 112, 114, 312
  layers of, 312–315

Skin, oiliness of, 316, 322
  in acne, 322–324
  in regulation of body temperature, 111,
    289, 312, 316
  secretory apparatus of, 315–316
  tone of, 315, 327
Skin color, 314–315, 326, 328
  abnormal changes in, 101, 111, 112, 160–
    161, 163, 172–173, 262–263, 267, 327–
    328, 346
  normal changes in, 88, 111, 326, 327
Skin tests, for allergy, 108, 219, 329–331
  in tuberculosis (tuberculin test), 215, 216
  in undulant fever, 270
Skull, 399–400
  articulation of, with spinal column, 398
  fracture of, 427
  olfactory bulbs in, 400
  organ of hearing in, 378, 399, 407
  pituitary in, 93, 400
  red bone marrow in, 394
  semicircular canals in, 399–400, 407
  sinuses in, 194
Sleeping sickness (epidemic encephalitis),
  132
Sling, triangular bandage, 426–427
Small intestine, absorption from, 252, 254
  digestion in, chemical, 254
    mechanical, 250–252
  effect on, of emotions, 256
  innervation of, 87, 89, 256
Smallpox (variola), 203
  vaccination against, 104, 105, 203
Smothering, 225
Sneezing, in colds, 201
  in hay fever, 109, 218
  as protective reflex, 92, 100
  in symptom complex, 112, 221, 352
  technique of, 223
Snellen, Hermann, 367
Snellen test chart, letter, 369–371
  symbol, 371–372
  vision testing with, 372–374
Social living, evading requirements of, by
    attack, 118–119
  by withdrawal, 118–120, 146
  learning to meet requirements of, 72,
    74–75
Sodium fluoride in prevention of dental
    caries, 283–284
Solitariness, 142, 146
Soma, 88
Sound, pitch of, 382
  producing sensation of, 381–382
  sensory receptors of, 380, 382

Sound, transmission of, in cochlea, 381–382
  by eardrum, 375, 381, 382
  by external ear, 374, 382
  by middle ear, 381, 382
  by ossicles, 381
  units for measuring intensity of, 384, 385
Speech, acquiring art of, 238
  difficulty in, 229, 240, 244
  in aphasia, 229, 239
  centers of, in brain, 87, 238–239
  defective, 228
  examination of, 228
  organ of, 229–230
  sounds of, consonant, 230–232
    vowel, 230, 233
  (See also Speech difficulties; Voice)
Speech difficulties, correction of, 228, 234,
    237–238, 244
  detection of, by teacher, 12, 228, 235, 236
  incidence of, 228
  in poor hearing, 383
  psychosomatic, 115, 142, 232, 234, 241–
    244
  varieties of, 228–229
Sphenoid bone, 396
  sinuses in, 207, 400
Sphincters, of alimentary canal, 250–251
    nervous control of, 95, 251, 255–256
  of urinary bladder, 304
Sphygmomanometer, 160
Spinal column (spine), 395, 398–399
  curvature of, 424
  curves of, 398
    body balance and, 411
    development of, 412, 414, 416
    in good posture, 414, 418
    in poor posture, 415, 418
  injury of, 427–428
  joints of, 394
  red marrow in, 394
Spinal cord, brain and, 86, 88, 89, 399, 400
  defecation center in, 255–256
  effects of infection of, 121, 136
    in meningococcal meningitis, 131
    in poliomyelitis, 123–124
  of injury of, 121, 136, 427, 428
  and reflex action, 91
  in spinal column, 395, 398
Spleen, circulation to, 157
  as graveyard of red blood cells, 167
  innervation of, 89
Splints, 425–426
Spores, of malaria parasites, 183
  of ringworm fungi, 338
  of tetanus bacilli, 344
Sporozoa of malaria, 183, 184

Sportsmanship, poor, 142, 147
Spotted fever, 183–185, 187–188
Sputum testing, 216
Squint (strabismus), 358
    correction of, 359–360
    detection of, 358–359
    latent, in reading difficulties, 366
Squinting of eyes, in eye testing, 374
    in nearsightedness, 364, 365
Stammering (see Stuttering)
Stapes, 376, 381
Staphylococci, 332
    in osteomyelitis, 422
    and streptococci in skin infections, 332–334
    toxin of, in food poisoning, 266, 269
Starches (see Carbohydrates)
Stensen, Nicolas, 277
Sternum (breastbone), 395, 396, 399, 401
    deformities of, 415, 423
Stethoscope, 159
Sties, 350
    in eye fatigue, 350, 365
    as furuncles, 334
Stimulus, physical, 90
    in producing pain, 112–113, 262
    psychic, 113, 137
Stomach, circulation of blood to, 157
    digestion in, chemical, 253
        mechanical, 250–251
    disturbances of, in symptom complex, 114, 122, 124, 221
    furred tongue and, 257
    gas in, in relation, to belching, 258
        to referred pain, 113
    heartburn and, 258
    innervation of, 87, 89, 100, 113, 256
    movements of, in hunger, 261
        in nausea, 260
        in vomiting, 259–260
    sensitivity of, to physical stimuli, 19, 100, 107, 257, 259–260
        to psychic stimuli, 88, 92, 100, 137, 256, 257, 260
    stretching of, as cause of pain, 262
    tone of, in relation to appetite, 261
Stomatitis, 275
Stool examinations, in dysentery, 268
    in hookworm, 274
Strabismus (see Squint)
Strangulation, 225
Streptococcal infections, respiratory, 211–213
    nephritis and, 203n., 306
    rheumatic fever and, 18, 161–163, 203n., 212

Streptococcal infections, respiratory, school absences and, 17
    of skin, 332–334
Streptococcal sore throat, 204–205, 211–213
Streptococci, 197, 199
    hemolytic (see Streptococcus hemolyticus)
    in osteomyelitis, 422
    and staphylococci in skin infections, 332–334
Streptococcus hemolyticus, 198, 199
    erythrogenic toxin of, 199, 203n., 211–212
    sensitivity of, to chemotherapeutic drugs, 162
    sensitivity to, in rheumatic fever, 161–162
    (See also Scarlet fever; Streptococcal sore throat)
Streptomycin, 197n., 217–218, 267
Stuart, Harold C., 53, 59
Stuttering, 240
    emotional disturbances and, 146, 241–243
    primary, 241–242
    secondary, 242–244
Subcutaneous fat, 290, 313, 315
    influence of, on body dimensions, 36–37, 44, 53
    measurement of, 53, 58, 59, 62
    (See also Adipose tissue)
Substandard health, posture and, 413
    resistance to infection and, 200
    rheumatic fever and, 163
Sugar, in blood plasma, 164
    decreased, in insulin reaction, 99
    in urine in diabetes, 97, 303, 307
    (See also Glucose)
Sugars (see Carbohydrates)
Sulfonamides (sulfa drugs), action of, on disease agents, 197–198
    medical uses of, 15, 17, 19, 131–132, 162, 164, 203, 205, 206, 210, 271, 335, 378, 422
Sun tan, 314
Sunburn, 314, 320
Sunlight, herpes simplex and, 275
    ultraviolet rays in, 294, 314, 423
Superego (conscience), 72
    in unconscious conflicts, 77
    (See also Conscience)
Suspensory ligament, 354, 360
    in accommodation, 361
Swallowing, of air, 258
    eustachian tube and, 375–376
    of food, esophagus and, 251, 258–259

Swallowing, of food, larynx and, 195–196
tongue and, 250, 276
Sweat, evaporation of, 111, 316
secretion of, autonomic control of, 87
nausea and, 260
psychogenic, 95, 113
in regulation of body temperature, 111, 316
in symptom complex, 99, 182, 184, 215
Sweat glands, 313, 316
autonomic control of, 87, 111, 316
infection of, 334
Sweating (see Sweat, secretion of)
Sweets, refined, dental caries and, 282, 283
Swelling (see Edema)
Sympathetic division, autonomic nervous system, 89
teamwork of, with adrenal medulla, 95–96
Symptom complex, 114, 220
Symptoms (see Signs and symptoms)
Syphilis in organic mental disease, 136
Systole, 155
and arterial blood pressure, 158
Systolic blood pressure, 158–160

T

Talus, 403
Tarsal bones, 396, 403
Tartar, 286–287
Taste buds, 274, 276
Tear glands (see Lacrimal glands)
Tears, functions of, as defense against infection, 101
in lubricating eyeball, 349, 351–352
secretion of, 351, 400
in eye irritations, 352, 356
in weeping, 352
Tectorial membrane, 380, 381
Teeth, 278–280
aching, in symptom complex, 207
calcification of, 291, 293
chattering of, 111, 318
cleaning of, by brushing, 282–283
prophylactic, 282, 286–287
decay of (see Dental caries)
deciduous, 279, 286
devitalized, 284–285
effect on, of calcium deficiency, 299
of vitamin-D deficiency, 301
enamel (see Enamel of tooth)
examination of, 285, 287, 288

Teeth, function of (mastication), in mechanical digestion, 250, 274, 278
impacted, 285
mottling of, 283
nutrition and, 281, 286
permanent, 279
defects of, by age, 279, 280
occlusion of (see Malocclusion)
sockets of, 279, 401
in speech, 230–232, 235–236
in speech difficulties, 229, 235, 236
Telebinocular, 372
Temper tantrums, 75, 137, 142
Temperature, body (see Body temperature)
of classrooms, 223
Temporal bones, 396, 397, 399
organ of hearing in, 399
semicircular canals in, 399–400, 407
Tendons, 395, 404, 417
Terramycin, 197n.
Testes, 94
inflammation of, in mumps, 205, 277–278
Tests, achievement, 65–66, 68
aptitude, 66, 68
intelligence, 64–65, 68
screening, for hearing, 12, 384–388
for orthopedic defects, 430
for speech, 12, 228
for vision, 12, 369–372
skin, for allergic reactions, 108, 219, 330–331
for bacterial allergy, 110, 216, 270
Tetanus (lockjaw), 344–345
immunization from, 105, 106, 345
Thiamine (B_1), body's need for, 292
crystals of, 292
daily requirements of, 295
effects of deficiency of, 292–293, 300
food sources of, 296, 300
Thighbone (see Femur)
Thighs, position of, in good posture, 414
in poor posture, 415
support for, in sitting, 418
Thirst, in diabetes, 97
reporting of, 305
Thorax (chest), 399, 401, 411
(See also Chest)
Throat, infection of, chronic, in hearing loss, 378
in Vincent's angina, 276
lump in, 258–259
sore, history of, as diagnostic aid, 163, 177

Throat, sore, septic, 213
  in symptom complex, 112, 124, 131,
    202–204, 221, 327
  (See also Pharynx)
Thrombin, 165
  in blood clotting, 166, 168
Thrombocytes (see Blood platelets)
Thumb, 402
Thumb sucking (see Finger sucking)
Thymus, lymphatic, 93, 94
Thyroid gland, 93, 94
  effect of, on growth, 34, 35
  enlarged, in simple goiter, 96–97
Thyroxine, 34, 96, 291
Tibia (shin bone), 396, 403
  in defective bone growth, 424
  infection of, 422
Ticks, precautions against bites of, 187–188
  removal of, from skin, 188
  in spread of spotted fever, 184, 187–188
Timidity, 142, 146
Tissue fluid, 173
  mineral salts in, 291, 406
  (See also Lymph)
Toenails, growth of, 318
Toes, bones of, 403
  position of, in clubfoot, 421
    in good posture, 414, 417
    in poor posture, 415, 417, 431
Toilet habits, change in, as danger signal,
    305
  unestablished, in maladjustment, 142,
    305
Toilet training, 73, 74
  unwise, 305
Tongue, 276
  attachment of, 401
  beefy (glossitis), 276, 300
  dry, in mouth breathing, 223
  furred, 276
  furrowed, 277
  geographic (mappy), 277
  in mechanical digestion, 250, 274, 276
  in speech, 229–232, 234–236, 238, 276
Tongue-tie, 234–235
Tonsillitis, middle-ear infection and, 377
  rheumatic fever and, 161
  streptococcal, 211–212
Tonsils and adenoids, 177, 195
  infected or enlarged, 177
    effects of, 38, 178, 222–223, 413
    removal of (tonsillectomy), 177
      poliomyelitis and, 127
      rheumatic fever danger signals and,
        163

Toothache, 285
Toothbrushing, 283–284
Torticollis (wryneck), 421–422
Tourniquet, 179, 181
Toxins, bacterial, 103, 104, 110
  of diphtheria, 204–205
  in edema, 174–175
  in fever production, 111
  staphylococcal, in food infections, 266,
    269
    in osteomyelitis, 422
  streptococcal, 204–205, 211–212
    erythrogenic (rash-producing),   199,
      203n., 211–212
  of tetanus, 344, 345
Toxoids, 104
  use of, in immunization, 15, 104–105,
    205, 345
Trachea (see Windpipe)
Trachoma, control of, 7, 8
Trauma (see Accidents)
Tremor, 121, 136
Trench mouth (Vincent's angina), 275–276
Triceps, 404, 405
Tropia, 359
Truancy, 75, 119, 142, 147
Trunk, body build and, 44
Tubercle bacillus (Mycobacterium tuber-
    culosis), allergic reaction to, 110, 215,
    217
  bovine type, 199
  formation of pulmonary lesions by,
    215n.
  human type, 199–200
Tuberculin, 216
Tuberculin test, 216
Tuberculosis, of bones and joints, 422–423
    posture and, 413
    prevalence of, 421
      in school children, 420, 422–423
  of cervical lymph glands, 177
  miliary, 214
  pulmonary, 200
    age incidence of, 14, 18, 214–217
    case finding in, 216
    death rates from, in school children,
      by age, 1930 and 1953, 14
        1950–1953, 214
    first-infection, 214–215
    hospitalization in, 217
    insidious development of, 4, 112, 214,
      215
    lesions of, 215n.
    progress in control of, 14–15, 18, 213,
      217–218
    rehabilitation in, 217

Tuberculosis, pulmonary, reinfection, 215
    danger signals of, 215
    medical diagnosis of, 215–216
    treatment of, 217–218
    vaccination against (BCG), 217
Turbinates, 194, 195, 400–401
    enlarged, 222
Turner, C. E., 63
Tympanum (see Eardrum)
Typhoid fever, 265, 267
    bacillus of, 265, 267
    immunization from, 105, 267
    progress in control of, 15, 265
Typhus, endemic, 184–187
    epidemic, 186–187, 265, 342

U

Ulna, 396, 402
Ultraviolet irradiation, 222
Ultraviolet rays, in sunburn, 314
    in tanning of skin, 314
    in vitamin-D formation, 294, 423
    in Wood's light, 339
Unconscious mind, 77
    in anxiety hysteria, 137
Unconsciousness (see Consciousness, loss
    of)
Underweight, 37–38, 43, 44, 327
Undulant fever (brucellosis), 267, 269–270
United States Public Health Service, 206
Urea, excretion of, 290, 304
    poisoning by, in nephritis, 306
    production of, 290, 304
Uremia, 306
Ureters, 304
Urethra, 304
Urinalysis, 5, 97
    value of, in diagnosis, 306–307
Urinary bladder (see Bladder)
Urination, frequency of, 97, 115, 305
    involuntary, 134
    voluntary control of, 304
Urine, 290, 294
    albumin in, 306, 307
    composition of, 303–304
    excretion of, 302, 304
    production of, 303–304
    red blood cells in, 306, 307
    sugar in, 97, 307
    variations in volume of, abnormal, 305,
        306
        normal, 304–305
Utricle, 407, 408
Uvula, 195, 236

V

Vaccination, 104
    (See also Immunization; Vaccines)
Vaccines, 104
    antirabic, 345
    search for, in colds, 206
    in influenza, 208
    in poliomyelitis, 127
    in tuberculosis, 217
    use of, in immunization, 104–106, 129–
        130, 203, 205, 210–211, 217, 267, 270,
        278
Vagina, pinworms in, 272
Vagus nerve, 89
Valves of heart, 155
    heart murmurs and, 159
Veins, bleeding from, 179
    pulmonary, 157
    tree of, 155, 156, 158
Ventilation of classroom, 223
Ventricles of heart, 155–157
Venules, 157
    in dermis, 326–327
Vertebrae, 395, 397–399, 411
    red bone marrow in, 394
    spinal curvature and, 424
    tuberculosis of (Pott's disease), 423
Vertigo (see Dizziness)
Vesicles, 320
Vestibular membrane of cochlea, 379
Vincent's angina (trench mouth), 275–276
Virchow, Rudolph, 171
Virilism, 35
Virus pneumonia, 210–211
    antibiotics in treatment of, 198, 210
Viruses, 197–198, 201
    as antigens, 103–104
    body's defenses against, 101–104
Vision, binocular, 357–358
    distant, accommodation and, 360
        in astigmatism, 364–365
        in nearsightedness, 364
        in squint, 359
    double, 358, 359
        in epidemic encephalitis, 132
    near, accommodation for, 361–363
        in astigmatism, 364–365
        in squint, 359
    prevalence of defects of, 361
    psychogenic disturbances of, 115
    sensation of, 90, 91, 356–357
Vision tests, administration of, 372–374
    farsightedness and, 363
    nearsightedness and, 364

Vision tests, preparation of children for, 372
  recording findings of, in form of fraction, 370–371, 373–374
  recording signs of visual disturbances, 374
  role of teacher in, 369, 372–374
  squint and, 359
  types of, 369–372
Visual acuity, in astigmatism, 364–365
  screening tests for, 369–374
  in squint, 359
Visual (seeing) center, 87, 356
  aphasia and, 239
  reading and, 238
Visual purple, 292
Vitamin A, body's need for, 200, 292
  crystals of, 292
  daily requirements of, 295
  effects of deficiency of, 292, 300, 324, 352
  food sources of, 292, 296, 300
Vitamin-B complex, 292
  deficiencies of, 276, 328–329
  food sources of, 296
  (See also Niacin; Riboflavin; Thiamine)
Vitamin C (ascorbic acid), body's need for, 293
  crystals of, 293
  daily requirements of, 295
  effects of deficiency of, 286, 293, 301
  food sources of, 293, 296, 301
Vitamin D, in calcification of bones and teeth, 33, 291, 293–294, 423
  crystals of, 294
  daily requirements of, 295
  effects of deficiency of, 34, 293–294, 301, 423
  sources of, 294, 296, 300, 413, 423
Vitamins, 249, 291
  use of, in body, 291–292
Vocal cords, 229–230
Voice, change in, during adolescence, 79, 232, 234
  falsetto, 232, 234
  hearing loss and, 229, 383
  production of, 230, 232
Voice and speech training, 228, 234, 235, 237–238, 244
Vomer, 400
Vomiting, 259–260
  psychogenic, 114, 137, 260
  as reflex act, 100, 259–260
  in symptom complex, 112, 124, 203, 221, 266, 267, 271
Vomiting center, 259
  excitation of, 260

W

Walking (see Gait)
Warts, 320–321
Watch-tick test, 387–388
Water, absorption of, from colon, 255
    in diarrhea, 264
    from kidney tubules, 303
  in blood, 164, 165
  in digestion, 250, 254
  drinking, as aid in elimination of body wastes, 264, 294, 296
    contaminated, in spread of disease, 265–267
    daily requirements of, 296
    fluorine in, 282–283
    safeguarding of, 15, 264, 266n.
  exchange of, between blood and tissues, 173–174
  excretion of, 294, 302, 406
  in food, 249, 294–295
  formation of, in oxidation, 289, 294–295, 406
  in tissue fluid, 173, 294
Weaning, 73
Weight, at birth, 38
  definition of, 43
  distribution of, in body balance, 410–411
    in standing, 416–417
    in walking, 417
  gain in, excessive, 63
    failure of, 62–63, 163
    rates of, 39
    slow, 177
    sudden, 351
  loss of, 5, 97, 214, 264, 272
  measurements of, 41, 43–62
    in classroom, 62–63
  range of, 6–7, 41
  segments of, 411
  sex differences in, 40–41
Weight-age curves, construction of, 44
  normal variations from, 44–48
  use of, 49
  (See also Height-weight-age tables; Height-weight-age-body-build tables)
Weller, Thomas H., 128
Wetzel, Norman C., 49, 51, 52
Wetzel's grid, 49–53
Wheals, 319–320
  in allergic skin reactions, 108, 109, 320, 331
Wheel chart for detecting astigmatism, 372

Wheezing, in bronchial asthma, 219
in bronchitis, 208
Whisper test, 386–387
White blood cells, increase of, in infection, 168, 335
in leukemia, 168, 171
as phagocytes, 101, 102, 167, 334–335
production of, 167
proportion of, to red cells, 165, 168
Whiteheads (milia), 320
in acne, 322
Whooping cough (pertussis), 204–205
bacilli of, 198, 204
immunization from, 18, 104, 105, 205
ruptured conjunctival blood vessels in,
352
school absences and, 18
Wiener, Alexander S., 169
Windpipe (trachea), 93, 192, 193, 195, 197,
207
foreign body in, 196
Wood, Robert William, 339
Wood's light, 339
Worms, intestinal, 271–274
Worry (*see* Anxiety)
Wounds, bleeding from (hemorrhage),
blood clotting in, 166, 168
first-aid control of, 179–181
in head injuries, 427

Wounds, tetanus and, 344
types of, 179
(*See also* Bites; Cuts)
Wrist, 394, 401, 402
sprained, 429
Writing, acquiring art of, 238
aphasia and, 239, 240
Wryneck (torticollis), 421–422
posture and, 413

X

X-rays, in determining skeletal age, 33
in chest examinations, 216
in examining teeth, 285
in treating ringworm of scalp, 338
Xerophthalmia, 292

Y

Yellowness, of eye whites, 353
of skin, 262–263, 327

Z

Zinnser, Hans, 265, 268